Community Public Health
in Policy and Practice

A Sourcebook

SECOND EDITION

Edited by

Sarah Cowley BA PhD PGDE RGN RHV HVT

Professor of Community Practice Development,
Head of Public Health and Health Services Research Section,
Florence Nightingale School of Nursing and Midwifery,
King's College London, London, UK

Forewords by

Angela Mawle BSc MSc PWTCert RHV RGN

Chief Executive, UK Public Health Association, London, UK

Cheryll Adams BSc(Hons) MSc PD(Nursing) RN RHV

Acting Lead Professional Officer,
Community Practitioners' and Health Visitors' Association,
London, UK

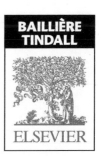

BAILLIÈRE
TINDALL

ELSEVIER

EDINBURGH LONDON NEW YORK OXFORD PHILADELPHIA ST LOUIS SYDNEY TORONTO 2008

BAILLIÈRE
TINDALL
ELSEVIER

An imprint of Elsevier Limited

First edition 2002
Second edition 2008

ISBN-13: 978-0-7020-2808-3

British Library Cataloguing in Publication Data
A catalogue record for this book is available from the British Library

Library of Congress Cataloging in Publication Data
A catalog record for this book is available from the Library of Congress

Note
Neither the Publisher nor the Authors assume any responsibility for any loss or injury and/or damage to persons or property arising out of or related to any use of the material contained in this book. It is the responsibility of the treating practitioner, relying on independent expertise and knowledge of the patient, to determine the best treatment and method of application for the patient.

The Publisher

Printed and bound in the United Kingdom

Transferred to Digital Print 2010

The Publisher's policy is to use paper manufactured from sustainable forests

Contents

Contributors

Jane Appleton BA MSc PhD RGN RHV PGCEA
Post-Doctoral Research Fellow Centre
Research in Primary and Community
Care, University of Hertfordshire,
Hatfield, UK;
Reader in Primary and Community
Care, School of Health and Social Care,
Oxford Brookes University, Oxford, UK

Helen Bedford BSc(Hons) MSc PhD FFPH FRCPCH
Senior Lecturer in Children's Health
Centre for Epidemiology and
Biostatistics, Institute of Child
Health, University College London,
London, UK

Christine Bidmead MSc RGN RHV
Training Facilitator, Centre for Parent
and Child Support, South London and
Maudsley, NHS Trust, London, UK

Jill Clemerson-Trew RHV RNA RNC
Health Visitor, Plymouth Teaching
Primary Care NHS Trust, Cumberland
Centre, Plymouth, UK

Sarah Cowley BA PhD PGDE RGN RHV HVT
Professor of Community Practice
Development, Head of Public Health
and Health Services Research Section,
Florence Nightingale School of Nursing
and Midwifery, King's College London,
London, UK

Pauline Craig BSc MSc RGN HV
Public Health Programme Manager,
Glasgow Centre for Population Health,
Glasgow, UK

Yvonne Dalziel BA MPhil RGN RHV
Public Health Practitioner, North East
Edinburgh Local Health Partnership,
NHS Lothian, Edinburgh, UK

Hilton Davis BA DipClinPsych CPsych
PhD FBPsS
Professor of Child Health Psychology,
Centre for Parent and Child Support,
South London and Maudsley NHS
Trust & King's College London, Guy's
Hospital, London, UK

Francesca Entwistle MSc PGCEA ADM RN RM
Programme Leader in Pre-Registration
Midwifery, Breastfeeding Co-ordinator,
Department of Health Eastern Region,
School of Nursing and Midwifery,
University of Hertfordshire,
Hatfield, UK

Moira Fischbacher BA PhD
Senior Lecturer, Department of
Management, University of Glasgow,
Glasgow, UK

Ruth Grant MSc RHV RGN
Health Visitor, Bath and Northeast
Somerset Primary Care Trust, Bath, UK

Peter Griffiths: BA(Hons) PhD RN
Director, Nursing Research Unit,
King's College London, London, UK

Sinéad Hanafin MSc PhD RGN RM DPHN SEANS
Health Research Board Fellow, School
of Nursing and Midwifery, King's
College London, London, UK

ix

Anna M Houston MA BSc RHV RM RN
Managing Director, Houston
Enterprises Ltd, East Grinstead, UK

Sally Kendall BSc (Hons) PhD RGN RHV
Professor of Nursing, Director,
Centre for Research in Primary and
Community Care, University of
Hertfordshire, Hatfield, UK

Pauline Pearson BA PhD DipSocRes DipThMin
RN RHV
Senior Lecturer in Primary Care
Nursing, School of Medical Education
Development, Newcastle University
Newcastle Upon Tyne, UK

Robyn Pound BA PhD RGN RHV FAETC
Health Visitor, Bath and North East
Somerset Primary Care Trust,
Bath, UK

Jean Rowe MSc RGN RHV PGCEA
Independent Public Health Specialist,
London, UK

Karen Whittaker BN MSc PGCE RGN RHV
Senior Lecturer, Department of
Nursing, University of Central
Lancashire, Preston, UK

X

Foreword by Angela Mawle

It is a privilege to write the foreword for a book that examines the policy and practice of community public health in such depth and with such clarity and expansiveness.

Never evading or avoiding the complexities of sustaining population health in present day Britain, *Community Public Health Policy and Practice* takes us through from the big picture perspective to the detail of working with communities, individuals and families.

It is a testament to the changing times in which we live that this book is in its second edition in 5 years.

First published in 2002 it coincided with the publication of the Wanless Report 'Securing our Future Health' which re-set the compass for public health. The Report was essentially an economic analysis which showed the extent of the burden of ill health on the Exchequer and the impacts on the quality of life of the UK population in 2020. Projections of NHS spending to 2020 showed that the health of the public was under severe threat from a dramatic growth in chronic disease largely rooted in unhealthy lifestyle patterns. Exploring this, the second Wanless Report 'Securing Good Health for the Whole Population' (2004) identified the need for major changes in the approach to improving public health. The public health workforce were challenged to demonstrate a 'fit for purpose' culture underpinned by a sound evidence base.

Unfortunately, although Wanless identified health inequalities as a major underlying obstacle that would prevent the achievement of a healthy and 'fully engaged' population, governmental attention and action has been largely focused upon the Report's call for lifestyle changes based on individual healthy choices.

Nevertheless the health of the public was put fairly and squarely on the Government's agenda and despite their concentration (diversion?) on to individual lifestyle choice the Wanless Reports paved the way for a re-examination of the whole philosophy of public health and the social, economic and environmental conditions in which it will thrive.

The sheer breadth and depth of all of the issues bound up in that one phrase 'public health' would daunt anyone lesser in character than the editor and authors of this encyclopaedic work. Taking as their working definition of public health Sir Donald Acheson's 'The science and art of promoting health, preventing disease and prolonging life through the organised efforts of society' they have picked up the gauntlet thrown down by Wanless and systematically worked through best practice in acquiring the evidence base applying the findings and evaluating the outcomes of public health programmes and initiatives. From one-to-one work with individuals and families through to community development and complex collaborative ventures the values of trust and mutuality are underscored time and time again. Partnership working often glibly referred to by PCTs and Local Authorities throughout the last decade, but equally often very poorly applied in practice, is now seen as a vital component in achieving the cultural and attitudinal changes vital to the improvement of public health. Whether it is one-to-one with a single parent or within and between organisations the quality and integrity of the relationships on which robust partnerships are built are crucial to achieving the changes that we seek.

This is nowhere more important than in working with individuals, groups and populations who are at the dangerous end of the health inequalities gap. If we are serious about addressing these inequities then we must ensure that the resources education and understanding core to a powerful and empowering community public health policy and practice are built into every element of local regional and national governmental planning.

The concept of public health is changing. As we advance further into the 21st Century it is up to all of those who are working to create a healthy and happy society to take up the challenge and put public health back where it belongs – in the families and communities of our Nation.

Foreword by Cheryll Adams

There has been no time in history when the importance of early intervention using a public health approach has been better supported by a research basis. We now have considerable understanding of the many links between early physical, social and emotional influences and the future disease profile not only of individuals, but also of our population as a whole. Whilst public health practice has its roots in the nineteenth century, it is constantly evolving, and there are new generations of practitioners needing to learn its complex and multifactorial skills.

This is why this book is so important. It provides both endorsement for the importance of public health practice and also the necessary platform from which that practice should evolve. The first edition has been updated, with the many recent advances in policy and research, so it will be of immense value to all public health professionals, policy makers and students of public health practice. The comprehensive review of the skills and knowledge required by 'grass roots' public health practitioners is particularly helpful. Equally important, though, is the discussion of the complexities of working in the public health field and why public health and health mean different things to different people. In each instance the reader is provided with both a theoretical explanation and evidence underpinning to the discussion.

I am pleased that the editor chose to set the book within the framework of the 'Principles of Health Visiting' which have proved useful to health visitors for thirty years and continue to be relevant (CETHV 1977, Cowley and Frost 2006). As shown in the recent review of health visiting, published as this book goes to press, successful public health practice includes work at the level of the population as well as for individuals (DH 2007). The 'principles' emphasise this, as well as the need to influence local and national change agents such as policy makers to bring about real health gain for the population. It gives a detailed analysis of these underlying principles and also makes clear the importance of the critical role of relationships in achieving successful health outcomes. These include not only the client–practitioner relationship but also the relationship between the practitioner and the wider community and those professionals and others working within it. Equally valuable is the detailed analysis of needs assessment; a very complex area, but critical to successful practice.

I would encourage anyone reading this book, or a chapter within it, to pause for at least a moment at the end of each chapter to reflect on the questions it holds. In so doing the value of your reading will be enhanced. Equally important are the topic-based chapters at the end of the book, providing an understanding of how the principles are applied to public health practice and the actions that may be necessary to produce the required outcomes. Particularly powerful here are the practitioners' own stories. They make clear that, whilst public health should be everyone's business, to bring about effective outcomes for individuals and communities, public health professionals require a sound theoretical and evidence base such as is provided by the preceding chapters.

References

Council for the Education and Training of Health Visitors (CETHV) 1977 An investigation into the principles of health visiting. CETHV, London

Cowley S, Frost M 2006 The Principles of Health Visiting: Opening the door

to public health. CPHVA & UKSC, London

Department of Health (DH) 2007 Facing the future. A review of the role of health visitors. DH, London

Preface

The first edition of this book was published at a time of considerable change across public health, health visiting and community nursing, so it began with an analysis of the differences and similarities between the three occupations (Cowley 2002). This showed that the key concepts of decisional control, professional and client autonomy, empowerment and consumer choice were prioritised differently by each occupation, according to their diverse public health purposes. Now, as then, all these are reflected in whether:

- the priority focus is on individuals or whole populations
- the service is mainly about the determinants of health or caring for people with established health problems
- the social or biomedical model of health is prioritised
- matters are considered the legitimate interest of publicly funded services or should remain private.

That chapter (Cowley 2002), like the whole first edition, emphasised both the important contributions made by all three occupations, and the essentially multi-disciplinary nature of public health and primary care; it suggested that the nursing profession, too, should begin to view itself as multi-disciplinary in nature. Instead of describing the roles of individual occupational groups, a focus on the three levels of public health functioning identified by the (then) Chief Medical Officer (CMO) seemed more useful. He explained:

1. Most professionals, including managers in the NHS, local authorities and elsewhere, e.g. teachers, would benefit from a better basic understanding of public health. Knowledge of how to gain access to more specialist input would be useful to strengthen their role in furthering health improvement goals in their daily work, a role they may not recognise as contributing to public health.

2. A smaller group of 'hands on' public health practitioners spend a substantial part of their working practice furthering health by working with communities and groups. They need more specialised knowledge and skills in their respective fields. This group includes public health nurses, health promotion specialists, health visitors, community development workers and environmental health officers.

3. A still smaller group are public health specialists, who come from a variety of professional backgrounds and experience, and need a core of knowledge, skills and experience. This core is in urgent need of definition so that generic public health specialists can be fully acknowledged for their contribution. This group includes professionals from backgrounds

such as the social sciences, statistics, environmental health, medicine, nursing, health promotion and dental public health.'

(DH 1998, p. 15)

Since that report, the skills and knowledge needed to operate as a public health specialist have been defined and refined into performance standards required for entry on to a voluntary professional register. However, far less attention has been paid to the skills and knowledge needed by the middle-sized group of 'grass roots' public health practitioners, who were the focus of the first edition of this book, and who remain central in this updated edition. Although their collective, substantial contribution to the public health was highlighted by the CMO's development project in 1998, this group of grass-roots practitioners occupy a contested and widely neglected professional space.

There are ongoing discussions about how best to represent the specific knowledge and skills of environmental health officers, health promotion specialists and other defined specialist groups within the new, multi-disciplinary public health register. Whilst public health is striving to promote and regularise notions of multi-disciplinarity, a more centralising, uni-disciplinary approach has gained ground within the nursing profession. Despite long-standing ambivalence between the distinct professions of health visiting and nursing, the Nursing and Midwifery Order 2001 formalised a decision to combine them by removing all reference to health visitors from the laws in which it had previously been mentioned, and to close their register in 2004. The new register held by the Nursing and Midwifery Council (NMC) includes a part for 'Specialist Community Public Health Nurses', with health visitors being incorporated under that title (NMC 2004). These widespread and highly contested changes in regulation, education and naming of professions have led to much confusion.

However, there has been a parallel, more positive and useful, emphasis on developing and describing all services in relation to their purpose and client/user group, rather than by the name of the professionals providing them. The title of this second edition was chosen to reflect this newer formulation, emphasising multi-disciplinarity and service focus rather than individual professions, whilst retaining the essential emphasis on policy and practice. At the same time, familiar occupational titles, such as health visitor, community development worker, midwife or nurse are still used within the chapters, recognising the continued division of labour and major contributions to public health made by specific grass-roots occupations.

This edition has been completely reorganised, expanded and updated, with 14 chapters in four sections. To keep up with the rapid progress and many changes across the field of community public health, seven new chapters are included and four chapters, despite having similar titles, have been completely rewritten for this second edition. The three remaining chapters have been substantially updated. Each chapter provides extensive research, conceptual critique and a breadth of information about sources and resources for further information.

Decisions about which aspects to leave in or take out of this second edition were as difficult as with the first; even though it is larger, it could easily have been twice the length! It is clearly impossible to encompass all possible aspects of public health concern within a single volume, and that is not the intention. Instead, details about underlying skills, knowledge, ways of working and methods for organising services to improve health are set out. As before, this is a sourcebook for students or established practitioners alike, especially those involved in either revamping existing services, or developing a focus on a new area of interest or topic of public health concern. I hope it proves useful.

London, 2007   *Sarah Cowley*

References

Cowley S 2002 Public health practice in nursing and health visiting. In: Cowley S (ed) Public health policy and practice: a source book for health visitors and community nurses. Baillière Tindall, London, pp. 5–24

Department of Health (DH) 1998 Chief Medical Officer's project to strengthen the public health function in England: a report of the emerging findings. DH, London

Nursing and Midwifery Council (NMC), 2004 Standards of proficiency for specialist community public health nurses. NMC, London

Acknowledgements

This book owes its existence to the foresight of Mairi McCubbin from Elsevier, who identified a need for a second edition, to the willingness of contributers who cheerfully updated, completely rewrote or developed new chapters to meet new demands of an ever-changing world, and to all the 'behind the scenes' people involved in the publishing process, notably Hannah Kenner and Jack Geddes. Thank you all for your patience and support.

Introduction

This book is about community public health. The World Health Organization (WHO 1998) adopted the definition of public health coined by Acheson (1988): 'The science and art of promoting health, preventing disease, and prolonging life through the organized efforts of society.' Further, the WHO describes public health as a social and political concept aimed at the improving health, prolonging life and improving the quality of life among whole populations through health promotion, disease prevention and other forms of health intervention. The 'new public health' is distinguished by its focus on understanding how lifestyles and living conditions determine health status. This includes recognition of the need to understand the socio-cultural context, and how this can influence the choices and behaviours adopted by individuals, families and communities. This context is central to the aetiology of health inequalities, which are a major, current public health concern. Professionals who work in community public health operate within this socio-cultural context, often aiming to influence and change this as much as the health-related activities of individuals, and this is the form of practice that is the subject of this book.

Specific diseases are, of course, central to public health. They are often best understood by identifying single causes, or at least risk factors that make them very likely; such as smoking or poor diet, which vastly increases the chance of cancer and heart disease, or the risky sexual behaviour that increases the likelihood of contracting Chlamydia or the human immunodeficiency virus (HIV). This kind of cause–effect information is extremely important in helping to improve the health of whole populations. However, it does not explain the more complex question of why some parts of the population are more likely to engage in hazardous activities than others. Nor does a focus on behaviour and lifestyles alone explain the extent of health inequalities witnessed across the world, between rich and poor countries and even within relatively wealthy, developed societies. The aim of community public health is to move beyond the circumscribed boundaries set by a focus on specific disorders and behaviours, to explore and influence the wider contexts in which they arise.

Often, activities directed at changing these contexts operate at a micro-level, such as within families or local communities. Cowley (2002) noted that this gives rise to a paradox, since public health cannot function solely at the level of individual care. Yet, public health progress is not possible without involving those people who make up the population, and whose individual states of illness or wellbeing are collectively described as the 'public health'. This raises questions about the nature of the work, particularly since some people regard public health as operating only at a population level. However, activities are justified as public health interventions if their main purpose is to contribute to the health of the whole population they serve, even if they meet the immediate health needs of individuals and families along the way (Cowley 1998, Keller et al 2004).

It is increasingly clear that socio-economic position and the socio-cultural context in which individuals, families and communities live, have a profound effect on people's health chances. Their influence is mediated by the psychological and physiological effects of fetal and early childhood experiences (Hosking & Walsh 2005, Shonkoff & Phillips 2000, Wadsworth 1999), through cultural norms within the families (Blane 1999) and communities, and re-affirmed across the life course, through generations and localities (Curtis 2004, Graham 2001, Marmot & Wilkinson 2006). The deep-seated and cumulative impact of these factors influence the likelihood of individuals developing particular diseases, of experiencing disabilities, violence or accidents, of living a long or a short life, and one that achieves its full potential or misses opportunities.

Factors that lead to adverse health conditions and risky activities are known as the 'determinants of health,' but these differ from the determinants of health inequalities (Graham & Kelly 2004). A great deal is known about the extent of health inequalities and, despite a comparative lack of rigorous information about how to reduce them, there is sufficient evidence to show the long-lasting benefits that can accrue from a strong focus on preschool years and pregnancy (Acheson 1998). This focus has been adopted in a great deal of policy (e.g. Department of Health 2003, Chief Secretary to the Treasury 2003, HM Government 2006). Many of the chapters in this book, therefore, focus on these early years. However, other age groups and the communities in which young children live are also very important. The extent of social exclusion or social capital in an area is a key influence in the extent of need experienced by young and old alike. Many of the practice approaches outlined in this book focus on developing partnerships, social cohesion or social networks, because of their potential to improve health in the long term.

This book includes many examples and discussions about how community public health services should be planned and delivered, which are familiar territory for the practitioners who working in this field. In the UK these are mainly, but not exclusively, the health visitors, school and occupational health nurses who are currently regulated through the third part of the Nursing and Midwifery Council (NMC) register. Other nurses, midwives and community workers, such as those employed in the multi-disciplinary public health partnerships in Scotland, or the Sure Start Children's Centres in England, are involved in this grass-roots community public health work, too. Elsewhere in the world, many other disciplines undertake activities that are similar, and have similar concerns and interests. This text is not exclusively intended for those on the NMC register, but it follows their lead in aggregating the content under sections linked to the principles of health visiting, first identified by the Council for the Education and Training of Health Visitors (1977). Since that time, health visitors have been clear that these principles underpin their work. They are not single performance standards or learning domains (Cowley & Frost 2006). Instead, the principles are a mechanism for aggregating the knowledge, philosophy and purpose of the work in community public health, and as such, they provide a useful framework for health visiting. It is hoped that the sections will provide a framework for organising the different chapters in this book, as well, in a way that is meaningful to both readers who are very familiar with the principles, and those who are meeting them for the first time.

References

Acheson D 1988 Public health in England: the report of the committee of inquiry into the future development of the public health function. HMSO, London

Acheson D (chair) 1998 Independent inquiry into inequalities in health. HMSO, London

Blane D 1999 The life course, the social gradient and health. In: Marmot M, Wilkinson R (eds.) Social determinants of health. Oxford University Press, Oxford, pp. 64–80

Council for the Education and Training of Health Visitors (CETHV) 1977 An investigation into the principles of health visiting. CETHV, London

Cowley S 1998 Public health: the role of nurses and health visitors. Health Visitor 71: 2–31

Cowley S 2002 Public health practice in nursing and health visiting. In: Cowley S (ed) Public health policy and practice: a source book for health visitors and community nurses. Baillière Tindall, London, pp. 5–24

Cowley S, Frost M 2006 The principles of health visiting: opening the door to public health practice in the 21st century. Community Practitioners' and Health Visitors' Association and UK Standing Conference on Health Visiting Education, London

Chief Secretary to the Treasury 2003 Every child matters (CM5860). HMSO, London

Curtis S 2004 Health and inequality: geographical perspectives. Sage Publications, London

Department of Health (DH) 2003 Tackling health inequalities – a programme for action. DH, London

Graham H (ed) 2001 Understanding health inequalities. Open University Press, Buckingham, UK

Graham H, Kelly M 2004 Health inequalities: concepts, frameworks and policy. Health Development Agency, London

HM Treasury, Department for Education and Skills 2005 Support for parents, the best start for children. HMSO, London

Hosking G, Walsh I 2005 The WAVE report: violence and what to do about it. WAVE Trust, Croydon, Surrey

Keller L, Stihschien S, Lia-Hoagberg B, Schaffer M 2004 Population-based public health interventions: practice based and evidence supported. Part 1. Public Health Nursing 21(5): 453–468

Marmot M, Wilkinson R (eds) 2006 Social determinants of health. Oxford University Press, Oxford

Shonkoff J, Phillips D (eds) 2000 From neurons to neighbourhoods: the science of early child development. National Academy Press, Washington

Wadsworth M 1999 Early life. In Marmot M & Wilkinson R (eds) Social determinants of health. Oxford University Press, Oxford, pp. 44–63

World Health Organization (WHO) 1998 Health promotion glossary. WHO, Geneva, Switzerland

Section 1

The search for health needs

The search for health needs describes a community public health approach to the surveillance and assessment of the populations' health and wellbeing. This is simultaneously more wide-ranging and more intimate than an epidemiological approach, being concerned with both recognised and unrecognised health needs, and with individuals and families as well as wider populations. Practice may include identifying and responding to health needs concurrently, or may involve collating information derived from individual assessments so as to inform service planning and community development approaches. To achieve this, it is necessary to understand both the range of approaches to health needs assessment set out in Chapter 1, and to be able to work in partnership with those whose needs are being assessed, as explained in Chapter 2.

The search for health needs is associated with the following performance standards (Nursing and Midwifery Council 2004, p. 10):

1. Collect and structure data and information on the health and wellbeing, and related needs, of a defined population.
2. Analyse, interpret and communicate data and information on the health and wellbeing, and related needs, of a defined population.
3. Develop and sustain relationships with groups and individuals with the aim of improving health and social wellbeing.
4. Identify individuals, families and groups who are at risk and in need of further support.
5. Undertake screening of individuals and populations and respond appropriately to findings.

1 Health needs assessments

Sarah Cowley

Key issues

- The nature of need and needs assessment is contested and controversial:
  - The policy background provides constraints and drivers
  - The questions is always, need for what?
  - Needs assessment as a basis for public health
- Community needs assessments:
  - Defined populations
  - Deciding the focus
  - Which data to collect and how
- Policy priorities: explain the reason for the focus on children and families
- Needs assessment approaches in these situations vary according to different circumstances and purposes:
  - Assessment for universal prevention: empowerment
  - Assessment for targeted services: indicated and selective needs:
    - Common Assessment Framework
    - Screening
- Needs assessments do not answer the moral question of who should receive public resources to meet their needs

Health needs

The idea of 'health need' is relatively recent, particularly in respect of health promotion or public health. The British National Health Service (NHS) was first established in 1948, in response to a wartime policy document, and focused largely on the need for social insurance to combat widespread poverty (Beveridge 1942). As one part of this, the Beveridge Report recognised the need for 'universal comprehensive medical treatment and rehabilitation' to be provided for 'all persons capable of profiting by it' (p. xi, para 19). Whilst this founding brief was largely achieved through the NHS Act 1946, two issues raised by the quotes were to recur through subsequent legislation.

First, it is clear that the NHS was originally conceptualised as a service to treat illness and disability, and to provide medical care. Public health and community health services (health visitors, school and district nurses, community midwives) were provided by local, rather than national, government until 1974. After this 'unification' of health services, the idea of prevention began to be formally incorporated into NHS policy, but even in recent primary legislation, the terminology remains quite limiting. The Health Act 1999 (Section 18.4) defines 'health care' as 'services for or in connection with the prevention, diagnosis or treatment of illness'. The legislation refers back to the NHS Act 1977, (Section 128 (1) c) for a definition of illness, which 'includes mental disorder within the meaning of the Mental Health Act 1959 and any injury or disability requiring medical or dental treatment or nursing; "medical" includes surgical'. It was assumed that the cost of health services would reduce once the backlog of disease had been dealt with, which would be a major contribution to public health. The idea of health as a positive state, or as an important function of the health service, is not, therefore, widely established in NHS legislation.

The second issue comes from Beveridge's qualifying remark that the service should be provided to 'persons capable of profiting by it', raising the question of who should decide whether profit is possible or not, and on what criteria? Similar subjectivity was incorporated into the NHS Act 1977, in which Section 34a (i) required provision of 'the number of medical practitioners required to meet the *reasonable needs* of their areas and the different parts of those areas' (added emphasis). Rising public expectations, rising costs of health care and different political views about what constitutes a 'reasonable need' have underpinned many subsequent policy changes.

Health and social care

The Health and Community Care Act 1990 was based on two separate White Papers. *Caring for people* (Department of Health (DH) 1989a) acknowledged the importance of providing support for people experiencing a range of needs that were regarded as 'social' rather than medical. This included people with long-term mental health needs and intellectual and physical disabilities in which (it was argued) help might be needed by family and friends, or be provided from local authority sources if informal support was not sufficient. Needs arising in old age, as part of a normal life course, were included, but support required by mothers and families with young children were not. Whilst the legislation stipulated that individuals had a right to receive care where an assessment showed that 'social needs' existed, the local authority could make a charge for the services they provided. This was distinct from *Working for patients* (DH 1989b), which concerned the provision of health services that were free at the point of delivery.

This legislation first introduced the notion of an 'internal market' into the NHS, stressing that services should be planned strategically within one organisation, then purchased from a different provider service to meet needs in the area. Medical Directors of Public Health led this activity. Whilst this planning requirement legitimised public health activities within the NHS, it tended to reinforce the earlier focus on illness and service provision, instead of wider factors that contribute to health, such as environment or lifestyle. Health and social care services were enjoined to collaborate to provide a seamless service, but distinguishing between 'health needs' and 'social needs' became a source of much confusion for care providers and service users alike (Bergen et al 1996).

Joint working

Collaborative working was stressed even more firmly within the Health Act 1999, which set out specific 'partnership arrangements' designed to overcome this confusion and improve flexibility between the NHS and local authorities in England. Although individuals could still be charged for services provided for 'social care', Section 31 of the Act allowed funding derived from different sectors (e.g. NHS and local authority) to be pooled to set up services in which more than one agency has an interest. This facility foreshadowed organisational arrangements

3

such as Children's Trusts, established under the Children Act 2004, which involved health, social and educational services, as well as the voluntary sector. Importantly, the Health Act 1999 required health authorities to set out a strategy to both improve the health of the people for whom they are responsible, and provide health care to such people. These policies stressed multi-agency working to address the wider determinants of health, although there was a paradoxical lack of emphasis on these wider elements within the NHS Plan (Secretary of State for Health 2000), perhaps reflecting its long association with illness and medical care, rather than public health and health promotion.

By this time, two things were happening. First, the impact of devolution was being felt, resulting in some quite marked differences in health policy between the four parts of the UK. Chapter 4, for example, explains the Community Health Partnerships (CHP) that are required in Scotland. Second, the government recognised the existence of wide and increasing health inequalities, and was developing policies to address them (DH 2003).

Need for what?

Given this background, it is clear that the notion of 'health need' is highly political, complex, value-laden and far from problem-free. However, there has been a burgeoning interest in the use of the term, and in different approaches to assessing needs. Needs assessment processes are considered an essential precursor to the planning of services, on both an individual and population-wide level. It is clear that needs must be assessed with the question in mind always, of 'need for what?' In clinical terms, this usually means making an assessment prior to prescribing a treatment; a population-wide assessment may lead to the 'prescription' of public health strategy, including the provision of general health services as well as prevention.

The definition of health needs in respect of health improvement is more complex than its clinical counterpart, as it concerns whole populations and determinants of health. The Beveridge ideal of being 'capable of profiting by it' might not apply to single person or individual, or the advantage may be so long term that it is hard to discern specific changes. The mechanisms used for both assessing needs, and evaluating services, in such circumstances, have to take a population-wide approach.

Need and needs assessment

Nature of need

Whether at a clinical or population-wide level, it is clear that the nature of 'need' is highly contested, and there is general agreement that need is a 'deceptively tricky concept' (Asadi-Lari & Gray 2005, p. 295). It is problematic as an operating concept (Sheppard & Woodcock 1999) and value laden, in that someone has to decide whether or not a need exists, which is an evaluative judgement (Endacott 1997). In a study carried out in the mid 1990s, the question of what the term meant to them was put to a series of focus groups of, first, service users, then professionals (district nurses and health visitors), then managers and those who commissioned and organised both NHS and local authority social services, then finally practice teachers and lecturers (Cowley et al 1996). They all had different views, and many found it very hard to think about what 'need' might mean, unless it was attached to something else, like 'health need', or 'needs assessment', or 'clinical need'. Most of the service users were somewhat unhappy with the term, as it had connotations of 'being needy', which they felt was stigmatising.

A detailed analysis across the focus group responses revealed many contradictions within the concept, and a conclusion was reached that need is a dual concept, in that it has some very contrasting meanings (Cowley et al 1995). It is possible to describe needs quite objectively, at least in part. Needs are recordable, and can be measured, observed and made explicit, to some degree. It is possible, for example, to assess someone's blood pressure, or their mobility, or whether they have postnatal depression, using a carefully developed and validated instrument. Such assessment tools give a good degree of what researchers call 'inter-rater reliability', which basically means that if two or more people take the measurement, they will reach the same conclusion. But needs are also very variable and personal, in that the same issue, for example, a child or young person's behaviour, or limited mobility in an older person, may result in different views of whether it is a problem or not. In this respect, needs are very subjective and changeable according to context. This is the polar opposite of inter-rater reliability, where completely different conclusions are reached about what, on the surface, may appear to be the same thing.

Some needs are very obvious, particularly those associated with clear physical diagnoses, perhaps with an obvious wound or a rash, or in a desperately run-down area that clearly displays its deprivation through graffiti, neglected or derelict buildings, and lack of facilities. Other needs – physical as well as social, emotional and mental health needs – are more hidden. Where genteel poverty and pride go hand in hand, where emotional distress is seen as a source of shame, or where the mental trauma is severe, clients may hide their needs from an assessor, or not reveal things that are worrying them simply because they cannot formulate the words. Indeed, people may experience a level of anxiety or difficulty without fully realising what lies beneath their worries. They may be quite genuine in stating that their childhood was happy, for example, because the 'family secrets' of sexual or emotional abuse that lay behind a façade are too deeply hidden for them to recognise themselves. Does that mean they are not needs? Or not needs until they are revealed, or only if experienced as problems? These were the kinds of very complex question asked in the study referred to above, about what constituted a 'need' (Cowley et al 1995, 1996).

Needs assessments

A whole taxonomy of needs assessment was developed after carrying out a series of observations in practice and interviews to develop the ideas voiced in the focus groups described above (Bergen et al 1996, Cowley et al 2000a, 2000b). Needs assessments can be considered under three main headings, each with different, interlinked elements. These are:

1. Ideals
   In policy – Discipline specific – Ascribed worth.
2. Timing
   Client issues – Service issues – Practice issues.
3. Types
   Purpose – Formality, specificity – Complexity.

Ideals

Formal policies and laws set out whose assessment counts in particular situations, and the rights and responsibilities that flow from the assessment. These constitute a specific set of values and ideals, agreed in the particular society that approves them and made real as they are enacted. The difference between health and social need, for example, is clear only in the duties placed upon different public services to meet identified needs. Expectations of the rights, responsibilities and choices available to service users are set out in policy, as well as the duties of service providers.

Despite the policy commitment, and frequent use of the terms 'need' and 'needs assessment', they tend to be used very differently by different disciplines, including economists, epidemiologists, policy makers and professionals (Billings & Cowley 1995, Lightfoot 1995, Robinson & Elkan 1996). Apart from differences when considering needs at an individual or service level, each profession has a distinct underlying philosophy, which influences their understanding of the term 'need'. For doctors, reaching a diagnosis is a central part of their professional work, which affects both their communication style (ten Have 1991) and their interest in disease-specific needs assessments (Asadi-Lari & Gray 2005). Nurses, too, tend to concentrate on deficits and difficulties, with Endacott (1997) also emphasising the importance of prioritising and the ability to meet needs. The social work literature highlights deficits, although Shephard and Woodcock (1999) argue that a more differentiated concept is needed for their work with children and families. Since health visitors focus on health promotion and positive health (Prime Research and Development 2001), to concentrate on deficits or problems would negate their main purpose (Cowley & Frost 2006). Community development workers, too, avoid focusing on deficits, preferring instead to highlight the capacity, strengths and resources found in the local population (see Chapter 5). The different uses of the term 'need' can create difficulties, for example, when a problem focus is used to determine needs assessment schedules for use by health visitors resulting in a medicalised approach to the work (Cowley et al 2004).

The extent to which an assessment is valued in an organisation varies according to who carries it out ('ascribed worth') and how important particular needs seem within an organisation. Where individual nurses and health visitors had assessed needs in their caseloads, for example, Bergen et al (1996) found their profiles tended to be disregarded, because they were not sufficiently senior in the organisation for their assessment to count for much. In contrast, local needs assessments made by senior public health doctors usually over-ruled everyone else.

Different perceptions about what constitutes a need vary between organisations, often in line with changing policies. Under the Childcare Act 2006, for example, English local authorities are all required to improve the wellbeing of young children and the reduce inequalities between them. Although the main emphasis is on provision of childcare so parents can work, and information that may be of benefit to them in bringing up their children, the Act also specifies local authorities' duties in providing 'early childhood services'. These include social services, health services relating to young children, parents and prospective parents and early years provision. There is an expectation that these services will generally be delivered through integrated Children's Centres, so it would be helpful to have an agreed understanding about the nature of needs to be met in order to improve children's wellbeing.

Timing

People need to be ready to talk about things that are bothering them, so timing is important from the client's perspective. Also, practitioners need the time to carry out assessments sensitively. Cowley and Houston (2003) found that clients were either bemused or offended when rushed practitioners read through a list of questions without listening to responses, because their organisation required the assessment form to be completed by the time an infant reached a certain age.

Services may introduce quality indicators suggesting that certain topics need to be introduced by a particular age; such requirements will influence the timing of when needs assessments are carried out as well. Indeed, time is one element of the model of service quality outlined in Chapter 13. The timing of an assessment is also related to the level of prevention; once a problem has become manifest, it is no use aiming to achieve primary prevention, nor to offer anticipatory advice about a developmental stage once it has passed. A policy focus on early prevention has been increasingly evident since the start of the 21st century.

Types

Some assessments are much more formal than others. Typically, the most formal assessments are those that have financial implications, such as those carried out at a strategic level to inform decisions about which services to fund or prioritise. At the grass-roots level, information may be gathered to feed into those decisions, either by collecting one or two particular types of information (perhaps the weight of school-aged children, for example, to feed into a strategy about obesity prevention) or may be collated into a community profile, considered further below.

The informal and non-specific assessments are no less important, and sometimes help to complete a complex picture; a mother struggling to introduce solids to a reluctant baby might make a throwaway remark about power battles in the home around mealtimes when she herself was a child, for example, that will be far more telling than a whole battery of behavioural tests. Also, the purpose of the assessment influences both how, and when, it is carried out.

In practice, assessments rarely fall neatly into a single format, with the different types and timing issues involved being intertwined with policy priorities and specific professional perceptions about what constitutes 'need'. Overall, needs assessments carried out on a well population, at the level of the community, child, family or individual for purposes of preventive care and health promotion, is less widely documented than approaches used for planning either services or treatment.

Assessing community health needs

The terms 'local health needs assessment' and 'health profile' tend to be used interchangeably. Billings (2002) distinguishes between them, regarding 'health needs assessment' as a broad term concerned with a description of factors that must be addressed in order to improve the health of the population. This definition allows for the delineation of a range of factors that make up the concept of need, whereas the health profile is a method by which needs are assessed (Billings 2002). It has been identified in its widest sense as: 'the systematic collection of data to identify the health needs of a defined population, and the analysis of that data to assess and prioritise strategies in health promotion' (Twinn et al 1990, p. 2). Health profiles use mainly quantitative health data, such as statistical information, but qualitative health data, such as individual assessments and client perceptions, can be incorporated to form a more holistic picture (Billings 2002).

Health profiling may be carried out as a search for specific, prioritised needs, which have been identified as important at a national, international or local level. Alternatively, a 'bottom up' approach may be used, to allow the local population to discern for themselves what they consider to be their own needs. This is a more common approach in community development and community practice work, as explained in Chapters 6 and 14. Often, the two are used to some extent in combination. Either way, the four questions to be considered before planning to assess needs at the level of grassroots practice are summarised in Box 1.1.

Box 1.1

Local health needs assessments

1. What is the population to be considered?
   Level: caseload, practice, neighbourhood?
   How is the population defined?
2. What is the purpose and scope of the assessment?
   Service planning?
   Evaluation?
   Multi-disciplinary and/or multi-agency?
3. Which data are readily available?
   Data from medical GP practice?
   Census data?
   Local public health department?
   Local, national and international statistics?
4. Which data must be collected specifically for the assessment?
   Local survey
   Rapid participatory appraisal?
   Audit and monitoring information?

Defined populations

The first stage of identifying health needs is to decide which population is under consideration. Public health practitioners usually have responsibility for working with a defined population of some kind, which is often called their 'caseload'. A public health caseload differs from one held by clinicians, where the numbers equate to the files held, indicating contact with a person. In terms of prevention and public health, it is necessary to be aware, even without having necessarily met a person, of what their needs might be. So, a public health caseload might include the whole school population, for example, even though a school nurse might never have the opportunity to meet all of the 10–20 000 children enrolled in the schools for which she has responsibility. In some places, the idea of 'whole school population' may include staff as well as children and their families, or specifically indicate enrolled children only. Similarly, an occupational health nurse may have responsibility for a defined population of employees, or this may extend to incorporate prospective staff (through pre-employment medical checks, for example), and ex-employees, such as those who have retired from an organisation, and possibly the local population, through staff clubs and family facilities.

Those working within primary care in Great Britain usually have their population defined in terms of the practice list defined by registration with a general medical practitioner (GP). Other services are defined by geographical area, particularly where they are either led by local authorities, or developed in collaboration with them. In either case, there may be subdivisions of the whole population, such as those living in a particular area, as well as being on a GP list, or belonging to a particular age range. In some places, for example, health visiting work may be restricted to pre-school children and their families, whereas in others it incorporates a wider age range.

Wider context

Some specialists may be appointed to focus on particular population groups, such as homeless families, the travelling community, refugees and asylum seekers or looked-after children. When planning services for a 'core population', it is preferable to look at the context within which they live, so as to determine the needs of the defined group more clearly. Focusing only on homeless families without looking at the wider population where they live, for example, would give no indication about the root causes of their housing problem. Seeing the needs of employees only whilst they are at work would limit the extent of preventive activities in which they might be engaged, whereas focusing on a wider community may give an indication of local leisure patterns, food behaviour and so on, all of which have an influence on health. Timelines are important, particularly for children. Eating patterns in the preschool years may set the scene for later obesity, or child behaviour at first school may indicate a risk of later delinquency, if help is not forthcoming.

This form of 'nesting' of information is used in community, neighbourhood and caseload profiles, with the overall title being determined by which level is foremost. These levels of health needs assessment are not separate from each other. Community profiles may include general practice and caseload information. Practice profiles will need some community-wide information for comparison purposes. At the level of strategic planning, there is an increasing tendency to try and match service boundaries, so they are coterminous. It helps if boundaries match electoral wards or boundaries, since most epidemiological data sources are collated in those formats. Figures are traditionally collected according to mortality (rates and causes), gathered mainly from birth and death certificates, and morbidity (see Box 1.2). Morbidity is the extent of illness and disease, gleaned from a range of sources, such as general practice or hospital data (attendance, admissions, investigations and treatments) and surveys and censuses (see Box 1.3). As far as possible, definitions are standardised nationally and internationally, so that comparisons can be made. International comparisons are particularly important when working with minority ethnic groups (to draw on home country information), to assess disease trends and treatment efficacy or service effectiveness.

Clarify purpose of assessment

Governments determine which services are to be funded through the public purse, which has a direct impact on the nature of needs that will be met, and which agency will meet them. In terms of public health, it is well recognised that multi-agency, collaborative services are necessary, since the root causes of health and illness are rarely the sole responsibility of the NHS, or any other single agency. It is important to have some idea of the scope of services that could be deployed to meet the needs that are identified, and to establish a joint planning group at the outset. When assessing local needs for a local children's centre, for example, will there be a representative from the local authority, who can speak on policy in respect of playgrounds and recreational facilities; or someone from the health service who can speak on the feasibility of a proposed clinic?

Which data to collect?

Readily available

Some data are readily available, such as the number of children in a school, or new births on a general practice list. Employers need and collect information about the number of staff with disabilities, which may prove useful when targeting groups for health promotion campaigns, for example. Census data are also readily available from the Office of National Statistics, and through local or Health Observatories. Ideally, demographic data collected in a local situation, such as a

Box 1.2

Gathering information: epidemiology basics

Definition

Epidemiology is the study of how often diseases occur in different groups of people and why.

Key features

- Epidemiology is the measurement of disease outcomes in relation to a population at risk.
- Epidemiological observations may guide decisions about individuals, but they relate primarily to groups of people.
- Clues to aetiology come from comparing disease rates in groups with differing levels of exposure.
- Epidemiology is concerned with monitoring or surveillance of time trends to show which diseases are increasing or decreasing in incidence and which are changing in their distribution.

Measurement

Measuring disease frequency in populations requires the stipulation of diagnostic criteria, sometimes known as 'defining the case':

- The International Classification of Diseases, Injuries, and Causes of Death, published by the World Health Organization, assigns a three-character alphanumeric code to every major condition. This is regularly updated, to ensure international consistency in data collection.
- For epidemiological purposes, the occurrence of cases of disease must be related to the 'population at risk' giving rise to the cases. Measures of disease frequency in common use are:
  - The *incidence* of a disease is the rate at which new cases occur in a population during a specified period (i.e. once a person is classified as a case, he or she is no longer liable to become a new case).
  - The *prevalence* of a disease is the proportion of a population infected with the disease at a point in time.

Mortality is the incidence of death from a disease

- Direct standardisation entails comparison of weighted averages of age-and sex-specific disease rates, the weights being equal to the proportion of people in each age and sex group in a convenient reference population (e.g. measures of testicular cancer related to males in the population).
- A comparable statistic, the standardised mortality ratio (SMR) is widely used by the Registrar General in summarising time trends and regional and occupational differences. To analyse time trends, as with the cost of living index, an arbitrary base year is taken.
- A crude incidence, prevalence, or mortality death rate is one that relates to results for a population taken as a whole, without subdivision or refinement. The death rate would be higher in certain populations, e.g. a retirement village where there is a higher elderly population, so standardised mortality rates adjust for such variation.

Some special rates (usually related to 1 year)

- Birth rate = Number of live births to mid-year population.
- Fertility rate = Number of live births to number of women aged 15–44 years.
- Infant mortality rate = Number of infant < 1 year deaths per number of live births.
- Stillbirth rate = Number of intrauterine deaths after 28 weeks compared with total number of births.

(continued)

- Perinatal mortality rate = Number of stillbirths + deaths in 1st week of life compared with total number births.
- Neonatal mortality rate = Number of stillbirths + deaths in 1st month of life (28 days) compared with total number births.
- Post-neonatal mortality rate = Number of deaths from 1st month of life (28 days) to end of 1st year, compared with total number births.

Source: Coggan D, Rose G, Barker DJP 1997 Epidemiology for the Uninitiated, 4th edn. British Medical Journal Publishing Group, London. http://bmj.bmjjournals.com/collections/epidem/epid.shtml

---

Box 1.3

Sources of information about health

International statistics

World Health Organization gathers and publishes statistics by country and by health topics. Also has a range of research and epidemiological tools, publications on key issues and monitors progress towards selected health improvement goals.

http://www.who.int/en/

UK national statistics

Demographic information from latest census, neighbourhood information about, e.g. deprivation, health inequalities and latest health surveys.

http://www.statistics.gov.uk

Country statistics

Information on key areas of immediate policy interest, including public health indicators, workforce and service provision.

England: http://www.dh.gov.uk/PublicationsAndStatistics/fs/en
Scotland: http://www.healthscotland.com/
Wales: http://www.wales.nhs.uk/
Northern Ireland: http://www.healthpromotionagency.org.uk/

Health Protection Agency

http://www.hpa.org.uk/

Umbrella organisation for each of nine Public Health Observatories in England: http://www.apho.org.uk/ and in Scotland http://www.scotpho.org.uk/

Public Health Departments and Health Intelligence Units based in local services are a most valuable source of information.

---

caselist, school roll or neighbourhood, needs to be compared to wider figures at the level of a borough, electoral ward or county; Box 1.3 provides sources.

Collected specifically for the assessment

Alternatively, information may be collected specifically for the assessment, perhaps through a local survey or rapid participatory appraisal. Grant (2001) (see also Chapter 12) describes the methodology known as Community Participatory Appraisal (CPA), which she used to investigate lay perspectives on health in her local area. This methodology uses a variety of methods to triangulate information gathered. It involves the local population in determining its own needs, through a process using a questionnaire survey, observations, interviews and focus

Box 1.4

A national framework for health information and intelligence

Data collection

- Data should be collected as a by-product of routine public- or private-sector activity as far as possible.
- Data should be of known validity and completeness.
- Available data should cover the causes of health and illness, including wider determinants, as well as health outcomes and quality of services provided.
- Sources of data should include primary, secondary and community NHS care, local public-sector sources, private-sector and voluntary-sector sources.

Data management

- Data should be efficiently shared, collated, validated, linked, anonymised and archived as appropriate, using secure systems.
- Person-level data should be handled in such a way that the rights and interests of the individuals concerned are acknowledged and respected, while striking a proportionate balance with the public benefit.

Analysis

Systems should allow a range of approaches to analysis, including:

- Ad hoc, query-based analysis
- The regular production of specified indicators
- Surveillance for unexpected trends and outcomes
- Modelling of health outcomes against targets
- Data feeds for disease registers including cancer registries
- Area-based analyses from national to small areas, with comparisons.

Interpretation in context

The results of the analysis must be interpreted in the context of:

- Statistical and methodological issues, including data quality
- Evidence from research
- Experience of practice
- Local knowledge.

Communication of messages

The messages derived from the interpretation of the information and evidence must be communicated to relevant audiences using a range of media appropriate to the target audience or audiences.

Source: Department of Health (DH) 2006. Informing healthier choices: information and intelligence for healthy populations. DH, London, p. 10

groups (Murray & Graham 1995). The approach has been used extensively across the world, with a general recommendation that the best methods are those that are easiest to use (Annett & Rifkin 1995, Ong & Humphris 1994).

Increasingly, health authorities are setting up 'health intelligence' units with a specific brief to gather this information (DH 2006). A national framework for health information and intelligence is proposed, which sets a standard for collating information (see Box 1.4). This is not to suggest that good health intelligence is automatically easy to achieve. A metaphor coined by Sir Muir Gray (cited in DH 2006, p.11) suggests, 'Information is like water. It must be gathered from where it falls, channelled, cleaned, treated and tested before being stored in reservoirs. It must then be made available on tap to those who need it, wherever and whenever they need it.'

Grass-roots public health workers are often in a position to gather information that is useful for health intelligence, but it is not ideal to make it 'routine' to ask everyone a series of questions about issues of concern to service commissioners rather than allowing clients the opportunity to discuss their health needs in their own preferred way. Instead, practitioners need time to analyse and synthesise the (anonymous) information they have to hand, before passing it on. It is not feasible to develop a single instrument suited to both family health needs assessment and the purposes of health intelligence (Cowley & Houston 2004), a point that is explained further below.

Need for prevention

Focus on children and families

The importance of maternal and child welfare as the basis for public health programmes is increasingly clear. Historically, and currently in much the developing world, this has been of direct importance, since high rates of mortality or morbidity during pregnancy, childbirth and in the early years of life inhibit the development of nations. The inception of a universal health visiting service, mainly focused on the health and welfare of women and young children, was an early response to high maternal and infant mortality rates in the UK in the late 19th and early 20th centuries. Similar services developed early in France, later spreading to various other countries, and are still needed where poverty is rife and basic health care lacking (World Health Organization (WHO) 2005). As mortality rates fell in developed countries, continued support for promoting the health of mothers and babies might, at first glance, seem less important. However, the links between a mother's health and that of her infant, and between children's health and their later health in adulthood, have become increasingly clear (Graham & Power 2004, Shonkoff & Phillips 2000, Wadsworth 1999). The impact of the child's early life course has a particular and strong effect, not only on an individual infant, but also on health inequalities across the nation (Graham & Kelly 2004, Independent Inquiry into Inequalities in Health 1998).

Universal or targeted services

Policy responses to evidence about the links between children's socio-economic circumstances and adult health can take two different forms (Graham & Kelly 2004), which have different implications for the assessment of needs. One approach is to focus on the most socially excluded, those with most risk factors and who are the most difficult to reach. These are often called 'targeted' approaches, and include the provision of various specialist services for named vulnerable or excluded groups, like the homeless population, asylum seekers or looked-after children; or geographically targeted measures, such as the provision of Sure Start Local Programmes or similar complex community initiatives (see Chapter 6). This kind of approach fits into the form of prevention called 'selective prevention' in the typology proposed by Gordon (1983) and adopted by Mrazek and Haggerty (1994), and the World Health Organization (2004) (see Box 1.5).

The second policy approach responds to the broader social gradient in health and the large numbers of people who, while they may not be formally regarded

Box 1.5

Definitions of universal, selective and indicated prevention

Universal

Universal prevention is defined as those interventions that are targeted at the general public or to a whole population group that has not been identified on the basis of increased risk.

Targeted: two forms

1. Selective prevention targets individuals or subgroups of the population whose risk of developing a disorder is significantly higher than average, as evidenced by biological, psychological or social risk factors.
2. Indicated prevention targets high-risk people who are identified as having minimal but detectable signs or symptoms indicating predisposition for disorder, but who do not meet diagnostic criteria for disorder at that time.

Adapted from Mrazek PJ, Haggerty RJ 1994 Reducing risks for mental disorders: frontiers for preventive intervention research. National Academy Press, Washington

---

as socially excluded, are relatively disadvantaged in health terms. This approach recognises the need for more universally available services, even if they are not delivered in a uniform way. All pregnant women in the UK, for example, are deemed to need midwifery support, starting early in the antenatal period and continuing through the delivery until after the birth. This universally available service also acts as a conduit through which women can access other primary and secondary care services if needed, whether by referral or through information-giving, following needs assessment, which is a form of 'indicated prevention' (see Box 1.5). This is another form of targeting, which is generally more individually focused and may be delivered in conjunction with a universal service.

A universal health visiting service has been available to all families with pre-school children since long before the NHS was established in the UK (Dingwall 1977). There is some debate about whether the universal service should continue, or be replaced with a selective one. Drawing on the work of the late epidemiologist Geoffrey Rose, Elkan et al (2001) emphasise the importance of retaining a universal focus for health visiting services, because 'the bulk of health and social problems occur in the large number of people who are not especially at risk, rather than in the few who are at high risk' (p. 117). If a universal service continues, there are questions about what form it should take; a reduction in staff numbers is driving much of the change. Both health visiting and school health services aim to promote health for all children through a personalised child health plan (DH 2004), and to reduce health inequalities by identifying other needs through individual child and family health assessments. The processes involved in needs assessment vary widely, depending on whether they are being used for targeting (whether through selective or indicated prevention) or for purposes of health promotion in a universal service (Cowley & Houston 2004).

Universal prevention: assessment for health promotion

Universal services focused on health promotion and prevention are delivered with three major aims in mind. First, they support the public health imperative

Table 1.1 Empowerment approach

Relevant health visiting research	Health visiting practice	Intent for client
Enabling relationships (Pearson 1991, Chalmers & Luker 1991, de la Cuesta 1994)	Health visitor as facilitator and resource	Client in the lead
Gaining access/entry work (Luker & Chalmers 1989)	Assessment is integral to practice	Promotes 'participatory competence'
Health promotion work (Chalmers 1992)	Flexible view of what constitutes 'need'	Non-prescriptive: permitted needs not predetermined
Client-centredness; 'fringe work' (de la Cuesta 1993)	Encourages client-centred approach to practice	Validation of client's perspective/opinion inclusive of contextual and socio-cultural issues
Development: changing expectations (Pearson 1991)	Allows professional judgement	
Shifting focus in conversation (Cowley 1991)	Fosters acceptance of the client view	Non-stigmatising
Unpredicted needs/therapeutic prevention (Cowley 1995b)	Proactive search for health needs	Assessment as an opportunity to discuss health, not a condition for receiving service
Actively promoting resources for health (Cowley 1995a)		

From: Houston & Cowley 2002

of improving health across the whole of the population to whom the service is delivered. Second, by destigmatising and normalising service provision, universality enables those who are the most disadvantaged, and usually hardest to reach, to accept initial offers of provision, which is key to the reduction of health inequalities. The third major aim is to jointly differentiate and target individuals, children or families who have a need for additional services, so they can have access to appropriate support and early interventions. Needs assessment processes are central to all of these three aims, and intertwined with delivery of a health-promoting service.

Health promotion draws strongly on the view that 'empowerment' is an essential basis for health, which can only be developed internally by individuals, families or community groups (Rissell 1994). It cannot be prescribed or dispensed by an outsider, but a facilitator might encourage or assist that development by working in a genuine, respectful partnership (Davis et al 2002). To achieve health, people need to own it themselves, in the sense of exercising full autonomy and choices in the way they live their lives (Rijke 1993). Universal services, therefore, use the assessment process as an opportunity to promote and develop 'participatory competence' on the part of the client, whose position Kieffer (1984) describes in terms of citizenship and empowerment. The assessment process should not inhibit their primary purpose of health promotion (Cowley & Houston 2004).

A great deal of qualitative research, summarised in Table 1.1, has been undertaken in respect of health visiting services, to show the key elements involved in this form of assessment (Houston & Cowley 2002a). Client-centredness, needs assessments and enabling access to services are all intertwined and interdependent rather than following a linear process (Appleton & Cowley 2003, Cowley & Houston 2004, Cowley et al 2000), as shown in Figure 1.1. Overall, the research paints a picture of assessment that is bound up with the whole of practice, rather than being a separate, preliminary stage, as occurs in selective prevention or when assessing needs prior to developing services.

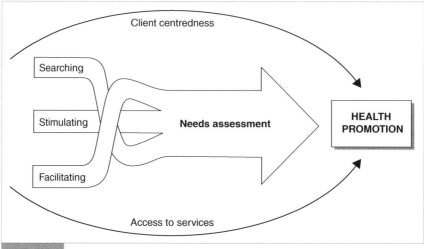

Figure 1.1 ● Needs assessment for health promotion (from Cowley & Houston 2004)

Luker and Chalmers (1990) detail the embedded processes and time needed to accomplish what they call 'entry work', treating problems as if they are 'normal' rather than 'deviant', which is an essential pre-requisite to the main body of activity, the 'health promotion work' (Chalmers 1992). This contrasts strongly with needs assessment protocols that list 'problem areas' for possible discussion, thus denying clients the opportunity to raise their own concerns, and placing firm boundaries around the remit of the service (Cowley et al 2004).

In an empowerment approach, practitioners do not go in with a fixed agenda or a closed choice of predetermined needs to be ratified by clients; they aim, instead, to explore how families can harness their own health-creating potential and capacity. Sometimes a trigger tool may be used, such as the validated Family-wise cartoon-based programme (Glover 2001). These have been developed and are available in a series of 'picture kits', as shown in Figure 1.2; the idea is that people might be shown the cartoon and invited to talk about it, which allows them to decide which elements to draw out or ignore. Alternatively, where literacy is sufficiently high, an aide-memoire, or various open instruments based on a list of words or sentences for completion may be used or left to one side if either practitioner or client feel its use is inappropriate at any particular time (Houston & Cowley 2002). More usually, an undirected and open conversational style is used to 'search for health needs', which is a foundation principle of health visiting (CETHV 1977, Chalmers 1993, Williams 1997).

Bearing in mind that health visiting is a proactive, unsolicited service, its practitioners need to be prepared to accept and follow shifts in the direction of conversation, responding to cues that may be quite minimal, and either verbal or non-verbal. This shifting focus follows and stimulates awareness of any health needs mentioned in the conversation (Cowley 1991). The shifting directions are purposeful, being used to maintain open agreement between health visitor and client about the purpose of the contact, enabling topics relevant to the client to be central. This approach may be equally relevant in other health promoting services that are offered, whether requested or not.

Proactive, health-promoting services need to be client-centred, requiring the 'fringe work' (de la Cuesta 1993) that lies outside normal organisational agendas,

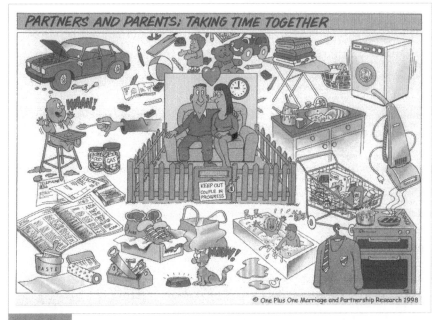

PARTNERS AND PARENTS; TAKING TIME TOGETHER

© One Plus One Marriage and Partnership Research 1998

Figure 1.2 ● Trigger cartoon for discussion

like arranging appointments at times to suit the client rather than the clinic and maintaining mobile role boundaries in order to maintain relevance of the service for clients. Relationship skills appear critical in determining the degree to which health visitors (Machen 1996, Normandale 2001) or any other practitioners are acceptable to clients (Davis & Spurr 1998, Davis et al 2002). Interpersonal relationships between clients and professionals are not generally regarded as a primary health outcome, or end, in themselves, but they are facilitative in that they enable health promotion work to be initiated and accomplished (Chalmers & Luker 1991, de la Cuesta 1994). Relationships form the basis for a great deal of public health work (see Chapter 2) and endure over time, whereas an assessment undertaken at one point in time is likely to yield quite different results if undertaken with the same family at another time (Elkan et al 2000).

The most effective services are multi-faceted and generalist in nature, so they are able to respond quickly and accurately to a wide range of health promotion needs (Bull et al 2004, Macleod & Nelson 2000). A versatile service helps practitioners to provide valued help in an acceptable or timely manner, perhaps with an apparently small query in the first instance, which helps to build trust in the service. A combination of trust in the professional as a person and in his/her ability to respond appropriately helps to build confidence and understanding about the purpose of the service (Collinson & Cowley 1998a). In turn, this helps clients to feel able to reveal and discuss otherwise hidden, possibly more relevant and deep-seated, health needs (Collinson & Cowley 1998b) (see Figure 1.3).

Assessments, therefore, often occur over a period time and at an unpredictable pace set by clients, as they come to recognise their own needs and seek support. This is the mechanism through which universal service provision achieves the major priorities of identifying and enabling access to services by those with specific needs, particularly by individuals and families who are traditionally the hardest to reach.

17

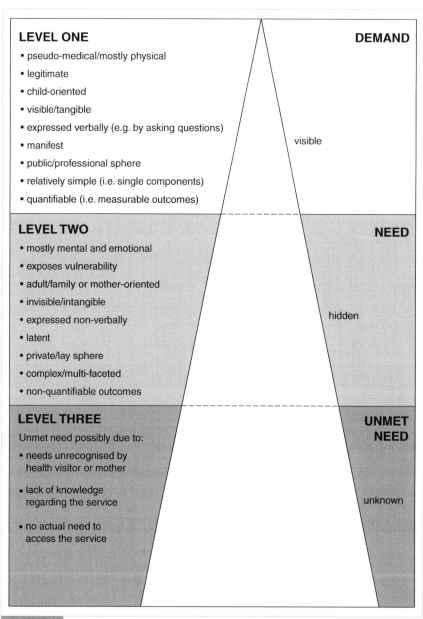

LEVEL ONE

- pseudo-medical/mostly physical
- legitimate
- child-oriented
- visible/tangible
- expressed verbally (e.g. by asking questions)
- manifest
- public/professional sphere
- relatively simple (i.e. single components)
- quantifiable (i.e. measurable outcomes)

DEMAND

visible

LEVEL TWO

- mostly mental and emotional
- exposes vulnerability
- adult/family or mother-oriented
- invisible/intangible
- expressed non-verbally
- latent
- private/lay sphere
- complex/multi-faceted
- non-quantifiable outcomes

NEED

hidden

LEVEL THREE

Unmet need possibly due to:

- needs unrecognised by health visitor or mother
- lack of knowledge regarding the service
- no actual need to access the service

UNMET NEED

unknown

Figure 1.3 ● Iceberg of need (family health) (adapted from Collinson & Cowley 1998a)

Assessment for targeted services

British government policy emphasises targeting as the preferred approach to redress inequalities, by directing resources towards those in greatest need (DH 1999a, 2001a, 2002a, 2003, Secretary of State for Health 2004). Needs assessment processes are increasingly invoked as the mechanism through which services can best be deployed, with nurses, midwives and health visitors all being expected to help identify service priorities and to target their efforts effectively and efficiently

(DH 1999b, 2001b, c, 2002b). In the face of this plethora of policy guidance, Cowley and Houston (2004) argued that, as a preventive approach, targeting is essentially driven by an organisational agenda. That is not to be understood as a criticism; effective and efficient organisations are central in driving forward the public health agenda and overall preventive effort; as long as the objectives serve a health improvement purpose.

Having an objective or a minimum result to aim at, which is what 'target' means, is immensely helpful in terms of organisational efficiency. Targeting the service, or aiming the resources more precisely, is not only a mechanism through which costs can be contained; it is also concerned with responding effectively to particular problems or causes of problems ('determinants of health') that have been identified as needing attention. In practice, this means an assessment that a specific need exists must take place; then a prescribed treatment or (to use terminology that is more familiar to nurses and health visitors) a 'programme of care' can be initiated.

Targeted prevention takes two forms; selective and indicated (see Box 1.5). Selective prevention is used with individuals or subgroups of the population with risks that are significantly above average; Eaton and Harrison (1998) cite the example of additional family support for young, poor, first-pregnancy mothers. In the USA, most home visiting services are delivered to selected subgroups, and most of the research showing the benefits of such provision is based on similarly targeted services (Bull et al 2004). In the UK, disadvantaged groups are scattered widely throughout the general population, and the long tradition of welfare provision has led to a different pattern of service delivery. Specialist services are appropriate for some of the most vulnerable groups, such as asylum seekers, homeless families, looked-after children or those with special/complex needs; specific assessment schedules are needed for each group. Generic, universal services reach out to vulnerable individuals and those with identified health needs, but it is not appropriate to routinely ask everyone questions that are suited mainly to a targeted subgroup.

Assessment for indicated prevention

Universal services are offered at a minimal level in the UK, working on the assumption that additional services will be offered to those individual children or families who are identified, through assessment, as needing an additional service over and above the minimum. This includes individuals who have minimal signs, symptoms or factors suggesting a risk may be present, even if they do not meet a threshold or diagnostic criteria for disorder at that time (see Box 1.5). In many cases, the need is such that a single professional, or a colleague working in the same sector, is able to provide sufficient support to meet the need. Most health visiting services, for example, include a range of group- or clinic-based activities to meet common needs, such as child behaviour problems, postnatal depression or breastfeeding support (Cowley et al 2007). School health services often incorporate drop-in facilities, including family planning or support for relationship problems, or run parenting groups (see Chapter 4). Alternatively, a referral may be made to a colleague from the same agency; a school nurse may refer a young person to a sexual health clinic, for example, or a health visitor may refer a child to a speech and language therapist. In such cases, collaboration (between two professionals working in the same agency, about a specific issue) is relatively straightforward and can help to ensure a seamless and appropriate service.

In more complex cases, when collaboration is needed across sectors and when several professionals need to be involved in providing the service, a single, common assessment framework (CAF) is available in England to promote integrated working. The idea is that, if all professionals and agencies use a similar assessment process, completing a standardised form in partnership with the child or

Box 1.6

Common assessment framework

1. Development of the infant, child or young person
   Health (including general health); physical development; speech, language and communications development
   Identity, including self-esteem, self-image and social presentation
   Behavioural development
   Emotional and social development
   Learning, including self-care skills and independence
   Family and social relationships (including participation in learning, education and employment), progress and achievement in learning and aspirations
2. Parents and carers
   Guidance, boundaries and stimulation
   Emotional warmth and stability
   Basic care, ensuring safety and protection
3. Family and environmental
   Wider family
   Family history, functioning and wellbeing
   Social and community elements and resources, including education
   Housing, employment and financial considerations

Adapted from Department of Education and Skills 2006a

family being assessed, this can form the basis for collaborative working and will avoid unnecessary, repetitive assessments each time a new worker is introduced. The process was widely piloted and evaluated during the development (Brandon et al 2006). A large information resource is available on the 'every child matters' website (*www.everychildmatters.gov.uk/caf*) and a national training and development programme introduced the CAF process in 2006.

It is intended that assessment, using the CAF process, should be a means of supporting earlier interventions. It aims to improve joint working and communication between practitioners by helping to embed a common language of assessment, need and a more consistent view as to the appropriate response. Box 1.6 summarises the three main areas (development of the infant, child or young person; parents and carers; family and environmental issues) for which detailed definitions are provided (DfES 2006a). A key aim is that the CAF will enable a picture of a child's needs and strengths to be built up over time and, with appropriate consent, shared among practitioners. To this end, assessors are directed to consider both strengths and needs, to ensure that a holistic picture is elicited, and to focus on an empowerment approach through the assessment process.

The CAF is designed to enable information to follow the child, for example, as they get older, change schools or move house (subject to controls to protect confidentiality). This is intended to help improve coordination and consistency between assessments, leading to fewer and shorter specialist assessments. The CAF form will support referrals where they are appropriate, although it is not a referral form (DfES 2006b). Once the CAF process is invoked, a lead professional is nominated, to act as a single point of contact for the child or family, coordinate the delivery of the actions agreed and reduce overlap and inconsistency in the services received (DfES 2006c). Also, an index of information is being developed (DfES 2006d), along with specific guidance about information sharing to help promote communication about all the children who have been assessed (DfES 2006e). The CAF is being used as a basis for universal assessments in some areas of high deprivation, where complex needs occur in the majority of families. However, in

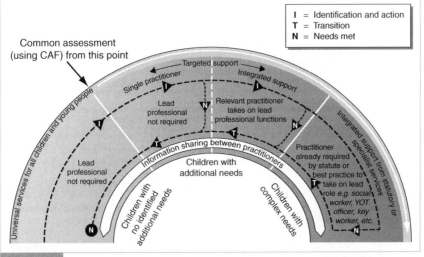

Figure 1.4 • The CAF as part of a continuum (from Department for Education and Skills 2006b)

most cases, the CAF process, along with the lead professional and child index of information, is a specific type of assessment that forms one part of a spectrum of needs and service provision (Fig. 1.4).

Assessment for selective prevention

At an individual level, assessment for selective prevention is a form of screening, aiming to achieve early interventions or offer programmes of care once a difficulty has been identified. To be valid, a needs assessment activity carried out for the purpose of targeting should have the same attributes as any useful diagnostic test. Such a test should be sensitive, picking up people who have the condition; be specific, excluding people who do not have the condition and be accurate, revealing the correct result (not false positives or negatives) (Greenhalgh 1997). In many instances, this will involve use of a structured instrument, validated for a particular condition.

The main reason for identifying the existence of a problem is so that it can be alleviated, so the availability of a known, effective treatment for the condition being targeted is important. One much cited example of a well-validated screening test for use by health visitors is the Edinburgh Postnatal Depression Scale (Cox et al 1987). This is a short, ten-item questionnaire that can be given to new mothers to assess their mood and, therefore, their likelihood of developing depression soon after the birth of the baby. If positive, a programme of care in the form of a short series of 'listening visits' can be offered, as this early intervention has been shown to be very effective in reducing the impact of postnatal depression (Holden et al 1989).

Use of the Sure Start Language Measure (SSLM) (Harris 2002, Sure Start Unit 2001) also highlights the benefits of the screening approach for evaluating organisational efficiency. The SSLM is designed to measure parental perceptions of a 2-year-old's language development as part of a national, ongoing comparative assay to assess over time whether the extra input leads to measurable gains in language for preschool children. Having discovered the extent of difficulties, some community health workers targeted the problem by developing child-focused, interactional opportunities for families to prevent communication delay, so they were able to demonstrate a timely response to a public health need (Turner et al 2004).

Introducing a general screening test for any specific condition is likely to have the effect of directing the service towards that area of interest, and away from others. In this respect, the process of targeting can be seen to overlap with that of prioritising at a population level, so the choice of which screening activities to use could be made in the light of anticipated health needs identified at an overall, neighbourhood or locality level.

In public health terms, it is a disadvantage that screening activities tend to focus attention on to individuals (whether mothers or children) with specified problems, instead of on the underlying social and contextual causes of the problems. If a need (such as delayed language development) has been deemed so prevalent in an area that all families are to be screened for this condition, some parallel community-wide activities are needed to challenge and change the underlying causes of the problem.

Conclusion

This chapter began by outlining changes in policy over decades, which have influenced approaches to health needs assessment, and the particular requirements for community profiling or assessing needs at the level of a caseload or neighbourhood. It then concentrated on describing the key features of needs assessments for individuals, children and families where preventive interventions are required. Despite its importance in terms of public health and improving health inequalities, there has been much less interest in this activity than in needs assessments for service planning, or for planning individual programmes of care once a diagnosis, deficit or problem has been identified. In part, this reflects the perceptions of need held by professionals delivering care, and how they view their responsibilities in relation to policy priorities.

Difficulties arise when the forms of assessment needed for health promotion and empowerment are overshadowed by those more suited to different situations, like service planning or prescribing treatments. Cowley and Houston (2003), for example, found that a schedule of questions drawn from instruments better suited to community profiling was unacceptable to clients and unhelpful in identifying needs at the level of the family. Well-developed communication skills and a commitment to working in an empowering way are both essential, as shown by two other studies where the assessment processes were considered unhelpful (Mitcheson and Cowley 2004, Roche et al 2005).

In most instances, an established relationship between client and professional helps to promote a positive atmosphere and fruitful assessment, although partnership working of the kind described in Chapter 2 can be developed at first meeting (Bidmead & Cowley 2005). If organisational requirements limit the assessor to asking only about predetermined needs, or to avoid identifying some needs because of service restrictions (perhaps because of lengthy waiting lists, or staff shortages) then practitioners become disempowered. In turn, their practice is more likely to be disempowering. Client perceptions need to be paramount and needs assessments should be open, not covert (Cowley et al 2004).

There is no single mechanism for needs assessment. It is not a purely technical task, but requires skill to negotiate the basically complex and contested nature of the concept of health need. Neither choosing a needs assessment approach, nor ensuring the skills to carry it out can answer the moral questions about which of many competing needs should be met by health services. But a good assessment of needs is the cornerstone of service provision, offering a sound starting point for universal and targeted prevention, integrated working and health improvement. The potential rewards are such that it is worth grappling with the complexity of the task.

DISCUSSION QUESTIONS

- What professional skills are most important for assessing health needs of communities?
- What professional skills are most important for assessing health needs of individuals and families?
- Can information about health needs in an area be used to plan service delivery and service configurations? How? What are the barriers?
- Consider how knowledge of health needs could be used to advocate for additional services, or to disinvest from specific provision. How are such dilemmas best resolved?

References

Appleton J, Cowley S 2003 Valuing professional judgement in health visiting practice. Community Practitioner 76(6): 215–220

Annett H, Rifkin SB 1995 Guidelines for rapid participatory appraisal to assess community health needs. World Health Organization, Geneva

Asadi-Lari M, Gray D 2005 Health needs assessment tools: progress and potential. International Journal of Technology Assessment in Health Care 21(3): 288–297

Bergen A, Cowley S, Young K, Kavanagh A 1996 An investigation into the changing educational needs of community nurses with regard to needs assessment and quality of care in the context of the NHS and Community Care Act, 1990. English National Board for Nursing, Midwifery and Health Visiting, London

Beveridge W 1942 Social insurance and allied services (cmnd 6404). HMSO, London

Bidmead C, Cowley S 2005 An evaluating family partnership training in health visitor practice. Community Practitioner 78(7): 239–245

Billings J 2002 Profiling health needs. In: Cowley S (ed.) Public health policy and practice: a sourcebook for health visitors and community nurses. Baillière Tindall, Edinburgh, pp. 113–143

Billings J, Cowley S 1995 Approaches to community needs assessment: a literature review. Journal of Advanced Nursing 22: 721–730

Brandon, M, Howe, A, Dagley, V, Salter, C, Catherine Warren C, Black J 2006 Evaluating the common assessment framework and lead professional guidance and implementation in 2005–6.

Research Report 740, Department for Education and Skills, London, http://www.dfes.gov.uk/research

Bull J, McCormick G, Swann C, Mulvihill C 2004 Ante- and post-natal home-visiting programmes: a review of reviews. Health Development Agency, London

Chalmers K, Luker K 1991 The development of the health visitor–client relationship. Scandinavian Journal of Caring Sciences 5: 33–41

Chalmers K 1992 Giving and receiving: an empirically derived theory on health visiting practice. Journal of Advanced Nursing 17: 1317–1325

Chalmers K 1993 Searching for health needs: the work of health visiting. Journal of Advanced Nursing 18(6): 900–911

Children Act 2004 HMSO, London

Childcare Act 2006 HMSO, London

Collinson S, Cowley S 1998a Exploring need: taking the marketing perspective. Community Practitioner 71: 244–247

Collinson S, Cowley S 1998b An exploratory study of demand for the health visiting service, within a marketing framework. Journal of Advanced Nursing 28: 499–507

Coombes L, Allen, D, Appleton J.V. 2007 Health Needs Assessment Theory and Pracice (2nd edition) Churchill Livingstone Elsevier Edinburgh

Council for the Education and Training of Health Visitors (CETHV) 1977 An investigation into the principles of health visiting. CETHV, London

Cowley S 1991 A symbolic awareness context identified through a grounded theory of health visiting. Journal of Advanced Nursing 16: 648–656

Cowley S 1995a In health visiting, the routine visit is one that has passed. Journal of Advanced Nursing 22(2): 276–284

Cowley S 1995b Health-as-process: a health visiting perspective. Journal of Advanced Nursing 22(3): 433–441

Cowley S, Bergen A, Young K, Kavanagh A 1995 Exploring needs assessment in community nursing. Health Visitor 68: 319–321.

Cowley S, Bergen A, Young K, Kavanagh A 1996 Identifying a framework for research: the example of needs assessment. Journal of Clinical Nursing 5: 53–62

Cowley S, Bergen A, Young K, Kavanagh A 2000a A taxonomy of needs assessment, elicited from a multiple case study of community nursing education and practice. Journal of Advanced Nursing 31: 126–134

Cowley S, Bergen A, Young K, Kavanagh A 2000b Generalising to theory: the use of a multiple case study design to investigate needs assessment and quality of care in community nursing. International Journal of Nursing Studies 37: 219–228

Cowley S, Caan W, Dowling S, Weir H 2007. What do health visitors do? A national survey of activities and service organization. Public Health doi:10.1016/j.puhe.2007.03.016

Cowley S, Frost, M 2006 The principles of Health Visiting: opening the door to public health practice in the 21st centry Community Practitioners' and Health Visitors' Association and UK Standing Conference on Health Visiting Education, London

Cowley S, Houston A 2003 A structured health needs assessment tool: acceptability and effectiveness for health visiting. Journal of Advanced Nursing 43(1): 82–92

Cowley S, Houston A 2004 Contradictory agendas in health visitor needs assessment. A discussion paper of its use for prioritizing, targeting and promoting health. Primary Health Care Research and Development 5: 240–254

Cowley S, Mitcheson J, Houston A 2004 Structuring health needs assessments: the medicalisation of health visiting. Sociology of Health and Illness 26: 503–526

Cox J, Holden J, Sagovsky R 1987 Detection of postnatal depression. Development of the 10-item Edinburgh Postnatal Depression Scale British. Journal of Psychiatry 150: 782–786

Davis H, Day C, Bidmead C 2002 Working in partnership with parents: The Parent Adviser Model. Wiley, The Psychological Corporation, London

Davis, H, Spurr P 1998 Parent counselling: an evaluation of a community child mental health service. Journal of Child Psychology, Psychiatry 39: 365–376

de la Cuesta C 1993 Fringe work: peripheral work in health visiting. Sociology of Health and Illness 15(5): 667–682

de la Cuesta C 1994 Relationships in health visiting: enabling and mediating. International Journal of Nursing Studies 31: 451–459

Department of Health (DH) 1989a Caring for People (Cmnd 849). HMSO, London

Department of Health (DH) 1989b Working for Patients (Cmnd 555). HMSO, London

Department of Health (DH) 1999a Saving Lives: Our Healthier Nation (Cmnd 4386). HMSO, London

Department of Health (DH) 1999b Making a difference: strengthening the nursing, midwifery and health visiting contribution to health and health care. DH, London

Department of Health (DH) 2001a Tackling health inequalities: consultation on a plan for delivery. DH, London

Department of Health (DH) 2001b Health visitor practice development resource pack. DH, London

Department of Health (DH) 2001c School nurse practice development resource pack. DH, London

Department of Health (DH) 2002a Tackling health inequalities: results of the consultation exercise. DH, London

Department of Health (DH) 2002b Liberating the talents: helping primary care trusts and nurses to deliver. The NHS Plan. DH, London

Department of Health 2003 Tackling health inequalities: a programme for action. DH, London

Department of Health 2004 National service framework for children, young people and maternity services. DH, London

Department of Health 2006 Informing healthier choices: Information and intelligence for healthy populations. DH, London

Department for Education and Skills 2006a Guide to definitions used in CAF form.

Department for Education and Skills, London, http://www.everychildmatters.gov.uk/caf

Department for Education and Skills 2006b Introduction to the common assessment framework (CAF). Department for Education and Skills, London, http://www.ecm.gov.uk/caf [April 2006]

Department for Education and Skills 2006c Fact sheet: the lead professional. Department for Education and Skills, London, http://www.ecm.gov.uk/leadprofessional [April 2006]

Department for Education and Skills 2006d Fact sheet: Information Sharing (IS) Index. Department for Education and Skills, London, http://www.ecm.gov.uk/index [April 2006]

Department for Education and Skills 2006e Fact sheet: information sharing guidance. Department for Education and Skills, London, http://www.ecm.gov.uk/informationsharing [April 2006]

Dingwall R 1977 Collectivism, regionalism and feminism: health visiting and British social policy 1850–1975. Journal of Social Policy 6(3): 291–315

Eaton WW, Harrison G 1998 Epidemiology and social aspects of the human environment. Current Opinion in Psychiatry 11: 165–168

Elkan R, Kendrick D, Hewitt M, Robinson J, Tolley K, Blair M, Dewey M, Williams D, Brummell K 2000 The effectiveness of domiciliary health visiting: a systematic review of international studies and a selective review of the British literature. Health Technology Assessment 4: 13

Elkan R, Robinson J, Williams D, Blair M 2001 Universal vs. selective: the case of British health visiting. Journal of Advanced Nursing 33: 113–119

Endacott R 1997 Clarifying the concept of need: a comparison of two approaches to concept analysis. Journal of Advanced Nursing 25: 471–476

Glover A 2001 Cartoon capers: an update on the Familywise programme. Community Practitioner 74: 60–62

Graham H, Kelly M 2004 Health inequalities: concepts, frameworks and policy. Briefing paper. Health Development Agency, London http://www.nice.org.uk/page.aspx?o=502453 [accessed July 2006]

Graham H, Power C 2004 Childhood disadvantage and adult health: a lifecourse framework. Briefing paper. Health Development Agency, London http://www.nice.org.uk/page.aspx?o=502707 [accessed July 2006]

Grant R 2001 A qualitative study to test the hypothesis that the population of Peasedown St John hold knowledge of their health and health needs that could be used to inform more accurate service provision and thereby improve their health. Unpublished MSc dissertation, Bath Spa Unversity College.

Greenhalgh T 1997 How to read a paper: the basics of evidence based medicine. British Medical Journal Publishing Group, Nottingham

Harris F 2002 The first implementation of the Sure Start Language Measure. Department of Language and Communication Science, City University, London

Health and Community Care Act 1990. HMSO, London

Health Act 1999 HMSO, London

Her Majesty's Treasury, Department of Health 2002 Tackling health inequalities: summary of the 2002 cross-cutting review. Department of Health, London

Holden J, Sagovsky R, Cox J 1989 Counselling in a general practice setting: controlled study of health visitor intervention in treatment of postnatal depression. British Medical Journal 298: 223–226

Houston A, Cowley S 2002 An empowerment approach to needs assessment in health visiting practice. Journal of Clinical Nursing 11(5): 640–650

Independent Inquiry into Inequalities in Health (chair, Acheson D) 1998 Independent inquiry into inequalities in health. TSO, London

Kieffer C 1984 Citizen empowerment: a developmental perspective. Prevention in Human Services 3: 9–36

Lightfoot J 1995 Identifying needs and setting priorities. Issues of theory, policy and practice. Health and Social Care in the Community 3: 105–114

Luker K, Chalmers K 1990 Gaining access to clients: the case of health visiting. Journal of Advanced Nursing 15: 74–82

Machen I 1996 The relevance of health visiting policy to contemporary mothers. Journal of Advanced Nursing 24: 350–356

Macleod J, Nelson G 2000 Programs for the promotion of family wellness and the prevention of child maltreatment: a meta-analytic review. Child Abuse & Neglect 24(9): 1127–1149

Mental Health Act 1959. HMSO, London

Mitcheson J, Cowley S 2003 Empowerment or control? An analysis of the extent to which client participation is enabled during health visitor/client interactions using a structured health needs assessment tool. International Journal of Nursing Studies 40: 413–426

Mrazek PJ, Haggerty RJ (eds) 1994 Reducing risks for mental disorders: frontiers for preventive intervention research. National Academy Press, Washington

Murray SA, Graham LJ 1995 Practice based health needs assessment: use of four methods in a small neighbourhood. BMJ. 310 (6992):1443-8, Jun 3.

Normandale S 2001 A study of mothers perceptions of the health visiting role. Community Practitioner 74: 146–150.

Ong BN, Humphris G 1994 In: Popay J, Williams G (eds). Researching the people's health. Routledge, London

Pearson P 1991 Clients perceptions: the use of case studies in developing theory. Journal of Advanced Nursing 16: 521–528

Prime Research and Development 2001 Developing standards and competences for health visiting. A report of the development process and thinking. UKCC, London

Rijke R 1993 Health in medical science: from determinism towards autonomy. In: Lafaille R, Fulder S (eds). Towards a new science of health. Routledge, London, pp. 74–83

Rissell C 1994 Empowerment: the holy grail of health promotion? Health Promotion International 9: 39–47

Robinson J, Elkan R 1996 Health needs assessment: theory & practice. Churchill Livingstone, Edinburgh

Roche B, Cowley S, Salt N, Scammell A, Malone M, Savile P, Aikens D, Fitzpatrick S 2005 Reassurance or judgement? Parents' views on the delivery of child health surveillance programmes. Family Practice 22: 507–512

Secretary of State for Health 2000 The NHS Plan. A plan for investment. A plan for reform (Cmnd 4818). HMSO, London

Secretary of State for Health 2004 Choosing health: making healthier choices easier (Cmnd 6374). TSO, London

Sheppard M, Woodcock J 1999 Need as an operating concept: the case of social work with children and families. Child and Family Social Work 4: 67–76

Shonkoff J, Phillips D (eds) 2000 From neurons to neighbourhoods: the science of early child development. National Academy Press, Washington DC

Sure Start Unit 2001 Sure Start Language Measure. Information Pack, October 2001. The Sure Start Unit, London

ten Have P 1991 Talk and institution: a reconsideration of the 'assymetry' of doctor–patient interaction. In: Boden D, Zimmerman DH (eds). Talk and social structure. Polity, Cambridge, pp. 138–163

Turner E, Houston AM, Mears P 2004 Implementation of the Sure Start Language Measure. Community Practitioner 77(5): 185–189

Twinn S, Dauncey J, Carnell J 1990 The process of health profiling. Health Visitors' Association, London

Wadsworth M 1999 Early life. In: Marmot M, Wilkinson R (eds). Social determinants of health. Oxford University Press, Oxford, pp. 44–63

Williams D 1997 Vulnerable families: a study of health visitors' prioritization of their work. Journal of Nursing Management 5: 19–24

World Health Organization (WHO) 2004 Prevention of Mental Disorders: Effective interventions and policy options. A Report of the World Health Organization, Department of Mental Health and Substance Abuse in collaboration with the Prevention Research Centre of the Universities of Nijmegen and Maastricht 2004. World Health Organization, Geneva

World Health Organization 2005 The World Health Report 2005: make every mother and child count. World Health Organization, Geneva, Switzerland.

Further reading

Coombes L, Allen, D, Appleton JV 2007 Health needs assessment theory and practice (2nd edition) Churchill Livingstone Elsevier Edinburgh

Annett H, Rifkin SB 1995 Guidelines for rapid participatory appraisal to assess community health needs. A focus on health improvements for low-income urban and rural areas. World Health Organization, Geneva, Switzerland

Basic guide available from: http://www.who.int/management/partnerships/community/en/index1.html

Department for Education and Skills 2006 Introduction to the common assessment framework (CAF), and guide to definitions used in CAF form. Department for Education and Skills, London

Both are available from the 'every child matters' website: http://www.ecm.gov.uk/caf. These are worth exploring, even for readers not in England, as they encompass a wide range of issues related to needs assessment.

Resources

One plus One Marriage and Partnership Research Organisation, from which the cartoon 'Picture kits' (e.g., Fig. 1.2 in this chapter) can be purchased. They pioneered the 'Brief Encounters' training programme, and provide resources to support professionals in their work with families: *http://www.oneplusone.org.uk/home.asp; http://www.theparentconnection.org. uk/index.asp*

Partnership working:
the key to public health

2

Christine Bidmead and Hilton Davis

Key issues

- Community practitioners and health visitors should work in a partnership relationship with clients in order to maximise healthy outcomes
- Public health policy for children and families underpins the need to work in partnership
- Working in partnership with clients must be defined, so that practitioners can be recruited for and trained in the required skills and qualities
- The Family Partnership Model provides a framework that enables practitioners to understand and fulfil the requirements of working in partnership

Introduction

The idea of working in partnership is a recurring theme in health care. Twenty-five years ago, the World Health Organization (WHO 1978) declared that 'people have a right and a duty to participate individually and collectively in the planning of their health care', inferring that health professionals needed to establish a partnership with clients based on their participation and involvement.

It has been suggested that initiatives fostering partnership with parents and personal self-reliance may be more effective in improving child health than much of the routine work done by health visitors (Goodwin 1991). The 'new nursing' also emphasises the importance of the relationship of the patient with the nurse for the improvement in health outcomes (Salvage 1990). The health promotion literature identifies the worker–client relationship as key to changes in producing healthier lifestyles (Tones & Tilford 2001). In psychotherapy there is evidence to suggest that therapist characteristics and the client relationship are major predictors of outcome (Martin et al 2000) and this may be true for all other areas of health care, where effective communication is related to diagnostic accuracy (e.g. Papadopoulou et al 2005), treatment adherence, staff stress, and physical and psychological outcomes (e.g. Davis & Fallowfield 1991). In Child and Adolescent Mental Health too, the therapeutic relationship is associated with positive outcomes (Green 2006, Shirk & Karver 2003). A recent paper from America also showed that the patient's perception of his/her relationship with the general practitioner was associated with a smaller risk of health status decline (Franks et al 2005).

The idea that the relationship is important to health outcomes is echoed in the work of Hall and Elliman (2003) who suggest that what works in terms of child health promotion programmes are: 1) that staff have the time and skill to establish a relationship of respect and trust with families and 2) that there is a sustained high quality and quantity of input and sufficient continuity to develop a relationship with the individual client. This may imply the need to commence a professional relationship during pregnancy rather than after the child is born. Almond (2001) found that positive health outcomes were reliant on the ability and skill of the health visitor to develop a positive relationship with the client. Tones and Tilford (2001) also argued that self-esteem, control and self-empowerment are all necessary features of health, and it would, therefore, seem evident that health visitors and other public health practitioners should have the skills to enhance these characteristics in their clients.

In spite of the importance of communication and relationship building, expertise of this type has been neglected in early preventive approaches, including health visiting. However, in recent UK policy documents there has been some acknowledgement of the importance of the relationship, not only with the client for healthy outcomes, but also between agencies. For example, the whole of chapter four of *Every child matters: next steps* (DfES 2004) is devoted to interagency partnership and collaborative working. The legislation that followed, the Children Act (2004), puts into place 'robust partnership arrangements to ensure public, private, voluntary and community sector organisations work together to improve outcomes' for children (p. 13). This acknowledges that at an organisational level working in partnership is effective in producing healthy outcomes. The Nursing and Midwifery Council (NMC), too, requires registrants on the Community Public Health part of their register to be able to 'develop and sustain relationships with groups and individuals with the aim of improving health and social wellbeing'(NMC 2004). This does not specify the kind of relationship that might be helpful, nor does it state how it is related to the aim of improving health and social wellbeing. We would argue that, at whichever level it operates, partnership working requires good inter-personal relationships, developed through the skills and qualities required for good communication.

The National Service Framework for Children, Young People and Maternity Services (Children's NSF) requires services to: 'give children, young people and their parents increased information, power and choice over the support and treatment they receive, and involve them in planning their care and services' (DH 2004, p. 9). There is also some importance placed upon working in partnership with children throughout the document with emphasis upon ensuring that 'children and young people's voices are heard and they are involved in the design and delivery of services' (p. 8). Primary Care Trusts (PCTs) have a duty to ensure that the Child Health Promotion Programme is 'delivered in partnership with parents to help them make healthy choices for their children and family' (p. 31). It appears to acknowledge that the relationship that is established is about empowerment through the giving of information and choice.

It goes on to state that planning is to take place 'in partnership with parents or carers' and is considered key to enabling a family to address their health and parenting needs. 'Planning identifies:

- The family's needs as they see them
- How they wish to address these needs
- Agreement with the family about the support to be provided by the midwife, health visitor and others, and
- What has been achieved?' (p. 39).

There appear to be elements of partnership here with a clear indication of working from the parent or child's agenda, taking note of their wishes and agreeing a way forward together and then reviewing what has been achieved.

The common core competencies and skills of the NSF are to include effective communication and engagement (listening to and involving children and working with parents, carers and families) (p. 115). Listening to parents is also identified as one of the most effective ways of improving support services for them

> ### Box 2.1
>
> ## Features of successful home visiting programmes
>
> - Initially there is early identification of need through universal services.
> - Onset is as early as possible, preferably in the antenatal period.
> - Interventions are multi-faceted and appropriately targeted to need.
> - Intensity of contact is high at first.
> - Parents and children's needs are considered as a priority.
> - Staff are selected carefully and trained appropriately.
> - Ongoing case management supervision.
> - Home-visiting needs to continue for a significant period.
> - Service needs to be integrated with other services.
>
> From: Bidmead & Whittaker 2004

(p. 84) and is given a high priority throughout the document. Although the inclusion of the need for effective communication and engagement is to be commended, the details of the skills, apart from listening and the personal qualities involved in this, seem to be omitted. The NSF itself acknowledges that its implementation is dependent upon having an adequately resourced, trained and motivated workforce. However, we would argue that without the skills to work in partnership little will be accomplished.

It has been suggested that management may not construe the forming of partnerships as 'real work' (Elkan et al 2000b) and researchers have called for further studies to 'demystify health visitor/client relationships in order to identify those aspects of the relationship that enable positive health outcomes' (Elkan et al 2000a). Although there is evidence that home visiting programmes can be effective, the effects are generally small and there are many studies that have shown no effects whatsoever, as discussed by Gomby et al (1999). An implication of this is that we need to know the effective ingredients and the processes involved, yet there is little information about either. This arises both from the absence of adequate research into the processes, but also because of the lack of adequate theory. Few interventions are based on explicit theory, and those that are describe mechanisms to do with children's development (e.g. parent–child interaction) and almost always ignore the equally important issues to do with the parent–helper interaction and the processes related to this.

Box 2.1 shows the kind of features that are suggested as ingredients of successful home visiting programmes. However, these do not elucidate the processes involved and fail to take account of the all-important relationship between the parent and home visitor.

Family partnership model for health and wellbeing

Given the urgent unmet mental health needs of children and parents in the population, existing service difficulties, current policy directives and the requirement for process research, the need for a model or theory of the processes of helping has never been greater. The Family Partnership Model has been developed over many years to meet this need (Davis 1993, Davis et al 2002a). It is intended as an accessible guide to the processes involved in helping families for all potential

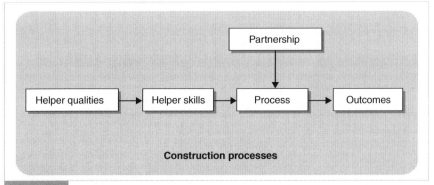

Figure 2.1 ● The Family Partnership Model (from Davis et al 2002)

helpers, to enable their practice, and as the basis of system design and training. The overall aim has been to provide an explicit, relatively simple and therefore usable understanding of the various aspects of the process of helping and to develop an associated and effective training programme that will increase workers' understanding and their skills in relating to and helping families.

The model is presented in Figure 2.1 as a set of five interconnected boxes within a rectangle. Each of the boxes and the rectangle represent a small number of related theoretical points. The model is intended to suggest that helping can be seen as a set of steps, stages or tasks (the Process box), which are required to produce a set of designated changes (the Outcomes box). It is assumed that the process starts with the establishment of a relationship between the client and practitioner and that there is a need to define the nature of the relationship (the Partnership box) that will be most effective in facilitating the process and hence achieving the outcomes. To enable a partnership relationship and, therefore, the process as a whole, it is further assumed that the practitioner must have a small number of basic human characteristics (represented by the Helper Qualities box) and a larger set of communication skills (designated by the Helper Skills box) by which these qualities may be demonstrated to the client. These interconnected boxes are encompassed in a rectangle intended to represent an overall model of human functioning that sees people as though they were scientists attempting to understand/anticipate the events of their world and to adapt effectively. We will outline the theoretical points encompassed within each of the boxes and the rectangle in turn below, beginning with the outcomes.

Outcomes of working in partnership with clients

To work effectively, it is argued that potential helpers need to be explicit about the changes they are attempting to produce. The outcomes suggested within the Family Partnership Model are intended to offset a narrow specialist focus and to represent a much more holistic view of people as thinking, feeling beings always operating within a social context. The outcomes are shown in Box 2.2 and are discussed below.

To do no harm

Mitcheson and Cowley (2003) found that using a health needs assessment tool meant that client participation was reduced and professional expertise emphasised so that clients were disempowered. The relationships that health visitors have with clients are complex and their professional power may inhibit the exercise of their supportive role particularly in the field of domestic violence, so there is considerable need for practice development in this area (Peckover 2002, 2003).

Box 2.2

Outcomes of working partnership with clients

- To do no harm
- To help clients identify, clarify and manage specific problems
- To enable parents/clients
- To facilitate wellbeing and development of children
- To facilitate social support and community development
- To enable access to appropriate services
- To help clients to be able to predict and manage future difficulties
- To compensate where necessary
- To change the system of care as necessary

Box 2.3

Using services related to psychosocial wellbeing

Incentives

- Supportive professionals providing advice, guidance and counselling.
- Professionals who listen, with whom one can talk openly and in confidence about difficulties.
- Feeling comfortable and not stigmatised or judged or belittled.

Disincentives

- Bad past experiences with professionals.
- Professionals not listening and being unsympathetic and insensitive.

Attride-Stirling et al 2001

What parents say they want is someone who will listen to them. In a recent paper, tellingly called 'Someone to talk to who'll listen', Attride-Stirling et al (2001) asked parents and adolescents what would deter them from using services related to psychosocial wellbeing and what would encourage them to do so (see Box 2.3). Overall findings indicated that parents needed to be valued and understood, treated as capable human beings and to be facilitated in their role as carers.

It is clear that harm can be done by practitioners who, though well meaning, may not listen to parents, who as a result may feel disempowered. This will undoubtedly affect the clients' access to services as previous bad experiences with professionals may mean that they are reluctant to engage with services that may potentially be of help to them and their children (Barlow et al 2005). Practitioners must attempt to make families' experiences of being helped highly respectful and closely attuned to the needs of the family, and not unpleasant and distressing. At all times the practitioner should try to ensure that clients feel completely involved in the process, and that their views are important and that they are in control. In this way harm will be minimised, as help will be sensitive to their explicit needs.

To help clients identify, clarify and manage specific problems

This requires sensitive exploration by the practitioner to help clients express what is relevant to them and their circumstances. It might mean discussion of issues pertaining to themselves, their children or their family generally, as they all may be closely related. Problems that are raised may be beyond the practitioner's expertise, and he/she will need to acknowledge this and help clients to become clearer about the problems themselves. It also enables the worker to gain a clearer insight into the client's circumstances and to seek out the most relevant and appropriate source of help for the client if this is necessary.

To enable parents/clients

Here the aim is to enable clients to take power and control and face life more confidently. This will help them to be more effective in meeting their own needs and that of their children. It is about working with them to reduce their vulnerabilities and working from their strengths. It is about raising their self-efficacy, self-esteem and enhancing their understanding of the helping processes and their own problem-solving powers. One of the most powerful ways of doing this will be through the respectful relationship that the practitioner establishes with client.

To facilitate the wellbeing and development of children

When working with parents, the wellbeing and development of the child will need to be kept in mind even if the main focus of the work is not upon the children and their problems. Whatever the work entails, parents can be helped to relate appropriately to their children so as to understand them more effectively and meet their needs.

To facilitate social support and community development

Social support has been found to be health enhancing (Oakley 1994). Therefore a major aim of working with clients should be to build on and enhance existing social support networks. Relationships between parents might be an important focus for the work but not to the neglect of other potentially supportive relationships with extended family, friends, neighbours and communities.

To enable access to appropriate services

Some families will require further support from other services. It is therefore important that adequate information is given to them to facilitate the use of these as appropriate.

To help clients to be able to predict and manage future difficulties

It is helpful to facilitate clients to be able to look to the future and to be able to predict their future needs. This will involve helping them to use a problem-solving approach to their difficulties in the here and now, which may be useful to them in the future. Enabling parents to look forward to children's transition points, for example, may be empowering in allowing them to anticipate future events and deal with them more effectively.

To compensate where necessary

Although it is always preferable to work with clients or parents to foster their own self-efficacy and self-esteem, occasionally it may be ineffective or even unsafe, for example when children are at risk of abuse and in need of protection. If parents or carers are unable to meet the child's needs for any reason, then the aims of the worker will need to include the provision of whatever support and resources are necessary in order to compensate.

To change the system of care as necessary

In order to make working in partnership most effective, service delivery systems need to be put in place that have two-way communication and partnership relationships built in at all levels (e.g. child–parent, parent–practitioner, practitioner–supervisor, etc.). However, it is argued that all workers should be responsible or have a right to attempt to change systems of care within any sector when they are inappropriate or inadequate. This is not just the responsibility of senior managerial staff and/or government, but of all personnel, who should be working in partnership with their managers and in two-way communication in order to facilitate service development.

Helping process

In order to be as effective as possible in helping anyone, all professionals should have a clear and explicit understanding of the process of helping. In the Family Partnership Model this is conceptualised as a simple series of eight steps, tasks or stages beginning with the establishment of a relationship between the client and the professional (see Fig. 2.2). It is assumed that the steps are sequential, with each subsequent stage dependent to a large extent upon the progress made in relation to the tasks preceding it. However, some clients may not need to progress through all the steps; it may be enough for them to explore issues that they have, come to a clear understanding of what they are about and then continue on their own without the need to involve the practitioner in any subsequent steps. As indicated in Figure 2.2 there may be a need to back-track to previous stages as continuing exploration brings into question conclusions drawn at previous stages. Of course, where there are multiple problems it may be necessary to loop through the whole process a number of times. We will now consider each of the steps in turn.

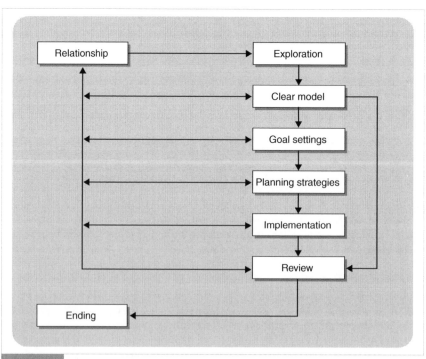

Figure 2.2 ● The helping process (from Davis et al 2002)

Relationship building

This is the process by which client and practitioner meet, get to know each other, and develop a working relationship. The rest of the process is based upon this relationship, which has as its foundation mutual trust and understanding. This may be accomplished within minutes with some people or hours with others, depending upon their previous experiences, including past encounters with professionals, and the qualities and skills of the worker. Facilitation of this process will be enhanced if there is explicit discussion and agreement about how the client and practitioner are going to work together. This will include negotiation of expectations, roles and responsibilities and agreement of a contract so that each knows what to expect. This relationship needs to be carefully maintained and built upon throughout the following processes.

Exploration of needs, problems/issues

The aim of this stage is for the client and practitioner to develop a clearer understanding of the problems and needs of the individual, child and/or family. The extent to which this happens is dependent upon the quality of the relationship that develops between them. The task for the practitioner is to enable the clients to come to an understanding of the particular way in which they see (or construe) their problems or their needs in the context of their world more generally (Kelly 1991). This can be done quickly when all that is necessary is for a client to have the opportunity to talk and self-reflect in order to gain a greater insight into his/her needs and to change accordingly. Here the practitioner's role will be to listen carefully, respecting the client, giving what Rogers called 'unconditional positive regard' (Rogers 1959). However, in more complex situations exploration may need to be more detailed. Here the skills of the practitioner in attentive and active listening will be of paramount importance to the development of a shared picture of the client's needs. Throughout the process the practitioner will be trying to see the situation through the eyes of the client, while at the same time generating his/her own view of the situation to allow for possible alternatives for comparison at a later stage. It is interesting to note that in a study of vulnerable women who chose not to take up the offer of an early intervention service in Oxford, one of the reasons given was differences in professional and lay perceptions of vulnerability and need (Barlow et al 2005).

Development of a clear understanding of needs, problems/issues

Careful exploration is likely to lead to the development of a clearer understanding of the client's problems. It may include the possibility of challenging the client to develop alternative constructions or explanations of the problems and to test them out. The implication throughout this stage is not that the client is wrong, but that there may be other more helpful ways of explaining a situation. The practitioner's suggestions may not be right always and, therefore, they should be made tentatively and with respect for the client. The clarification of the issues at this point forms the basis on which the work may progress through the following stages of formulating goals and agreeing plans of how to attain them.

Setting agreed aims and goals

Explicit aims and goals can be negotiated and agreed once a clear and acceptable understanding of the problem is available. Where problems are complex, this stage will involve a process of prioritising which issues to address and in which order, necessitating the need for defining multiple goals. Goals are the outcomes the client is hoping to achieve and to be useful need to be Specific, Measurable,

Attainable, Realistic, within a Time-frame, Explicit and Agreed (SMARTEA). One small goal achieved is likely to enhance considerably a client's feelings of self-efficacy.

Development of planned strategies for attaining goals

The next stage is to help clients decide the steps they must take to achieve their goals. The practitioner's task is to enable clients to discover all the possible strategies that might help them and to explore and evaluate these, considering the advantages and disadvantages of each approach. As a result, the client should be in the best informed position to know what to do next.

Implementation of plans

The next stage is for the client and practitioner to implement the plans, when they have been clearly formulated and obstacles anticipated as far as possible. The practitioner's role is one of support, monitoring what is happening, encouraging the client's efforts and helping them to deal with unanticipated problems. Even the smallest success deserves praise and encouragement so that clients do not become discouraged and tempted to give up.

Review of outcomes

This is an extremely important part of the process. The practitioner's role is to enable the clients to examine what they have done and what has been achieved. Understanding the reasons for their success and their part in it may shed light on the problem and help them deal with future difficulties. Alternatively the practitioner's task may be to enable clients to learn all they can from their experiences, particularly if goals were not or only partially achieved. This involves returning to earlier stages in the process, possibly to re-clarify the problem, and to reformulate goals and to work through the process again.

Possible ending of relationship

Providing all is well, it may be possible to bring the helping relationship to a close. This needs to be done carefully as some clients may find this particularly difficult. However, if the practitioner has been working in partnership with the client throughout, then the client should feel enabled and empowered to seek solutions to his/her own problems should they arise in the future.

Partnership relationship

Given that the first stage of the helping process is the establishment of a relationship, gaining an explicit understanding of the exact nature of the relationship one is attempting to develop is essential. Although the concept of partnership is proposed in many UK government policy documents, it is a term that is ill-defined. However, within health visiting there have been recent attempts to outline what working in partnership might mean (Bidmead et al 2002, Normandale 2001). Bidmead and Cowley (2005a) defined partnership in the context of health visiting as: 'a respectful, negotiated way of working together that enables choice, participation and equity, within an honest, trusting relationship that is based in empathy, support and reciprocity. It is best established within a model of health visiting that recognises partnership as a central tenet. It requires a high level of interpersonal qualities and communication skills in staff who are, themselves, supported through a system of clinical supervision that operates within the same partnership framework' (p. 208). Whilst this definition has been derived from nursing and health visiting literature, it may be useful in other settings also, given that public health is about the 'organised efforts' (Acheson 1998) of the whole of society not just those designated as health workers.

It is important to understand exactly what the characteristics of partnership relationships are, so as to know what it is that is aimed for and whether or not it has been achieved. For these reasons we will try to set out here exactly what we mean by working in partnership with clients.

Within the Family Partnership Model, it is assumed that a partnership between the practitioner and family is the most effective relationship to enable change. An attempt has therefore been made to define the concept by an explicit set of characteristics, against which what is achieved with a particular client can be evaluated. These characteristics are listed in Box 2.4 and will be described below.

Working together/participation

It is assumed that the most effective relationship is one in which both client and practitioner are participating, actively involved and working together. It is not possible for either the client or the practitioner to carry out the work alone. Collaboration is required, where both partners bring their own resources to the situation and their commitment to positive outcomes.

Complementary expertise

Working in partnership does not deny professional knowledge and skills; these are vital. However, such expertise can only be effective if it is understood that the expertise of the client is equally important for understanding and ameliorating problems. The Model acknowledges, therefore, that clients and professionals have different expertise and that it is the complementary nature of the two that is most effective in helping families, parents and their children. This needs to be openly acknowledged at the beginning and throughout the relationship that is established with clients. The stage is then set for a true power-sharing relationship.

Power sharing

It is argued that true partnership can only exist when neither partner is in overall control of the situation. It is assumed that there is a partnership when professionals and clients have the power to make decisions, and share this power. In reality, the balance of power is likely to shift between them over time, but given the practitioner is there to provide a service, one might assume that the client or parent should in most circumstances be the senior partner.

Agreed aims and process

If the practitioner and client are working in partnership, then they will be attempting to agree every step of the process together. There needs initially to be an

Box 2.4

The characteristics of a partnership relationship

- Working together/participation
- Complementary expertise
- Power sharing
- Agreed aims and process
- Mutual trust and respect
- Open communication
- Negotiation

explicit agreement to work together and then continual agreement about what they are trying to achieve and how.

Mutual trust and respect

Partnership will exist when the participants in the relationship have mutual trust and respect. Practitioners should work to earn this and not assume it by virtue of their profession. This means that practitioners will need to approach each relationship with complete respect for the client, valuing their expertise and their ability to change.

Open communication

The hallmark of partnership is clear and open communication. Both partners need to share all relevant information in ways that maximise the understanding between them and minimise misunderstandings. This also involves sharing the processes of helping, so that the client is as aware of the process as the helper and learns how it works. Openness also implies the need for each partner to be as honest as possible, paving the way for each partner being able to challenge the other as necessary.

Negotiation

No relationships are without a degree of disagreement or conflict at times, even though one attempts to work with openness, honesty and respect. Disagreements have to be managed. This means that sources of conflict have to be identified and deliberate attempts made to resolve them. Agreement is sought by respecting the client's views and indicating acceptance and a willingness to explore all possibilities with the aim of negotiating a way forward. If the practitioner is gentle, tentative and invitational in proposing alternative views, conflict will be minimised.

By working in partnership it is assumed that there are a number of benefits to be derived (see Box 2.5). Among these is the suggestion that the task of helping becomes less stressful for practitioners, as it may relieve them of the burden of needing to have all the answers to everyone's problems. Evidence for positive effects upon professional satisfaction and stress are suggested by Davis and Fallowfield (1991).

Box 2.5

Working in partnership

Benefits

- Clients are more likely to engage
- Realistic acknowledgement of the power of the client
- Accords explicit power/control to clients, with positive consequences for the self-esteem and self-efficacy
- Allows clients to express their views openly, improving the quality and accuracy of information shared
- Allows clients' expectations to be expressed, explored and negotiated
- Clients are involved in an understanding of the helping process
- This may optimise outcome for them in terms of their own abilities to problem-solve and adapt positively to new situations
- Enables clients to take the credit for their contribution
- Less stressful for the worker and more rewarding

Practitioner qualities necessary for working in partnership with clients

The Family Partnership Model assumes that the process of helping as a whole is dependent upon the core qualities and skills of the practitioner. We will describe the personal qualities needed by practitioners to facilitate relationship building and the process as a whole. These qualities may be understood as general intra-psychic characteristics, which orientate the practitioner appropriately to the helping situation and the person with whom they are working, and must be demonstrated in ways that are perceived by the client. These qualities are assumed to be additional to a body of professional knowledge that the practitioner must bring to the situation, including an in-depth and explicit understanding of the processes and ingredients involved in helping. The six qualities, highly influenced by the work of Rogers (1959), are shown in Box 2.6.

Respect

Respect is fundamental and involves a general belief that the client is valuable and important, able to cope and to change. Professionals can communicate this in many ways, such as by being punctual, introducing themselves, and being courteous at all times. Perhaps the most powerful demonstration, however, is by being interested in and concerned for, and by listening to, clients and children.

Empathy

Empathy involves a willingness and ability to try to enter the other's world and see it from his/her point of view. If successfully demonstrated it gives the client a sense of being understood and valued. Developing a clear understanding of the thoughts, feelings and behaviour of another person requires in-depth concentration and careful listening, both to what the person is saying and to what he/she is implying.

Genuineness

Genuineness or congruence is a complex quality that was used by Rogers (1959) to denote the importance of openness to one's own and others' experience. It is crucial, when exploring clients' problems or difficulties, that their ideas are not coloured too much by one's own experiences, constructions and prejudices. Practitioners need to know their strengths and their weaknesses and be at home with themselves so they can remain objective. Being oneself within the relationship implies openness and honesty in all communications.

Box 2.6

The qualities

- Respect
- Empathy
- Genuineness
- Personal integrity
- Humility
- Quiet enthusiasm

Personal integrity

This is closely related to genuineness and refers to the practitioner's capacity to: 1) be strong enough emotionally to support those who are vulnerable; 2) tolerate the anxieties of the helping situation; 3) retain an objectivity that enables careful thought about people; and 4) be able to challenge or disagree with clients when it is thought to be to their benefit.

Humility

This involves practitioners developing a realistic assessment of their own strengths and weaknesses, knowing their limitations, and acknowledging the differences between themselves and others without assuming that they are superior by virtue of being a professional. It includes an accepting, non-judgemental attitude and an explicit acknowledgement that they do not have all the answers, but will try to work with clients to facilitate their strengths and expertise.

Quiet enthusiasm

This is important as it is the basis for conveying warmth and positiveness to clients. Anyone who enjoys his or her work conveys enthusiasm, which is infectious in client interaction, adding warmth and spontaneity to the relationship. Enthusiasm that is excessive is inappropriate as practitioners may be working with clients who are dealing with very real and distressing difficulties. However, it is possible for the practitioner to take pride in a job well done and, although a practitioner's needs must not take precedence over those of the client, they must derive satisfaction from their work or they will suffer compassion fatigue or burn out.

Skills of working in partnership

In the Family Partnership Model it is assumed that the qualities of the practitioner are demonstrated via a set of communication skills that, in turn, enable the process of helping, including relationship development. There are many of these skills, but we will briefly describe the major groups below (see also Box 2.7).

Attending and active listening

The bases of all help are the skills of attending to the client and actively listening to him/her, i.e. showing respect for the client, developing the relationship and enabling the process. The practitioner needs to concentrate fully on the client, removing all other distracting thoughts from beyond the immediate situation, and to indicate this through eye contact, responsive facial expression, body orientation, openness of posture, and all other aspects of verbal and non-verbal

---

Box 2.7

The skills

- Attending and active listening
- Prompting and exploring
- Empathic responding
- Enabling change/challenging
- Problem management

behaviour. It entails being visibly tuned into clients with the heart, mind and body. Attending carefully can encourage clients to be more open and to explore problems in a way that they have not done in the past. If, however, the practitioner is only partially present, with his or her mind on other things, then this will communicate itself to the client who will be less than willing to trust and be open. This is the basis for listening, which is not a passive process. It involves actively processing all the information the client provides verbally or otherwise, including what is omitted. The intention is to make sense of it from the client's perspective, trying to discern what the client really means, and checking out this understanding with constantly. This is a demanding task, requiring the practitioner to think about the client in a holistic way, attempting to register his/her thoughts, feelings and behaviour while at the same time being conscious of his/her own reactions to them.

Prompting and exploring

Attending and listening are the bases of the skills for exploring the issues, concerns or problems raised by clients. However, there are additional skills that are needed to enable clients to talk, elaborate and structure their thoughts and feelings and to derive a clearer understanding of their situation. These include the skills of questioning, appropriate use of pauses, highlighting significant issues by reflecting them back to the client and, for example, summarising. The practitioner's task is to help clients tell their story (Egan 1998). Some clients will need little prompting and will tell a coherent tale and all practitioners have to do is to summarise from time to time to ensure that they have grasped the detail. However, other clients may not be so forthcoming, for many possible reasons (e.g. embarrassment, anxiety, depression), and will need time, patience and considerable skill to help them talk about their concerns. For some clients there may be no resolution to the problems encountered (e.g. bereavement), but the role of the practitioner in these situations is to listen carefully and to indicate that he/she clearly with or alongside the client in his/her distress.

Empathic responding

This is an extremely important skill for facilitating the relationship with clients, indicating listening and enabling change. It involves showing in words or in behaviour what the client is feeling, thinking and/or doing. Many people who enter the caring professions do so because they care about others and want to help them with their problems. This sometimes means that they attempt to take the problem away or make it better with immediate advice, without acknowledging the client's feelings and at the cost of minimising the problems and ignoring the client's own role in dealing with the issues confronting them. However, it may be more helpful to begin by indicating an understanding of the client and his/her situation, so as to build trust, on the basis of which the resources of both client and practitioner can be brought to bear.

Enabling change/challenging

There are times when clients are fixed upon an understanding of their situation that may not be helpful to them; they may, for example, view themselves negatively unnecessarily, attribute inappropriate feelings to their children, or have a limited understanding of their children's development and needs. In such circumstances, there is a need to help them change their perceptions, even though there may be extreme resistance to change and even feelings of considerable threat and conflict. Working in partnership, therefore, means that practitioners may need the strength to acknowledge unhelpful constructions in their clients and the skills to challenge these (i.e. invite the person to change). These skills include the ability to request permission to consider such difficulties, to negotiate a way of tackling them, and to do so using a tentative, invitational style, which is non-judgemental, does not put the client down, acknowledges the client's strengths, and elicits these in dealing with the issues involved. A variety of potential skills and techniques may be used here, including sharing the model of helping with the client and particularly the process and the notion of construing (see below), providing new information, using advanced empathy (e.g. drawing unacknow-ledged conclusions or implications from what the client has said), or immediacy (i.e. using the practitioner–client relationship itself to make points about how the client relates to others and the difficulties that might be involved in this). The use of these skills, within the context of a respectful and trusting relationship, and a strong concern for the good of all the family is more likely to enable the client to change without alienating her/him.

Problem management

There are a set of skills that are related to the problem management steps in the helping process (i.e. setting aims and goals, planning strategies, implementation and review). These include, for example, the skills of sharing the model with the client, involving her/him in the decision-making processes, prioritising the problems, negotiating aims, generating and evaluating goals and strategies, and exploring the outcomes. Such skills are the essence of problem-solving/manage-ment, but are also crucial in motivating clients, increasing compliance, increasing their own skills and understanding of the processes involved and raising the cli-ent's sense of self-efficacy and their self-esteem.

Construct theory

The final aspect of the Family Partnership Model to be described is intended to provide an understanding of human functioning and adaptation. This is funda-mental to the whole model with implications for all parts of it and uses Kelly's theory of personal constructs (1991). For the purposes of this chapter, the major assumptions are as follows:

- All people develop in their heads a model or set of constructions of their world.
- This is to help them make sense of their world by enabling them to anticipate and hence adapt to all aspects of their world.
- Each person's constructions are unique to them, although they may overlap with those of others.
- The constructions are derived from experience and therefore change over time to accommodate new events.
- Our social interactions are determined by our understanding of the construc-tions of those with whom we interact.

These ideas are extremely helpful in enabling an understanding of all aspects of the processes of helping already elaborated. There is not the space here to explore this in depth, and a couple of illustrations will have to suffice. For example, the practitioner–client relationship may be understood in terms of the constructions that each person has of the other. The client's previous good or bad experiences of professionals will colour their expectations and will affect the success of the whole process. The development of a partnership is a process in which the client begins to construe the practitioner as of value and to be trusted and they begin to make explicit and agree constructions (or the rules) governing how they work together and why.

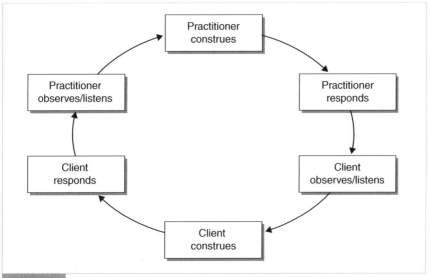

Figure 2.3 ● The client–practitioner cycle of interaction (from Davis et al 2002)

As another example, the process of exploration includes an attempt to elicit and understand the client's existing constructions and to enable him/her to develop a clearer, more helpful model of their problems or concerns within the context of his/her life. The skills involved must include careful listening, because the client has a unique picture (or set of constructions) of his/her situation, which the practitioner must try to elicit, make explicit, think about and, hopefully, clarify without necessarily imposing the practitioner's constructions (see Fig. 2.3). This has to involve the practitioner in checking out or testing whether he has understood the client's constructions, because it is so easy to make false assumptions.

Clients' constructs determine how they will act or react in a given situation, and the process of helping may require that clients change their picture of the world as there are always alternative ways of construing situations. Sometimes simply allowing clients to tell their story in their own ways brings them clarity and allows them to change their constructions as they see the situation more clearly. However, sometimes it may be necessary for practitioners to gently challenge clients to change. This may involve the practitioner comparing his or her own picture of the client's situation with the picture he or she thinks the client has and enabling alternative views to be considered. This is never an easy process as central constructs that may need to change can be strongly held beliefs that powerfully determine the rest of the picture. It may only be achieved through a strong and trusting partnership relationship built on mutual respect.

Clearly the aims of the helping process are a function of the constructions of the participants. An obvious consequence of this is the need for careful negotiation of the expectations of each: the client and the practitioner. They may have different agendas (i.e. constructions), and this needs to be clarified and negotiated at the outset. For further development of these ideas, please refer to Davis et al (2002a, b).

Evidence base of the family partnership approach

We have presented a broad outline of the Family Partnership Approach, which is intended as a useful guide to practice. However, prior to implementing such a model, it is important to consider its validity in terms of evaluative research in relation to processes and outcomes.

Evidence of the effectiveness of the Family Partnership Approach is gathering momentum. Outcomes of the research carried out to date will be described under three general headings: 1) the effects on people trained in the Family Partnership Model; 2) the effects on the parents of having a practitioner trained to work in partnership; and 3) the effects on children of parents working with people trained in the Family Partnership approach.

Effects of the Family Partnership training on practitioners

Regular feedback on the Family Partnership course from those trained is consistently highly positive in relation to overall satisfaction, learning and relevance to their work (Brocklehurst et al 2004, Davis et al 1997). For example, Papadopoulou et al (2005) trained 52 primary care professionals to work on a preventive project (Davis & Tsiantis 2005) with families in five different European countries and found close to maximum ratings for overall satisfaction (mean 4.5; maximum 5) and professional relevance (mean 4.3; maximum 5). The process of the training was also validated by highly positive rating (mean 3.6; maximum 4) of the style of teaching, which is intended to mirror the helping situation (e.g. listening to participants and treating them with respect).

Improved helper self-efficacy has consistently been found in participants of the course (Davis et al 1997, Lea et al 1998, Rushton & Davis 1992), using the Constructions of Helping Questionnaire, which involves participant ratings of the qualities and skills they bring to helping parents (e.g. empathy). McArdle and McDermott (1994) similarly found significant improvements in nursing staff in relation to their perceived ability to work in partnership and communicate effectively.

Understanding of the helping processes has also been shown to increase significantly as a result of the Family Partnership training using measures of theoretical knowledge (Davis et al 1997, Rushton & Davis 1992).

Significant improvements in the qualities (e.g. empathy) and skills of helping have been demonstrated in a number of studies as a result of the course as assessed, for example, by ratings and observational measures taken from videotaped interactions (Bidmead & Cowley 2005b, Davis et al 1997, Lea et al 1998, Rushton & Davis 1992).

Course participants have been shown to improve in terms of their sensitivity to family need (Puura et al 2002) and in the accuracy of their assessments (Papadopoulou et al 2005) in a prevention programme known as the European Early Promotion Project. By inference this indicates improved helper–parent relations and communication, and, therefore, a greater likelihood of providing appropriate intervention in promoting parent–infant interaction and preventing psychosocial problems in children.

Parental psychosocial outcomes

A number of studies have shown increased parental self-esteem as a result of intervention by trained personnel (Davis & Spurr 1998, Davis et al 2005, Rushton & Davis 1991):

- Evidence of decreased parental stress has been found in families where workers were trained in the Family Partnership approach (Davis & Spurr 1998, Davis et al 2005).

- Maternal anxiety and depression have been shown to improve in parents working with staff trained in the model (Davis & Rushton 1991, Davis & Spurr 1998, Davis et al 2005).
- Several studies have shown improved parent–child relationships and actual interaction, as a result of intervention by trained personnel, as measured by how positively parents construe their children, the HOME Inventory (Bradley & Caldwell 1979), and other observational measures (Davis & Rushton 1991, Davis & Spurr 1998, Puura et al 2005).
- Primary care workers trained in the Family Partnership approach have also been shown to enhance parental perception of support and to increase their satisfaction with services (Davis & Rushton 1991, Davis & Spurr, 1998, Davis et al 2005).

Child outcomes

There are huge problems for specialist services in trying to meet child and adolescent mental health needs (e.g. Audit Commission 1999) in the populations. This requires collaboration between services, and partnership between service providers and their clients. However, if the need is to be met, preferably by prevention and promotional approaches, then all who work with families and children must understand the processes of helping and have the skills to provide a first line of support.

Although workers trained in the Family Partnership Model may not necessarily focus specifically on the behaviour and development of the children in the families with whom they work, studies have shown both improved developmental progress as measured by the Griffiths (Avon Premature Infant Project 1998, Davis & Rushton 1991) and the Bayley Scales (Davis et al 2005), and improvements in behavioural and emotional functioning (Davis & Rushton 1991, Davis & Spurr 1998, Davis et al 2005).

The evidence presented indicates that it is the relationship with the client that is key to producing effective outcomes. Partnership working at both organisational and client level, using good interpersonal qualities and skills, is, therefore, fundamental to working in public health.

Continuing research with vulnerable families

A further study (Oxford Home Visiting Study) is currently being conducted to consider the effectiveness of the Family Partnership approach in relation to the prevention of child abuse and neglect (Barlow et al 2003) using health visitors working with families from pregnancy onward. The final results are yet to be published, but preliminary qualitative data from the home visitors (Brocklehurst et al 2004) support the Model in terms of the training, enabling improved relationships between the mothers and their home visitors, as well as benefits for the mothers, their children and their relationships within the family and with other professionals.

Conclusion

There is evidence of considerable psychosocial need in children and families in the community. Although this has important implications for children's development and for society as a whole, services are neither meeting this need effectively nor providing obvious preventive measures. Service changes are occurring and there is a general acknowledgement by government and service models that the relationship between clients and those needing help is important for outcomes and that the nature of the relationship should be a partnership. However, the lack of an adequate theoretical basis is hindering the helping processes, service development (including staff selection and training) and research. In an attempt to ameliorate this situation, this chapter has presented an explicit and relatively simple model of the helping processes, based upon an elaboration of the meaning of partnership in this context. This approach, entitled the Family Partnership Model, is accompanied by a detailed training package and has been implemented in a number of settings worldwide. The results of a number of studies so far conducted indicate that when professionals are trained to work in partnership, the results are beneficial both in terms of their own functioning and that of the clients served. Important implications of the Model are that, to be effective, staff need to be selected for the personal qualities and skills described within the model (e.g. empathy) and to be trained specifically in understanding the helping processes and in the skills of implementing it. However, there is also a need to support practitioners from all disciplines with skilled supervision, which is assumed to mirror directly the processes of helping. If they are supported within a respectful partnership with their managers, then practitioners working in public health and all other services are less likely to burn out, and are much more likely to show the qualities and skills that will be of benefit to their clients. They will be able to form relationships with their clients that will have direct benefits (e.g. on client self-efficacy) and also indirect effects of modelling how they should be with their own families. If self-esteem, control and self-empowerment are all qualities necessary for health (Tones & Tilford 2001), then it is of paramount importance that practitioners working in public health should have the qualities and skills to work in partnership, so as to enhance these qualities in their clients. If practitioners do not have these qualities and skills, little will be accomplished as partnership working is the key to public health.

DISCUSSION QUESTIONS

- Partnership working may take more time initially but may save time in the long run. How will you be able to implement this approach in your daily working?
- According to Bidmead and Cowley (2005a), practitioners working in partnership with their clients need support and supervision. Does a system of clinical supervision exist where you work? How will you implement one if not?

References

Acheson D 1998 Independent inquiry into inequalities in health. The Stationery Office, London

Almond P 2001 Partnership in health visiting: client health outcomes. MSc. King's College University, London

Attride-Stirling J, Davis H, Markless G et al 2001 'Someone to talk to who'll listen': addressing the psychosocial needs of children and families. Journal of Applied Social Psychology 11: 179–191

Audit Commission 1999 Children in mind: child and adolescent mental health services. Audit Commission Publications, London

Avon Premature Infant Project 1998 Randomised trial of parental support for families with very preterm children. Archives of Disease in Childhood, Fetal and Neonatal Edition. Fetal & Neonatal 79(1): F4–F11

Barlow J, Brocklehurst N, Stewart–Brown S et al 2003 Working in partnership: the development of a home visiting service for vulnerable families. Child Abuse Review 12: 172–189

Barlow J, Kirkpatrick S, Stewart-Brown S et al 2005 Hard-to-reach or out-of-reach? Reasons why women refuse to take part in early interventions. Children and Society 19: 199–210

Bidmead C, Cowley S 2005a A concept analysis of partnership with clients. Community Practitioner 78(6): 203–208

Bidmead C, Cowley S 2005b Evaluating family partnership training in health visitor practice. Community Practitioner 78(7): 239–245

Bidmead C, Davis H, Day C 2002 Partnership working: what does it really mean? Community Practitioner 75(7): 256–259

Bidmead C, Whittaker K 2004 Positive Parenting: a public health priority. CPHVA, London

Bradley R, Caldwell B 1979 Home observation for measurement of the environment: a revision of the preschool scale. American Journal of Mental Deficiency 84: 235–244

Brocklehurst N, Barlow J, Kirkpatrick S et al 2004 The contribution of health visitors to supporting vulnerable children and their families at home. Community Practitioner 77: 175–179

Davis H 1993 Counselling parents of children with chronic illness or disabilities. British Psychological Corporation, Leicester

Davis H, Day C, Bidmead C 2002a Working in partnership with parents: the Parent Adviser Model. Harcourt Assessment, London

Davis H, Day C, Bidmead C 2002b Parent adviser training manual. Harcourt Assessment. London

Davis H, Dusoir T, Papadopoulou K et al 2005 Child and family outcomes of the European Early Promotion Project. International Journal of Mental Health Promotion 7: 63–81

Davis H, Fallowfield L 1991 Counselling and communication in health care. John Wiley, Chichester.

Davis H, Rushton R 1991 Counselling and supporting parents of children with developmental delay: a research evaluation. Journal of Mental Deficiency Research 35: 89–112

Davis H, Spurr P 1998 Parent counselling: an evaluation of a community child mental health service. Journal of Child Psychology and Psychiatry 39: 365–376

Davis H, Spurr P, Cox A et al 1997 A description and evaluation of a community child mental health service. Clinical Child Psychology & Psychiatry 2(2): 221–238

Davis H, Tsiantis J 2005 Promoting children's mental health: the European Early Promotion Project (EEPP). International Journal of Mental Health Promotion 7: 4–16

Department of Health 2004 National service framework for children, young people and maternity services. The Stationery Office, London

Department for Education and Skills 2004 Every child matters: next steps. DfES Publications, Nottingham

Egan G 1998 The skilled helper. A problem management approach to helping, 6th edn. Brooks/Cole Publishing, Pacific Grove, CA

Elkan R, Blair M, Robinson J 2000a Evidence-based practice and health visiting: the need for theoretical underpinnings for evaluation. Journal of Advanced Nursing 31(6): 1316–1323

Elkan R, Kendrick D, Hewitt M et al 2000b The effectiveness of domiciliary health visiting: a systematic review of international studies and a selective review of the British literature. Health Technology Assessment 4(13)

Franks P, Fiscella K, Shields C G et al 2005 Are patients' ratings of their physicians related to health outcomes? Annals of Family Medicine 3(3): 229–234

Gomby D, Culross P, Behrman R 1999 Home visiting: recent program evaluations – analysis and recommendations. The Future of Children 9: 4–26

Goodwin S 1991 Breaking the links between social deprivation and poor child health. Health Visitor 64(11): 376–380

Green J 2006 Annotation: the therapeutic alliance – significant but neglected variable in child mental health treatment studies. Journal of Child Psychology and Psychiatry 47(5): 435–435

Hall D, Elliman D 2003 Health for all children, 4th edn. Oxford University Press, Oxford

Kelly G 1991 The psychology of personal constructs. Volume 1: A theory of personality. Routledge, London

Lea S, Clarke M, Davis H 1998 Evaluation of a counselling skills course for health professionals. British Journal of Guidance and Counselling 26: 159–173

Martin D J, Garske J P, Davies M K 2000 Relation of the therapeutic alliance with outcome and other variables: a meta analytic review. Journal of Consulting and Clinical Psychology 68: 438–450

McArdle G, McDermott M 1994 From directive expert to non-directive partner: a study of facilitating change in the occupational self-perceptions of health visitors and school nurses. British Journal of Guidance and Counselling 22: 107–117

Mitcheson J, Cowley S 2003 Empowerment or control? An analysis of the extent to which client participation is enabled during health visitor/client interactions using a structured health needs assessment tool. International Journal of Nursing Studies 40: 413–426

Normandale S 2001 A study of mothers' perceptions of the health visiting role. Community Practitioner 74(4):146–150

Nursing and Midwifery Council 2004 Standards of proficiency for specialist community public health nurses, NMC, London

Oakley A, Rigby A, Hickey D 1994 Life stress, support and class inequality. European Journal of Public Health 4: 81–91

Papadopoulou K, Dimitrakaki C, Davis H et al 2005 The effects of the European Early Promotion Project training on primary health care professionals. International Journal of Mental Health Promotion 7: 54–62

Peckover S 2002 Supporting and policing mothers: an analysis of the disciplinary practices of health visiting. Journal of Advanced Nursing 38(4): 369–377

Peckover S 2003 'I could have done with a little more help': an analysis of women's help–seeking from health visit-ors in the context of domestic violence. Health and Social Care in the Community 11(3): 275–282

Puura K, Davis H, Papadopoulou K et al 2002 The European Early Promotion Project: a new primary health care service

to promote children's mental health. Infant Mental Health Journal 23: 606–624

Puura K, Davis H, Mantymaa M et al 2005 The outcome of the European Early Promotion Project: mother–child inter-action. International Journal of Mental Health Promotion 7: 82–94

Rogers C 1959 A theory of therapy, personality and interpersonal relation-ships as developed in the client–centred framework. In: Koch S (ed.) Psychology: a study of science, 3rd edn. McGraw Hill, New York

Rushton R, Davis H 1992 An evaluation of the effectiveness of counselling train-ing for health care professionals. British Journal of Guidance and Counselling 20: 205–220

Salvage J 1990 The theory and practice of the new nursing. Nursing Times 86: 4

Shirk S R, Karver M 2003 Prediction of treat-ment outcome from relationship variables in child and adolescent therapy: a meta analytic review. Journal of Consulting and Clinical Psychology 71: 452–464

Tones K, Tilford S 2001 Health promotion effectiveness, efficiency and equity, 3rd edn. Nelson Thornes, Cheltenham

WHO 1978 Primary health care: interna-tional conference on primary health care. World Health Organization in conjunction with United Nations Children's Fund, Alma Ata, USSR

Further reading

Dale N 1996 Working with families of children with special needs: partnership and practice. Routledge, London

Davis H, Day C, Bidmead C 2002 Working in partnership with parents: the Parent Adviser Model. Harcourt Assessment, London

Egan G 1998 The skilled helper. A problem management approach to helping, 6th edn. Brooks/Cole Publishing, Pacific Grove, CA

Fransella F, Dalton P 2000 Personal construct counselling in action. Sage Publications, London

Section 2

The stimulation of an awareness of health needs

Working in a collaborative way to achieve health and wellbeing is central to all public health. In community public health, this involves not only collaboration with other agencies, but also a finely developed ability to work with and for communities and social groups, including families, to improve their health and wellbeing. Many of the key skills are similar, whether collaborating with professional colleagues, or with clients or local residents. Colleagues and clients alike may be unaware of the links between social determinants of health, or of the impact of difficulties encountered by individuals and families, particularly those living in disadvantaged circumstances. Understanding these links is a necessary prerequisite to collaborative work. The long-term developmental impact of early family life, and the extent to which services and residents can work together to ameliorate the worst effects of disadvantage, are explored in the four chapters in this section.

The stimulation of an awareness of health needs is associated with the following performance standards (Nursing and Midwifery Council 2004: p. 11):

1. Raise awareness about health and social wellbeing and related factors, services and resources.
2. Develop, sustain and evaluate collaborative work.
3. Communicate with individuals, groups and communities about promoting their health and wellbeing.
4. Raise awareness about the actions that groups and individuals can take to improve their health and social wellbeing.
5. Develop capacity and confidence of individuals and groups, including families and communities, to influence and use available services, information and skills, acting as advocate where appropriate.
6. Work with others to protect the public's health and wellbeing from specific risks.

Collaborating for health

Pauline Craig and Moira Fischbacher

Key issues

- The development of collaboration and integration in health and social care is the mainstay of ongoing public sector reform
- Examples are given of integrated services in Scotland and England
- Integration of planning for improving health is explained, along with working through networks:
  - Concepts and principles
  - Characteristics
  - Network types
  - Practice and strategic level networks
  - Managing and sustaining networks

Introduction

Collaboration within health services and between health services and other partners is assuming increasing importance as integrated planning and service delivery takes root in the public sector. Collaborating takes place at all levels. It might be used informally for individual service users, such as when community practitioners organise the provision of a combination of local services for a single client, or it could be adopted for more formal processes, such as in creating new national structures for joint funding and management of health and social services. The evidence base is growing for approaches and processes that can support good collaborative practice, and for articulating the benefits of working in partnership. However, collaboration between different agencies or professional groups is rarely straightforward, and the consequences of engaging in a collaborative network are not always fully understood.

This chapter examines two manifestations of collaborating to improve health and wellbeing. The first is policy development for integrated health and social service planning and provision, arguably now the mainstay of ongoing public sector reform, much of which assumes that effective collaboration will reap many benefits for service delivery as well as for the service users. The second manifestation discussed here is the notion of working through networks. A network is described as ongoing collaboration between organisations where information is shared, joint working practices developed, cultures adapted and delivery of services integrated. Both the benefits and difficulties of engaging in a network are examined and the chapter concludes by considering the implications for health practitioners that arise from networking.

Development of collaboration and integration in health and social care

Integration of health and social care is not a new phenomenon. Public health departments in local authorities, overseen by Medical Officers of Health (MOsH), provided hospital, primary and community care services from the end of the 19th century. For example, between the first and second world wars public health departments in local authorities had a remit to provide maternal and child welfare services; school medical services; TB clinics and treatment; infectious disease, ear, nose and throat, and VD services; health centres; regional cancer schemes; and to run the old Poor Law hospitals (Lewis 1991).

The MOsH tripartite system of prevention, family practitioners and hospital services was transferred to the NHS in 1974, although local government retained social care and environmental health services. This split is believed by some commentators to have had a long-lasting impact on the ability of health and social care services to work together (McClelland 2003). In addition, allowing general practitioners to remain as independent contractors rather than salaried employees has resulted in the need to introduce complex incentives to ensure service delivery and distribution of staff.

Collaboration between, and integration of, health and social services, therefore, have a long history spanning different degrees of working together and apart, but the last two decades have seen concerted efforts to merge health and social care structures and functions. One of the first specifications for this move came in the 1990 NHS and Community Care Act, which required local authorities to produce community care plans in partnership with health boards and other local agencies. The main objective of this Act was to keep people requiring care in their own homes rather in institutions, but also to create a 'mixed economy of care', which was chiefly aimed at involving voluntary and private sector service provision to meet the growing need for care for older people.

In 1997, *The NHS: modern, dependable* (Department of Health (DH) 1997) and *Designed to care* (Scottish Executive 1997) were the English and Scottish White Papers, respectively, which introduced a modernisation programme for the NHS of dismantling the internal market and working towards a system of integrated care. In England, Primary Care Groups were set up not only to commission services but also to have more influence with acute care; their aims included promoting the health of the local population in partnership with other agencies and better integrating primary and community health services. Primary Care Groups were to develop further into freestanding Primary Care Trusts, totally responsible for commissioning and delivering services but remaining accountable to Health Authorities.

In Scotland, primary care was to be delivered through Primary Care Trusts (PCTs) and Local Health Care Co-operatives (LHCCs). Scottish PCTs had fewer budget-holding responsibilities than their English counterparts, but provided staff such as nurses, allied health professionals and health centre management, and were later (from 2002) merged with NHS Boards. LHCCs were to work in association with general practitioners (GPs), dentists, pharmacists and opticians, who remained independent contractors, but were encouraged to be given places on boards of LHCCs. LHCC objectives were described as providing services to patients, working with public health to plan for meeting the defined health needs of the LHCC population, clinical governance and developing population-wide approaches to health improvement and disease prevention (Scottish Executive 1997).

Both sets of polices clearly set out moves towards working in partnership and integration between primary care and both acute and social care services. They also introduced the need for primary care to begin to take a population approach to improving health as well as to deliver services to individual patients.

The move towards integration between health and social services in Scotland was supported by a national collaborative group, called the Joint Future Group. This was set up by the Scottish Office in 1999 (Joint Future Group 2000) to find ways of improving joint working to deliver modern and effective person-centred services, to identify options for charging for home-based care and sharing good practice. The focus was initially to be on older people, but to eventually move onto other client groups, including children. The Group produced a number of recommendations in 2000, including:

- Local authorities (social work and housing), health boards, NHS trusts and Scottish Homes should draw up local partnership agreements, including a clear programme for local joint resourcing and joint management of community care services collectively or for each care user group individually.
- Agencies locally should have in place single, shared assessment procedures for older people and for those with dementia by October 2001, and for all client groups by April 2002.
- The Scottish Executive should, by 2002, offer a strategic lead on the development of community care information, information sharing and systems integration.

A survey of LHCCs across one-third of the Health Boards in Scotland found that local working between LHCCs and social work, particularly in relation to community care, had developed substantially since the introduction of LHCCs, although joint working between primary and secondary care was less developed (LHCC Best Practice Group 2000). Recommendations from this report influenced the objectives of the next re-structuring of LHCCs as they were further developed into Community Health Partnerships.

The process of integration and further reform in Scotland continued in the next NHS White Paper *Partnership for care* (Scottish Executive 2003a). LHCCs were to evolve into Community Health Partnerships (CHPs), but the new bodies would have statutory underpinnings instead of being voluntary groupings, and would be part of the NHS Boards. CHPs were to establish a substantive partnership with local authorities (social work, housing, education and regeneration this time), patient involvement through establishing Patient Partnership Forums for patients and staff, have more devolved budgetary responsibilities and a duty to promote health improvement (Scottish Executive 2003a). The White Paper also required health boards to work with local authorities to ensure more effective working with social care in appropriate locality arrangements, and to integrate the management of primary and acute services. However, CHPs were expected to play an increasingly central role in integration of services locally as they matured into their partnerships, in order to improve the health of local populations as part of an ongoing programme of development and modernisation in public services (Scottish Executive Health Department 2004a).

Further integration of services

Greater Glasgow NHS and Glasgow City Council took the CHP national guidelines a step further in 2006 in to create fully integrated Community Health and Care Partnerships (CHCPs) (Greater Glasgow NHS 2005). CHCPs brought together primary care and social work services under a single management structure, with associated accountability and governance arrangements, and with similar aims for integration to that of England's Care Trusts (see below). They also propose substantial involvement of (and credibility with) elected members and intend to develop structured links to housing, regeneration and employment. With these proposals, the Glasgow Scheme of Establishment for CHCPs stated that its aims were to add value to existing programmes for integrating and improving services, particularly children's services, and was notable as the first integrated NHS and social care services structure for children and families in Scotland.

Integration of services for vulnerable population groups

Following on from the work of the Scottish Joint Futures Group for services for older people, the drive towards integration in Scotland was developed in other services. At first, reform focused on services for people with learning disabilities and for people with alcohol and drug problems, with the development of co-located health and social care services including with joint funding and joint management (Joint Future Group 2000).

A similar process was undertaken in England, with the introduction of Care Trusts in the NHS Plan as a mechanism for integration of health and social services. Care Trusts were to be established on a voluntary basis in partnership, with a joint agreement at local level regarded as the best way to offer services, rather than forcing a partnership where no relationships existed. Different models for Care Trusts could be developed, but it was envisaged that they would mostly be based around existing Primary Care Trusts, focusing on commissioning and providing services for older people and mental health services initially. They aimed to bring together existing staff from health and social care services within one local organisation, and were to be governed by a mixture of local councillors, health managers and patient and user representatives (DH 2002).

Children's Trusts in England

Children's Trusts, based on similar principles as Care Trusts described above were introduced in England in *Every child matters* (HM Government 2004). They were to bring together local education authorities, health and social services in order to establish greater strategic coherence, better integration of services and improved access to services. The main driver for this model for children's services was said to be the Laming inquiry into the death of Victoria Climbie, which made extensive recommendations for raising standards and improving the monitoring of social care staff and services. The Laming inquiry demonstrated that frontline social services staff were working in departments that were struggling with poor management supervision, unfilled posts and substantial underfunding. Commentators at the time of the report being published hoped that the new codes of conduct and the emphasis on evidence-based practice would give social workers greater clarity of their roles and responsibilities in multi-agency working. Concern was also expressed in that the impact of structural reform on a service already very stretched, was thought to have the potential to further undermine the services.

Children's Trusts were duly created, but using a stepped approach. Thirty-five pathfinder Children's Trusts were initially set up in 35 of the 150 local authorities in England, and their early implementation reviewed as part of a national evaluation (University of Anglia and NCB 2004). Most of the pathfinders aimed to achieve all five of the outcomes stated in *Every child matters*, that is of being healthy, staying safe, enjoying and achieving, making a positive contribution, and economic wellbeing (although the latter had a lower priority). By 2004, most pathfinders had pooled budgets already in place, or planned, along with written partnership agreements; most were establishing processes for sharing information about individual pupils, clients or patients; most had brought together front-line professionals from across health, education and social services sectors; and most had incorporated views of children, young people and their parents and carers in the development of the trusts.

The evaluation reported that integration and collaboration was said to have been facilitated by joint training, maintaining a stable workforce, commitment to integration at all levels and a history of joint working. Barriers were identified where there were complex service interfaces, insufficient funding, lack of time, changes in management personnel and problems recruiting and retaining staff.

Integrated Children's Services in Scotland: Starting Well

Starting Well is a Scottish demonstration project that has developed an integrated approach to children's health and social care services, in a similar way to England's Children's Trusts.

Demonstration projects were first announced in the Scottish Public Health White Paper, *Towards a healthier Scotland* (Scottish Office 1999) and were designed to develop and demonstrate good practice in the areas of child health, coronary heart disease, sexual health and colorectal cancer. Glasgow won its multi-agency bid for the child health project for £3 million over an initial 3-year period and Starting Well was duly launched in November 2000. Extensions of the funding were later granted and continued until 2006, at which point plans were in place to roll out the model of working throughout Glasgow (Wallis 2006).

Starting Well aimed to demonstrate that child health can be improved by a programme of activities to support families, coupled with access to enhanced community-based resources for parents and their children. It was developed through a multi-agency partnership and assumed a collaborative approach in its design and delivery. The project focused on two of the most deprived areas in Glasgow and drew heavily on the US literature on home visiting, which demonstrated significant impacts on a range of child- and family-health-related outcomes. The main programme for Starting Well in its first phase encompassed an augmented programme of home visiting for all families of newborn babies in the two areas, the development of enhanced local community supports and structures within the areas, and the development of integrated organisational services within the areas and across Glasgow (Mackenzie et al 2004).

A project team was established in each area with a health visitor co-ordinator, Starting Well health visitors and health support workers (from a voluntary organisation), a bilingual worker in one of the areas, community nursery nurses and a community support facilitator in each team. Linked social workers and midwives were identified for the teams, although were not co-located in the first phase. Training was provided to the teams on a range of topics, including child development and protection, domestic violence, and the Triple P Programme (an Australian parenting programme). The project managed to engage almost all eligible families across the two areas.

In the last year of the project, Starting Well re-focused to target the most vulnerable children in the intervention areas and extended the multi-disciplinary teams drawn initially from health and voluntary sectors to include professionals from social work and education. The approach they took to integrated working was to recognise that it was not just the staff working directly with families who needed to work together, but that the whole system within which services are planned, funded and managed must integrate together to ensure that families health and social care needs are met (Wallis 2006).

Integration of planning for improving health

Alongside the development of integrated health and social services, collaborative approaches to improving health and wellbeing are becoming well-established. These approaches link primary care into the planning structures for other public service provision, and provide the mechanism for collaborating to work towards population health improvement.

Health improvement and health inequalities in Scotland

In addition to improved integration of health and social service delivery, the Community Health Partnerships (and Community Health and Care Partnerships) in Scotland also aimed to have stronger roles in health improvement and to reduce health inequalities. Collaboration through partnership working is regarded as an important focus for this work. For example, the Scottish Executive's Guidance document (Scottish Executive 2004a) for establishing Community Health Partnerships (CHPs) states that the focus for health improvement should be on:

- Population health
- Influencing Boards through needs assessment
- Working with disadvantaged communities
- Health promotion
- Taking a wide perspective on health
- Working with partners
- Improving wellbeing, life circumstances and lifestyles especially in disadvantaged communities.

This focus reflects Scottish public health and health improvement policy documents, that is, *Towards a healthier Scotland* (Scottish Office 1999) and *Health improvement – the challenge* (Scottish Executive 2003b), and arguably builds on years of public health, health education and health promotion research and practice. It also reflects that health improvement, as a move on from health promotion, is increasingly understood as a partnership activity between health, local authority, voluntary and community sectors, rather than residing only in the 'health' domain.

The focus in the CHP guidance for health inequalities is also stated as being to work in partnership to address the needs of the full range of community groups (Scottish Executive 2004a). While partnership is again reinforced as the appropriate approach to take, there is otherwise a lack of clarity as to what is expected of CHPs in relation to addressing health inequalities. However, the Scottish targets for reducing health inequalities are included as a section in the Scottish Executive's regeneration policy (Scottish Executive 2004b), which is delivered through the mechanism of community planning. CHPs and Community Planning Partnerships (CPPs) are now linked through legislation, policy and emerging practice, and provide an example of where integration within the public sector has become irreversibly established within planning structures.

Community planning

The mechanism for improving health and wellbeing across the UK is embedded in the development of collaborative structures for strategic planning, which bring together public, voluntary, community and private sector agencies and interests, in umbrella partnerships for social, economic, health and environmental planning. Such partnerships in the four UK countries have different names, as follows:

- Community Planning Partnerships in Scotland
- Local Strategic Partnerships in England
- Local Strategy Partnerships in Northern Ireland
- Community Strategy Partnerships in Wales.

However, their aims are broadly similar, with small differences between countries, such as in accountability mechanisms, and differences between and within countries in the configuration of the structures. Community planning in Scotland is highlighted here as an example of integration of strategic planning.

The Local Government in Scotland Act 2003 provided the statutory basis for Community Planning in Scotland, which is now the key overarching partnership framework for coordinating the planning and development of public service provision.

Community planning in Scotland has two main aims:

1. To make sure that people and communities are genuinely engaged in the decisions made on public services that affect them.
2. A commitment from organisations to work together, not apart, in providing better public services.

Community Planning Partnerships aim to integrate both vertically and horizontally, as described above. In the local community planning process, local authorities are expected to engage with a wide range of interests including:

- Community and voluntary organisations, whether delivering services or representing a specific area or interest. They might be locally, regionally or nationally based. This could include young people and youth-work bodies; environmental bodies, rural bodies, consumer bodies and sports and cultural bodies.
- Community councils as representatives of their local area.
- Equalities groups and interests.
- Business, through representative organisations or businesses themselves.
- Trade unions as representative and democratic agencies.
- Professional interests.

In addition, they are said to also act as a 'bridge' to link national and local priorities better by influencing national direction, but also helping to co-ordinate the delivery of national priorities in a way that is sensitive to local needs and circumstances. Local or neighbourhood priorities should also be able to influence the priorities at the Community Planning Partnership, or local authority level. Integrating vertically should ensure a balance between the local authority level, localised or neighbourhood level, and collaboration between community planning partnerships when an issue warrants a more strategic consideration. However, community need should be the central focus, with the main community partnership being at local authority level. This level is linked to themed partnerships, such as for health improvement, and supported by other local, regional or international structures as required (Scottish Executive 2004c).

The Act also gave the NHS and other public bodies a 'duty to participate' in the community planning process, reinforced by the NHS Legislative Reform Bill of 2004, and participation was specified in relation to health improvement by char-ging NHS boards and local authorities with responsibility to work together to produce local health improvement plans.

In addition, amongst other powers, the 2003 Local Government Act gave local authorities a power of wellbeing. This power enables local authorities to take a creative and innovative approach to improving wellbeing as well as providing statutory services, such as carrying out an assessment of what is needed to advance wellbeing in an area. The guidance for local authorities for the power of wellbeing recognises a number of key factors that might contribute to promotion or improvement of wellbeing as follows:

- Economic factors, such as the availability of jobs, support for local small businesses, transport links, lifelong learning, training and skills development, information and communication technologies, etc.

- Social factors, such as good-quality and affordable housing; safe communities; the encouragement of the voluntary sector; looking after the needs of children and young people, particularly the most vulnerable; access to the arts, leisure, education, etc.
- Health-related factors, such as the promotion of good physical, social and mental health, and developing and promoting policies that have a positive impact on health outcomes, especially on health inequalities.
- Environmental factors, such as clean air, water and streets, the quality of the built environment, the removal of offensive graffiti, protecting communities against the threat of climate change and flooding, improving and promoting biodiversity and accessibility to nature.

Clearly, for the local authority to take action on any of the above wellbeing issues, it would have to work in an integrated way with other statutory and voluntary organisations at local and national levels (Scottish Executive 2004d).

Why collaborate?

Integration and closer collaboration is generally thought to bring benefits relating to reducing management costs and this is likely to be the main motivation for the policy imperatives for integration. For example, the move towards integration was stated in 1997 as a means of improving quality and reducing costs (Department of Health 1997). Simeons and Scott (2005) outline the different dimensions of integration that can take place for integrated primary care organisations (IPCOs), such as England's Primary Care Trusts or CHPs in Scotland. IPCOs can be vertically integrated, co-ordinating primary, secondary and tertiary care, or they can be horizontally integrated, with greater co-operation across primary care providers. They can also be a combination of both. CHPs provide an example of a combined model, with greater influence over health boards' resource allocation (although not commissioning secondary services directly) and a strong emphasis on greater collaboration between health and social care professionals, the voluntary sector and the general public. PCTs in England are similar to CHPs, although they have these emphases inverted, that is, they have a strong emphasis on vertical integration with a lead commissioning role, and collaboration comes secondary. However, some English PCTs were identified as beginning to merge some functions in order to integrate for reasons of reducing management costs and sharing professional expertise (Regen et al 2001).

While current UK policies emphasise the reduction of costs as a reason for increasing integration, this might not be enough to motivate the health and social care professionals to carry integration through. For example, the focus for health care professionals tends to be on the patient's journey, and integration can be interpreted as better co-ordination between services or teamwork between health and social care providers, rather than a concern for management costs being the driver. Research evidence shows that the development and operation of IPCOs is likely to be determined by the behaviour and attitude of primary care providers, and that integration can be encouraged by changing the features and remits of IPCOs to take account of the interests of providers (Simeons & Scott 2005). However, a great deal of professional time is required to achieve integration, as found during the development of LHCCs in Lothian (Hopton & Heaney 1999), and the process itself might be unattractive to clinicians who are aware that research has not yet identified what might be the benefits to patients of integration of services.

From policy to practice: the case of networks

Public policy in the UK since 1990 has offered a vision for integrated health and social care services and it is clear that a lot of ground has been covered in the last two decades, but that full integration has not yet been achieved. The move towards integration is thought to be supported by policy as a means of improving quality and reducing costs. In the current climate of concern for the spiralling costs of the NHS and the media focus for questioning quality of public services, it is argued that these aims are unlikely to be fulfilled at least in the near future.

However, it is clear that at practice level, at least, there are many potential benefits to be had from public sector services working in collaboration, such as better communication, shared aims and less duplication. It is argued that it would appear to be counterproductive to attempt to reverse moves towards integration at this stage without a better understanding of the full costs and benefits of integrated service planning and delivery. The following section offers pointers towards an understanding of collaboration through an examination of the practice of working through networks.

Concept and principles of interorganisational networks

The practice of networking has grown in recent years in a range of sectors and industries and, as this chapter has shown, is now in widespread use across the public sector and, in particular, within the health sector (Williams 2002). In some respects, the increasing adoption of networks reflects a perception that collaboration brings mutual reward and can enhance the quality and efficiency of services. It is also the case, however, that networks are thought to be a more efficient way of organising. There are typically three models of how the provision of a service can be organised: markets, hierarchies and networks.

Markets typically fit within a commercial (private sector) setting. Products and services are exchanged at a price. The price customers are willing to pay reflects their view of the quality of that product/service and their need for it. Where there is a choice of products/services, sellers will compete to offer the best combination of quality and price. Markets are often regarded as highly efficient, but also inequitable. They ensure that consumer tastes are met using the resources available (efficiency), but do so only where consumers have the ability to pay, and this ability is not something that is equitably distributed.

Hierarchies are single organisations (commonly referred to as bureaucracies). Many public sector organisations are, or were, hierarchies. Here, products/services are planned and delivered through a centrally administered system that governs service planning and control of service delivery. In this system, efforts are made to ensure consistency across all service areas and an equitable distribution of resources. In contrast to markets, hierarchies are often thought to be equitable in that they can plan for a fair, non-competitive distribution of resources according to need. They are, however, thought to be inefficient due to size (which results in delayed decision making and often loss of information) and thus burdensome. The emphasis on procedures can be restrictive, with bureaucracies being slow to respond to internal or external change. It is this problem of inefficiency that has given rise to the NHS seeking to find new ways of organising health services.

Networks are sets of interorganisational relationships where parties engage in long-term agreements. These agreements are usually formalised, though not always legally, and are based on mutual interests and inputs. Networks may involve some buying and selling of services (as in a market), but principally involve a shared understanding that parties will work for their collective interest in the long term and may need to forgo short-term interests. The expectation is that there is an advantage in working together. Parties can share information, encourage innovation, integrate services, and be flexible to external and internal events (unlike a hierarchy) without the short-term, competitive ethos of the market place.

Organising in the NHS

The current political impetus behind networks has followed from implementation of both the hierarchy and market form of organising. When the NHS was first created in 1948, it was done so as a hierarchy. For many years services were centrally planned and were subject to direct intervention from government at all levels from strategic through to operational levels. Accountability for service quality and performance (albeit these were at that time measured in a rather rudimentary fashion) was through layers of district and regional administration. During the period of Conservative government in the 1980s, however, the wisdom of this NHS hierarchy was called into question. The NHS was experiencing rising costs leading to increased demands on public sector funding and a new way of running and organising the service was sought.

The solution introduced in *Working for patients* (DH 1989) reflected a partial adoption of the market model described above. Providers of health care were expected to compete for patients. GPs and health boards/authorities were to buy services through contracts that specified quality and price. There was mixed evidence as to suitability of a market in health care with some research pointing to improvements in patient care and service quality, and with research elsewhere raising concerns about adverse affects of the market system.

Whether the abolition of the market following the entry to government of the Labour Party reflected an evaluation of research evidence, or a predominantly political decision to move away from Conservative market-based models, is not for consideration here. That the 'new' way of working endorses the network model is of significance. This is because, although networks offer the promise of great benefit, there are difficulties with them:

- the concept of networks is difficult to define
- structural relationships are complex
- network processes (e.g. building trust) are complex and take time
- network outcomes are difficult to measure.

Characteristics of networks

Within the health sector there are various types of network. Policy networks are formed by the coming together of groups and individuals that have an interest and input into the development of a particular policy (e.g. drugs, public health or mental health). Research networks form where academics, policy makers and practitioners with an interest and/or expertise in a particular research area coalesce in order to bring their collective knowledge and experience to bear on a new research problem or the development of a research agenda. Social and professional networks form often quickly and automatically. Through training and career progression, individuals within occupational disciplines (e.g. medicine, nursing, physiotherapy, dentistry) will increasingly identify with others in the same occupational discipline. University education, mentoring schemes and Royal College membership are just some of the means through which that identity and an often close-knit professional network are developed and nurtured.

Service delivery networks, which we concentrate on in this chapter, are built upon the range of providers who collectively make an input into meeting the needs of a particular group of customers or, in the case of public services, members of the public. They usually involve informal and formal structures and processes between several agencies/service providers, including service agreements, joint planning statements and/or protocols for partnership working. They are, therefore, multi-agency and multi-disciplinary (see Huxham & Vangen 2005 for examples).

Network types and their properties

There are many different definitions of network and the literatures examining the concept and practice of networks are extensive and varied. They include perspectives from political science, economics, management, health services research, marketing and sociology. The definitions of networks offered from these academic disciplines emphasise different aspects of networks and networking, each sensitised to particular discipline-specific theories and insights (see Laing et al 2002). However, some common themes emerge from these literatures when considering the characteristics of networks.

Complementarity

It is important that if two or more organisations are to work together, they must bring to the relationship complementary skills, knowledge and resources. For example, in the holistic treatment of an individual or group of patients with a common illness or condition, a range of practitioners will be needed. Each will have expertise in a different aspect of the illness/condition, each will have behind them a slightly different set of organisational resources. This is evident in the coming together of health and social care service providers in the support of a patient who is being rehabilitated and needs adaptations in the home, occupational therapy, counselling, physiotherapy and so forth. That no one organisation or practitioner can serve all patient needs demonstrates the nature of complementarity.

Interdependence

Having established a complementarity amongst network members, it follows that these members are often interdependent in that the success of one organisation's attempts to meet a particular agenda depends on co-operation with the others in the network. It is often the case that health improvement for an individual or patient group cannot be attained without the input from several organisations. Further, the success of each individual organisation, in terms of the performance targets it must meet, is likely to be in part dependent on other organisations effectively offering their service. The patient in need of rehabilitation, for example, cannot remain in the home if social services are unable to put in place the adaptations required in the home. This in turn raises the possibility of readmission to hospital, which would have a negative effect on the availability of hospital beds and other hospital performance targets.

Mutual or 'collaborative' advantage

The principle of interdependence underpins the notion of mutual or 'collaborative' advantage (Huxham 2003). As Huxham writes 'to get the real *advantage* out of collaboration ... something has to be achieved that could not have been attained by any of the organisations acting alone' (p. 403). Huxham's point is that it is not just that two organisations might need to work together but rather there is an added advantage in their doing so. Managed Clinical Networks (MCNs), for example, represent collaboration between organisations in order to improve patient journeys and to improve information available to practitioners involved in the treatment of particular condition. This information sharing has the potential to grow to a point of knowledge creation that derives from practitioners working more closely together. Networks that bring together academics and practitioners offer academics access to study sites (empirical data) and live case studies, so as to provide state-of-the-art research and knowledge. They offer practitioners more immediate access to research findings as well as an opportunity to shape the research agenda.

Trust

Whilst recognising interdependence and the opportunity for collaborative advantage is important, a further element invariably regarded as being crucial to the success of a network is trust. Trust is often referred to as the 'glue' that holds network members together. Whilst collaboration may be set out in broad terms in strategic agreements, at the level of the individual health practitioner or social worker, collaboration needs to be negotiated between individuals. Some researchers suggest that there has to be a level of trust already in place for networks to function (i.e. trust is a precondition). Others, however, emphasise that trust grows through successful collaboration and develops over time (i.e. trust is an outcome). The issue of trust is complex because it is tightly related to issues of professionalism, expectations of and from employers, professional hierarchies and the politics within and between organisations. If, however, networks are to be successful, they require 'give and take' between individuals and this can be done only as individuals trust one another to fulfil their promises.

Formality and informality

Health services have long been provided not only through official (or formal) structures, but through good working relationships on the ground where health service, social work and voluntary sector staff have established effective, informal working relationships. Networks incorporate and, to some extent, depend on this type of relationship. They also require a degree of formality to cement interorganisational (or interagency) working. This is likely to come in the form of the joint planning and shared protocol initiatives mentioned earlier. Formal arrangements should take effect at strategic levels, to ensure coordination between agencies, and also at operational levels, to allow those dealing with patients to work effectively with staff in other agencies particularly where no previous informal ties exist.

Creativity and conflict

In any situation where individuals come together within and between organisations, there is the potential for creative interaction as their different perspectives and experience stimulates ideas and new ways of working. Where work relies on the exercise of individual, professional judgement, then there is increased opportunity for a range of perspectives that are, in fact, simultaneously a source of creativity and a source of conflict. The culture of the organisations members involved in networks belong to (see below for more) will, in part, determine whether individual and organisational differences become a source of conflict alone, or lead to a creative environment in which practitioners embrace different ways of working with, or thinking about, a client/patient group.

Culture and norms

Organisational culture is an aspect that cannot be ignored in any network, organisational structure or change management discussion. Organisational culture is generally understood to be the way in which things are done within the organisation: the stories told, the 'rituals' observed, the principles that underpin staff interactions, etc. Every organisation has a culture (and in fact many subcultures) that exerts a significant influence on how practitioners think, behave, engage witin the organisation and relate to those outwith the organisation. NHS practitioners, for example, have a shared language, a common tacit understanding of hierarchy and often a strongly held belief in the importance of the NHS as a comprehensive service. Culture often works at a subconscious level and is represented in taken-for-granted assumptions that are not often understood by, or even recognised by, those outside the organisation. When two or more organisations come together they will each be influenced by their own cultures. This again can result in conflict and creativity. It is important to recognise these different cultures and to try and ensure that underlying assumptions about working practices, service philosophies (e.g. in drugs a harm reduction or abstinence philosophy) and priorities are aired. Moreover, it is crucial that network members seek to develop a shared language that is inclusive in nature.

Practice and strategic level networks

The features or properties of networks discussed above will be found to varying degrees within different network settings, but should all be present to some extent. They will also exist at different levels within organisations. Many practitioners believe themselves to have been part of an interagency network throughout their working lives. District nursing staff have, for example, long since liaised with general practitioners and health visitors. Community psychiatric nurses (CPNs) have worked closely with hospital and community practitioners, such as social workers, psychiatrists and voluntary agency project workers. Throughout the lifetime of the NHS, these practice-level relationships have existed, grown and been sustained often without formalised interagency protocols or agreements and despite the organisational barriers that exist between health care, social care and voluntary care providers.

In many respects, then, these informal practice networks pre-date recent formalised network relationships between agencies formed through Managed Clinical Networks, Joint Futures working and other such initiatives. The strategic level of networking represented by high level agreements (e.g. through NHS Board/Health Authority commissioning) and joint planning arrangements can therefore be seen in some respects as supplementing, reinforcing or even recognising the value of practice-level networking.

Benefits of networked organisations

As we explained earlier, networks are thought to be efficient ways of organising services, allocating and using scarce public sector resources. This would be reflected in an enhanced ability to direct resources to where they are most needed, to remove waste or duplication from the system. Where networks are well designed and managed, this organisational efficiency can be coupled with improving the effectiveness of service delivery that in turn yields a range of benefits to service providers and patients alike (see Box 3.1 for examples).

Perhaps one of the most widely cited benefits of networks is that of sharing information. In a health setting, this may mean greater sharing of patient information between services – in some cases, with much of the information being collated in a patient-held record. Shared databases between agencies, such as the police, the probationary service, the prison service and other law-enforcement

Some potential benefits from networks

- Sharing information
- Making the best use of resources and expertise
- Integrating services and removing unnecessary duplication
- Involving and responding to key stakeholder interests
- Creating 'win win' situations (i.e. everyone in the network gains in some way without losing)

agencies, allow an electronic database network to underpin greater co-operation and intelligence sharing both to solve and prevent crime. Information sharing can be used to underpin protocols for working between agencies. Clinical or care pathways, for example, may be underpinned by much more open sharing of patient data between agencies.

Interagency networking of this nature can also remove the service gaps that previously existed. Where health and social care services, for example, have insufficient information sharing and understanding of one another's ways of working, they cannot work effectively together. A patient discharged from hospital may, therefore, experience delays in community follow-up, rehabilitation or primary care support.

Costs of networked organisations

As with any organisational arrangement, there are costs associated with creating and managing networks. These costs can be both direct and indirect. The direct costs are obvious and include the time required to work out interagency protocols and agree joint targets or objectives, resources to fund team co-ordinators, training courses to facilitate team or multi-disciplinary working relationships. The indirect costs are potentially less obvious. Opportunity costs are typically those that are most frequently recognised and cited. Where partnership or network arrangements take time to develop, practitioners become increasingly concerned with the opportunity costs involved, i.e. whilst spending time in meetings to agree interagency objectives and ways of working, caseloads are neglected or colleagues pressurised to cover for those involved in network meetings. Monitoring costs also have the potential to become burdensome. For every network that is established, particularly where it has attracted additional funding, there is the need to account for the resources used in support of the network. The use of these resources will be justified where the network is found to have met its targets. These targets might be expressed in terms of improving waiting times, health outcomes, patient satisfaction, community involvement and/or treatment of particular conditions (e.g. the cancer networks). Time and effort are therefore required to monitor interagency targets, ensure they are achieved and take remedial action where they are not.

There can be several other types of cost associated with networks, particularly those costs incurred where network relationships break down. During the period of the NHS market, a number of network relationships formed alongside contractual (fundholding) relationships between GPs and acute hospitals (see for example

Fischbacher 1998, 2001). In these cases, GPs and acute trusts would share the cost of a new MRI scanner or other piece of equipment. If, however, the relationship between the GP practice and the acute trust broke down, the GP practice and its patients no longer reaped any benefits from their financial investment.

A more common cost, or loss of investment, arises from people-related 'investments'. As practitioners work together (e.g. a CPN and a voluntary sector project worker), they develop a shared language and understanding, and individuals, their patients and the employing agencies can benefit from this working relationship. However, if that interagency relationship changes (another voluntary organisation becomes involved or the geographical boundaries for the health worker are changed) then this investment is lost and cannot be recovered.

The final cost worth noting here is more of an organisational or personal cost. Any attempt to set up a network of agencies involves time, effort and goodwill. It may also involve considerable degrees of change in working practice at the individual and organisational level. Change within the public sector is in some respects the only constant! However, where change programmes fail, they can create apathy or reluctance to engage in further change. Failed network relationships can create similar apathy or resistance to future change or networks.

This selective account of the types of costs that may be incurred whilst not depicting the whole range of costs, illustrates how important it is for practitioners and agencies to be fully aware of the consequences of engaging in network arrangements. They may yield significant benefits, but where they fail to do so, the costs can be considerable.

Managing and sustaining networks

Networks can involve a large number of service organisations and other stakeholders. As a result, there can easily be ambiguity about the expected role each network member will play, and about the ways in which members are willing to work together in the longer term.

The reality is that establishing and successfully managing a network is complex, time consuming and more than likely to suffer from what has been called 'collaborative inertia' (Huxham 2003), i.e. the problem of failing to achieve all that the network promised, and all that its members so enthusiastically worked towards, despite high-level strategic commitment to the network.

Having already established that networks can yield significant benefits and costs, one final aspect to emphasise is the long-term nature of network relationships and network development. It is inevitable that when several agencies come together they bring their own agendas, they have shared agendas, and they must recognise not only their own and collective interests, but also the interests of a range of further stakeholders who affect, or are affected by, the services the network delivers. Problems of 'collaborative intertia' arise despite commitment to the network, so efforts need to be continually made to overcome inertia and keep the network on track. These efforts need to include:

- a clear assessment of each organisations goals, capabilities and short- and long-term contribution(s) to the network
- identification of some quick wins for the network (as a means of encouragement that effective joint working can be established)
- shared understanding of one another's working practices
- a common language, particularly where organisational cultures vary considerably
- establishing and developing trust between network members
- agreement about how resources will be used.

These and other such considerations can be explored more fully in Huxham and Vangen (2005).

It is likely that many network benefits will be realised over the long term, and that there will be many early hurdles to overcome before the network sees the full result of network-development efforts. It is important, therefore, that network members remain clear about the objectives of the network, set realistic performance targets and take stock of what has been achieved.

Conclusion

Health practitioners' challenge

Health practitioners and others reading this textbook may encounter networks in a number of different ways. Some may be network facilitators; some may be involved in working with a range of organisations at the service level, while others may have some responsibility for setting up new service networks. It is likely that in practice, the willingness to network will be present among many with whom you are to be working. However, it is also likely that many of the issues raised in this chapter will be particularly challenging and difficult to disentangle.

We have tackled a number of aspects here that relate to the structure and strategy of organisations. These will be of significance to readers who have a role in designing and setting up networks. Also considered here are the issues associated with developing and sustaining networks, such as building trust between organisations and developing a common language. At the level of the individual practitioner, working in a network context calls for particular skills, some of which overlap with those commonly associated with teamworking.

The need for information sharing, negotiations and adaptations between organisations heightens the demand for network players to deploy not only communication skills and interpersonal skills, but also more developed skills of negotiation and managing across organisational boundaries. These involve an ability to understand and engage in political game playing where it takes place, and also to influence the behaviour of those over whom one has no direct line authority. For example, if a health services practitioner is seeking financial or staff resources from practitioners of other agencies, this cannot be done by direct compulsion, incentive or reward. Rather, it must be achieved through skilled negotiation, lateral thinking and an ability to envisage and shape future relationships and long-term benefits to all parties. This may be particularly difficult where there are power differences between network members. In an MCN, for example, negotiations will take place between clinicians, nurses, therapists, managers, counsellors and other disciplines where there will be significant differences in individuals' direct power base. Understanding the range of stakeholders involved (directly and indirectly), the nature of their interest, the nature and extent of their power (exhibited, for example, through control of resources or ability to influence) become crucial skills and abilities for all within a network setting and must clearly be the subject of staff training within organisations as networks ways of working become more common.

A fuller discussion of the skills and training aspects of working practice in networks is beyond the scope of this chapter. However, as a means of bringing together some of the practice-level implications of working in networks, some key questions are presented below that network members should consider individually and discuss collectively at the outset, and during the development of the network. Also presented are some considerations for network members to address again at an individual and collective level, as network relationships form between individuals within multiple organisations.

DISCUSSION QUESTIONS

- What is the purpose of the network (short term, long term, to create a new organisation/centre)?
- What kind of network is it intended to be (e.g. policy or strategy formation, knowledge exchange, research commissioning, project management, service restructuring/integration)?
- What is the intended nature of the network relationships or connections (formalised or informal interorganisational links; tightly managed or relaxed, largely social exchange)?
- How is the network perceived (or likely to be perceived) by other key stakeholders in the sector/locality?
- How will the success of the network be measured (e.g. stimulating and funding research projects, spawning further networks, integrating services, overseeing consultation, reaching agreed strategy amongst member organisations)?

Points to consider

It is relatively easy to get broad agreement on the purpose of the network and difficult to get **agreement on details** and operational considerations. Members will need to make conscious decisions about when to 'move on' in order to achieve something (hoping agreement will follow).

Those who identify the need for the network need to consider carefully **who best to involve**. Too many players will slow down the development. Network members need to be able to make commitments on behalf of their organisations, and need to be able to attend the meetings (rather than send representatives), particularly at the early stages of network formation. Careful consideration also needs to be given to the **power balance between the players** (organisational power and individual power). Such power may come in many forms: political 'weight'; access to financial resources; control over staff and/or data; access to related networks/key players; ability to delivery what the network hopes to achieve.

Chairmanship of the network is fundamental to success. Who is selected says something about the direction, nature and profile of the network.

Focused, detailed discussion about **network aims** should take place otherwise members will assume they know what others are expecting in terms of contribution, outcome, process and success.

There needs to be open acknowledgement and agreement about the different **types of contribution** to, and return from the network that members may experience and the timeframe during which they may be expected to make a contribution.

Explicit reference needs to be made to the **nature of relationships** between members. Are they to be formalised through clear and accountable systems/procedures? Are there to be legal contracts or are relationships more 'open-ended'? If open and informal relations are desired, then the development of trust between network players (individual and institutional trust) will be crucial and will take time.

Members also need to be clear about how the make-up, direction and achievements of the network will be **viewed by key stakeholders** (policy makers, practitioners, etc.) and what this might mean for the future of the network and any projects/organisations is spawns/oversees.

References

Department of Health (DH) 1989 Working for patients. Government White Paper, HMSO, London

Department of Health (DH) 1997 The new NHS: modern, dependable. The Stationery Office, London

Department of Health (DH) 2002 Care Trusts background briefing. Department of Health website: http://www.dh.gov.uk/

Fischbacher M, Francis A 1998 Purchaser provider relationships and innovation: a case study of GP purchasing in Glasgow. Financial Accountability & Management 14(4): 281–298.

Fischbacher M, 2001 Improving secondary care efficiency: motives & mechanisms in Scotland. Public Money & Management January–March: 15–19

Greater Glasgow NHS 2005 Scheme of establishment. Scottish Executive CHP website: http://www.show.scot.nhs.uk/sehd/chp/

HM Government 2004 Every child matters: change for children. The Stationery Office, London

Hopton J, Heaney D 1999. Towards primary care groups: the development of local healthcare cooperatives in Scotland. British Medical Journal 318: 1185–1187

Huxham C 2003 Theorizing collaboration practice. Public Management Review 5(3): 401–423

Huxham C, Vangen S 2005 Managing to collaborate: the theory and practice of collaborative advantage Routledge, London

Joint Future Group 2000 Community care: a joint future. Scottish Executive, Edinburgh

Laing A, Fischbacher M, Hogg G, Smith AM 2002 Managing and marketing health services. Thompson Learning Europe, London

LHCC Best Practice Group 2000 Connecting communities to the NHS. Scottish Executive, Edinburgh

Lewis J 1991 The public's health: philosophy and practice in Britain in the twentieth century. In: Fee E, Acheson RA (eds) History of education in public health. Oxford University Press, New York

Mackenzie M, Shute J, Berzins K, Judge K 2004 The independent evaluation of 'Starting Well' final report. Scottish Executive website: http://www.scotland.gov.uk/

McClelland S 2003 Health and health services in Wales: a Plaid Cymru – The Party of Wales discussion paper. Plaid Cymru

Regen E, Smith J, Goodwin N, McLeod H, Shapiro J 2001 Passing on the baton: final report of a national evaluation of primary care groups and trusts. Health Services Management Centre, Birmingham

Scottish Executive 1997 Designed to care. Scottish Executive, Edinburgh

Scottish Executive Health Department 2003a Partnership for care. Scottish Executive, Edinburgh

Scottish Executive Health Department 2003b Improving health in Scotland: the challenge Scottish Executive, Edinburgh

Scottish Executive Health Department 2004a CHP statutory guidance. Scottish Executive, Edinburgh, p. 20

Scottish Executive 2004b Closing the opportunity gap. Scottish Executive website: http://www.scotland.gov.uk/

Scottish Executive 2004c The Local Government in Scotland Act 2003 Community Planning: Statutory Guidance. Scottish Executive, Edinburgh

Scottish Executive 2004d The Local Government in Scotland Act 2003: Power to Advance Well–Being Guidance. Scottish Executive, Edinburgh

Scottish Office 1997 Designed to care Scottish Office, Edinburgh.

Scottish Office 1999 Towards a healthier Scotland – a White Paper for health. Scottish Office, Edinburgh

Simeons S, Scott A 2005 Integrated primary care organizations: to what extent is integration occurring and why? Health Services Management Research 18: 25–40

University of East Anglia and National Children's Bureau 2004. Children's Trust: developing integrated services for children in England. Department for Education and Skills, London

Wallis L 2006 Starting Well phase two report. Greater Glasgow and Clyde NHS Board, Glasgow

Williams P 2002 The competent boundary spanner. Public Administration 80(1): 103–124

Parenting and family support:
a public health issue

Christine Bidmead and Karen Whittaker

Key issues

- Why are parenting and family support 'public health' issues?
- How is that support to be provided and who should provide it?
- Is government policy sufficiently robust in making this a key role of professionals working in public health?
- Are there effective evidence-based interventions to provide universal parenting and family support services?
- What are the implications for practice for health visitors, school nurses and midwives and other professionals working for public health?

Introduction

Public health can be defined as, 'the science and art of preventing disease, prolonging life and promoting health through organised efforts of society' (Acheson 1998). Health visitors have a long history of working with families (Malone 2000) and have always seen their work as having a public health focus, although this has not always been acknowledged. The government-sponsored health visitor development pack defines the public health role of the health visitor as working through a continuum with individuals, families, groups and communities (Department of Health (DH) 2001). Families are the basic building blocks of our society or, in Bronfenbrenner's (2005, p. 260) words, 'the heart of our social system' into which children are born and parented. Supporting families is crucial to enabling parents to nurture their children into mature, emotionally secure adults capable of initiating and sustaining their own relationships and meeting their own personal potential. This will undoubtedly have a positive impact on communities and society as a whole. However, parents' efforts need to be complemented by action at a community level so that families feel supported by an environment where they can ask for help when they meet with difficulties.

In this chapter we will consider in more detail family support and its necessity for family health. We will explore the psychosocial health needs of parents and of children and consider some of the difficulties that services face in meeting these needs. It is clear that the UK government agenda is seeking to address these needs and so we will think about the latest policies put in place to support parents and children. This will lead us finally to look at how policy can and is being implemented in practice with a range of interventions.

Family and parenting support

What constitutes family and parenting support?

The term family support, when used within UK culture, can immediately rouse ideas about responding to problems and it is a common misconception to assume that inadequacy must exist if support is required. Within health and welfare services, The Children Act (1989) particularly lent credence to this view with its emphasis on the implementation of family support becoming synonymous with identified need. This legislation required local authorities to respond to a child as deemed in need and make available 'family support' to compensate for that need. Arguably this paved the way for the undesirable identity of family support that resulted from associations with neediness and inadequacy. This history, however, distorts perceptions and blinds us to the full extent of family support and thereby an understanding of it not just as a response system, but also as a fundamental component of a healthy society that actually needs to exist to maintain human development.

In order to appreciate what constitutes family support it is perhaps first helpful to consider what we understand of the modern family and hence parenting roles. Bronfenbrenner developed a bioecological understanding of human development, where environment plays a part in person development. He explains in a recent edited collection (Bronfenbrenner 2005) that there now exist new family forms that operate in an era where the family retains moral and legal responsibilities for children, but often lacks the opportunity to do the job properly. This, Bronfenbrenner argues, is due to the changed conditions of life, where children and parents spend little time together and instead each is in the company of peers. Indeed, current political drives to encourage increased paid employment (HM Treasury & Department for Work and Pensions 2003) is being supported by strategies that will extend the school day with the provision of breakfast and after school clubs (HM Treasury 2004b), where parents and children will continue to spend more and more time in their separate worlds. The existence of economic migration, secular adult partnerships, young motherhood and longer life span are some of the influences affecting the contemporary family that exists in various sizes, gender, ethnic and age combinations. With change comes an altered parental role where, for example, the loss of one parent may force the other to become breadwinner and carer, or, indeed, the loss of both parents may bring grandparents back into primary caregiver roles for children. Such situations exist with or without different types of family support and as Sheppard and Gröhn (2004) found, some have become so much a part of day-to-day existence that they are in danger of not being properly recognised as support. Moreover, the giver and receiver of support may have very different views about what and when it is needed and what purpose it is primarily serving.

Family support can be easily misunderstood, especially when it is so well integrated into daily patterns and, sadly, may only be recognised when it disappears. Clarity is needed to avoid what Quinton (2004) describes as never-ending circles of discussion on the topic and help with this comes from Ghate and Hazel's (2002) study of parents' experiences when living in economically harsh circumstances. They identified a three-fold model of social support comprised of:

- informal support arising from pre-existing personal social networks
- semi-formal support arising from community organised activities
- formal support made available by statutory services, sometimes in partnership with the voluntary sector (Ghate & Hazel 2002).

This model fits with Bronfenbrenner's notion of human ecology (Lerner 2005), which identifies the existence of social structures, sitting within one another as if nested like Russian dolls. Each nested structure is influenced by and, indeed, influences the other. When applied to Ghate and Hazel's model, the informal support is nested around the immediate environment of the person. Semi-formal supports are an extension of informal support, but have more order to them. Within the model, semi-formal support influences the personal social network used by the person as opposed to the person directly. Likewise, formal support structures organised by statutory and officially sanctioned agencies operate as part of public policy and culture shaping the environment within which community-organised activities (semi-formal structures) take place. Thus, each affects the other and trickles down to influence the individual at the centre of the nest.

This conceptualisation usefully encourages questioning about our understanding of the relationships between the levels of support and, indeed, the consequences when deficiencies exist. For example, if the semi-formal support is absent, can the person at the centre of the informal support reach support at the formal level; is semi-formal support, in fact, a mediator or a gateway to formal services? This is a question pertinent to the debate about social capital and whether, indeed, social capital as a commodity can be generated by formal support systems.

In recent years there have been major initiatives introduced by government to address family needs and in particular support child development and child health (Department of Health 2004, Department for Education & Skills 2004a). This includes the Treasury's increased investment in the delivery of Sure Start programmes and Children's Centres. Those bidding to secure funding for these initiatives need to demonstrate how new programmes will not only work alongside statutory services, but also in partnership with the local community to develop supportive networks for vulnerable children and families. Changes of this kind have influenced a tide of interest in parenting and with greater financial resources there has been growth in support facilities at various levels. An illustration of the diversity of arrangements is provided in the flow chart shown in Figure 4.1. Like Ghate and Hazel (2002), we identify existence of formal and informal support systems, but particularly draw attention to their coexistence through shared settings, which include intimate home environments, public community venues and virtual spaces accommodated by information technology and media facilities. Working alongside statutory service provision provided by professionals from health, education and local authority services, some are organised as part of Children's Trusts (Department for Education & Skills 2003), Sure Start programmes (Department for Education & Employment 1999), Children's Centres (Department for Education & Skills 2004b), and other independent bodies, operating with perhaps a national charity (e.g. Barnardos, Homestart & NSPCC) or with a local perspective (e.g. Ferries & Port Sunlight Family Groups in the Northwest of England, Enfield Parents Centre in North London, Parent Network in Caerphilly, the Parents Advice Centre in Belfast and the Aberlour Child Care Trust, which has a number of strands to its work, but is funded through local authorities to provide family centres in Scotland).

The purpose of the flow chart is to highlight the multi-faceted nature of parenting education and support, and the inextricable links between formal and informal care structures. The parent who meets others through attending a formal group at the health centre may on other occasions meet these same people opportunistically. In addition, he or she might use self-directed parenting resources for advice by regularly reading the popular press, watching the latest parenting television programme or by 'logging-on' to parent advice websites for information. Parenting as a source of media entertainment has grown out of all proportion in recent years (Brooks 2005, Crawford 2005, Woods 2005). The point is that each person accessing formal interventions delivered by professionals will also be exposed to less formal ideas, advice and explanations about parenting whether through personal social networks or the

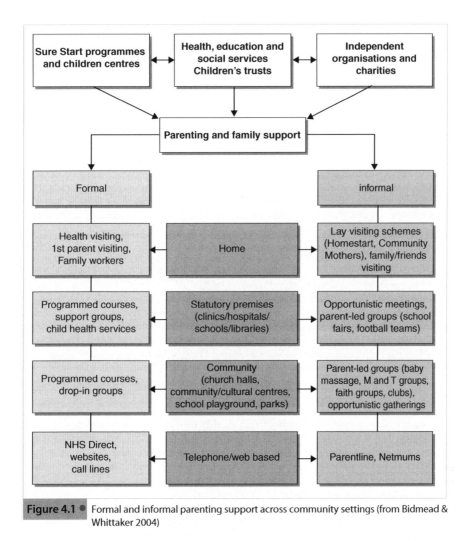

Figure 4.1 ● Formal and informal parenting support across community settings (from Bidmead & Whittaker 2004)

popular media. Suggestions offered about individual experiences could be perceived as criticism or praise and hence could either undermine or encourage a willingness to commit to formalised programmes of education and/or support. This means that to understand any local parenting and family support service there needs to be an appreciation of the wider community context because the unpredictable features of a community could be important determinants in the success of formalised strategies.

Why family and parenting support are a necessity for family health

Bronfenbrenner, in article 18 of his edited collection, reintroduces his 1988 paper on 'Strengthening family systems'. Through the theme of caring, he uses the analogy of the heart and the body to describe the importance of the family to a society to assert the need for nurturing the family in order to keep society healthy. This perspective recognises that the development of a child will be influenced not just by the immediate family, but also by the community within which the family is located.

Community factors to some extent determine the manner and organisation of routines within the family. These factors include educational and employment opportunities that will shape the economic status of the family, which in turn impact on the availability of material resources important for maintaining health. Equally, beliefs held within the family will influence what goes on within the community. For example, parents' perceptions about personal safety in the local community may influence their decisions about those routine activities that have a bearing on how and whether children socialise with other community members. Activities can include walking to school, playing outside or joining clubs. Thus, the two are closely connected. For Buchanan (2000), Bronfenbrenner's ecological perspective offers a helpful way of understanding how the impact of family disadvantage on child health can be minimised through the artificial introduction of protective factors in the community setting. Examples include the availability of school milk and fruit for physical health or home-visiting play workers for child psychological health when mothers are postnatally depressed. Both support the parenting role and offer some level of compensation for either impoverished childhood diets or social interactions with adult caregivers.

Compensatory factors such as these are presumed to be important for the generation of resilience and reducing vulnerability when exposed to challenges later in life (Werner 1995). Parenting, because of its ability to influence new directions and experiences in a child's life, then becomes one of the most significant means of affecting both resilience and vulnerability. The ability to parent and do so sufficiently is an ability to positively influence the health of children and thereby the next generation of adults. When understood in this way, parenting can be recognised as an important public health activity.

Stewart-Brown (2000) also builds on Bronfenbrenner's work and helps explain the connection between parenting and health through the development of the wellbeing model, setting the emotional wellbeing of children and adolescents centre stage. The model presents a flow of relationships between parents and their children who grow into young adults facing new social situations in communities and workplaces. In Stewart-Brown's view, healthy parenting involves showing respect, empathy and genuineness to growing children, who are then capable of learning how to appropriately relate to others and face challenges in adult life.

This model sits comfortably beside a growing body of the life-course research demonstrating relationships between adult health, early family experiences (Bifulco et al 2002, Russek & Schwartz 1997, Sweeting & West 1995), and childhood socio-economic disadvantage (Davey Smith et al 1998, Galobardes et al 2004, Kuh et al 2002, Kuh et al 2004, Richards et al 2001). Indeed, Davey Smith and Lynch (2004) explain that many of the risk factors for cardiovascular disease (a significant problem for health care systems worldwide) are 'socially patterned' and are evident across the entire life course. This means that the risks accrue from pre-conception, antenatally and then through infancy and childhood, dependent upon the parental circumstances. Negative socio-economic circumstances faced by parents and hence their children, contribute to mechanisms of risk for vascular disease through the reinforcement of behavioural or biological pathways (Davey Smith & Lynch 2004). Childhood states listed as contributing to risks for such pathways include: the experience of sustained stress, poor diet, obesity and poor growth. Equally, childhood social experiences have a part to play in determining future outcomes impacting on:

- child growth (Montgomery et al 1997)
- educational attainment (Hertzman & Wiens 1996, Sweeting & West 1995)
- adult physical health (Kuh & Ben-Schlomo 2004, Lundberg 1993)
- mental wellbeing (Bifulco et al 2002, Wadsworth 1996)

- propensity to crime and violence (Farrington & Welsh 1999, Stattin & Romelsjo 1995, West & Farrington 1973)
- future parenting practices (Polansky et al 1981).

Similarly, when placed with evidence illustrating the connection between social relationships and physical health (Brunner 1997, Chandola et al 2004, House et al 1988, Power et al 1996, Russek & Schwartz 1997, Whiteman et al 2000), the importance of emotional wellbeing to individuals, families and communities becomes increasingly apparent. So much so that emotional health (alongside mental health) is now identified as an integral part of the being healthy outcome within the Every Child Matters: Change for Children programme (Department for Education & Skills 2004a).

The unpleasant consequences of early socio-economic disadvantage have been important drivers behind the development of the current Every Child Matters: Change for Children programme. There are good reasons for this, as research studies continue to reveal the damaging effects of poverty on children (Attree 2004) and parents (Attree 2005, Ceballo & McLoyd 2002). Being poor matters to children as it places an extra strain on family life. Nurturant parenting is compromised and the benefits that would normally be derived from strong social ties in a community are reduced (Ceballo & McLoyd 2002). Being parented and then becoming a parent in poor circumstances introduces a cumulative effect that limits the availability of material resources otherwise accessible through social networks and, therefore, the capacity for social ties to compensate for economic disadvantage (Attree 2005). Despite this, social relationships and the informal supports derived from these do have a crucial part to play in the wellbeing of children and parents (Attree 2004, 2005, Cochran et al 1990). Cochran et al (1990) explored the nature, purpose and value of social networks for parents and children in some detail within an international programme of research across four, Western, industrialised nations. Here they highlighted processes of social exchange, comparison, socialisation, care giving, modelling and stress buffering that provides children and their parents with rich learning opportunities. Outcomes derived from such processes included the chance to develop skills in respectful communication with others and be exposed to what Bandura (1995) would identify as the positive sources of self-efficacy. These include vicarious experiences, verbal persuasion and a chance to practice and master new behaviours. However, it is argued that because informal systems of support can be so fragile (Llewellyn & McConnell 2002), formal social support needs to be carefully balanced and take account of existing strengths within families and communities (Kirk 2003).

A decade ago, Oakley et al (1994) argued that social support was in fact, health promoting and particularly important to those who are more at risk from adverse life-events through living in stressful circumstances with little income, poor housing, and a lack of supportive relationships. It is in these circumstances that the 'stress buffering' effects that Cochran et al (1990) mention can come into force, by moderating the impact of difficult material circumstances. This is achieved by a strengthened capacity to manage challenges as a result of improved knowledge and information about external resources and a greater sense of self-esteem and confidence fuelling a personal inner resource to act. These internal and external resources are regarded as resources for health (Cowley & Billings 1999) and if harnessed through social support should, indeed, be helpful mechanisms that enable parents to promote the health of their children.

More recently, Oakley has with colleagues tested these ideas to determine the effectiveness of social support when offered to women living in areas of deprivation. This research involved a three armed randomised controlled trial located in two London boroughs (Austerberry et al 2004, Turner et al 2005). The trial compared a support health visitor (SHV) service, community group support (CGS) and standard services, with the last acting as the control. The social support provided by the

SHV involved monthly supportive listening visits whereas the standard service involved only one routine home visit during the early postnatal period and thereafter women could only access health visitors through child health clinics. The CGS arm of trial offered women contact with one of eight locally based community groups that were predominantly staffed by volunteers. The most successful arm of the trial was the SHV intervention, which provided women with a sense that they were being listened to and an opportunity to discuss personal issues. These women also reported less anxiety about their parenting, had fewer concerns about their child's development and, interestingly, altered their style of health service use. The change was in a manner that the authors felt was more favourable (Austerberry et al 2004) and in keeping with seeking advice concerned with maintaining health as opposed to managing illness. The main challenge for the CGS arm was the engagement of women in the activities offered by the community groups. One in five women claimed that their non-use of services was because they were too busy or had a full social life. For the small proportion (19%, 35) that did use the CGS some positive views were expressed about the value of getting out and meeting other parents, but equally attention was drawn to the subtle features of the group sessions (e.g. sense of disorganisation or missed opportunities to welcome newcomers), that can act as turn-offs and feed reasons for non-attendance in the future (Turner et al 2005). A clear message from this study is that the provision of social support services does not guarantee that needs will be met, especially if service use requires special efforts on the part of the parent. Involvement in community groups essentially involves making some level of investment, such as time, personal organisation to get there and not least an ability and willingness to engage socially with others. Social support offered by health visitor home visits asks less of the parents before they have witnessed the investment made by the health visitor. This is perhaps, therefore, a more conducive means of encouraging more marginalised parents to make better use of social support services that can evolve as important sources of emotional and practical help. Llewellyn and McConnell (2002) discuss the significance of parenting social support with special reference to parents with learning disabilities, illustrating how these parents are especially vulnerable if supportive relationships fail.

Children living in families with insufficient social support will feel the effects through the social and, thereby, educational opportunities available to them (Cochran et al 1990), which shape how they are socially programmed (Wadsworth 1999). Social programming results from the experiences that infants and children are exposed to through family life. This includes the family circumstances (economic prosperity, educational opportunity) and family function (cohesion, accord and positive regard, parental self-esteem), which collectively impact on child educational attainment and opportunity to develop self-control and skills in managing one's own behaviour. Wadsworth (1999) explains that these features of early social life generate vulnerability or resilience to subsequent life stressors. This is likened to Barker's (1998) model of biological programming for fetuses *in utero*, infants and children when exposed to biological hazards, such as parental smoking, poor nutrition or early infection. These hazards interfere with subsequent maturation of cells and organs, and create vulnerability in adults if later exposed to biological stressors, such as a high-fat, -sugar and -salt diet, smoking or infectious disease.

The significance of parenting as a social programming activity can be realised in the evidence that is emerging from the previously acknowledged life course research and, in particular, that which illustrates the relationship between the quality of nurturing and nourishment provided during childhood years and the development of coping and competence skills in adult life (Bartley et al 1999). A recent addition to this body of work is the life course framework published by the Health Development Agency (Graham & Power 2004). This identifies pathways towards poor adult health originating from conception and right through childhood. What is evident is the powerful force parental disadvantage has on childhood and the expectations young people have of themselves as they enter adulthood.

Graham and Power (2004) indicate how children with limited social and educational opportunities have greater reason for investing in identities that do not require school achievements and, instead, sources of self-affirmation are found through identity with peers and family. In essence they become socially programmed to follow certain life patterns. These identities, Graham and Power (2004) explain, typically involve sexual relationships that result in early cohabitation and parenthood for females and other activities that offer instant excitement and interest that can involve young males in law breaking and criminal activities. If experienced, these factors become life limiting, impacting on a young person's ability to manage new challenges in the education system and, later, the labour market. This may influence personal economic destinies and resilience or vulnerability to physical, mental and social stressors (Montgomery et al 1996). The secondary outcome from this unhappy chain of events is the self-perpetuating nature of such life patterns that tend to be repeated through generations if parental disadvantage is not addressed (Bartley et al 1999, Graham & Power 2004). Once more, future generations of parents are reliant on the scenarios played earlier on in their lives, since the task of parenting is learnt from the parenting previously received. Wilkinson (1999) identifies this cyclical situation as a disastrous recipe for health which, when combined with weakened social bonds, raises stress experiences and chronic anxiety. These states then act as precursors to other health-limiting behaviours, such as smoking and alcohol consumption, that increase the risk of coronary heart disease (Kuh & Ben-Schlomo 2004). The task then is to help children and young people become resilient to such life risks, by improving early social experiences.

From this basis, we argue that parenting support is an essential ingredient in improving public health overall. But before we turn to how public policy can assist with this we will look at where it all starts, in infancy, and consider the legacy that a lack of parenting and family support creates for future generations.

Family and parenting support: impact on life trajectory from infancy

Both our physiological and psychological systems are developed in relationships with other people and this is never more true than in infancy (Gerhardt 2004). The intensity of interaction between a baby and its carers has enormous consequences for:

- infant brain development
- child mental health, physical wellbeing and development
- adult mental and physical health.

Infant brain development

Gerhardt (2004) describes the newborn baby as a seedling that develops strong roots and good growth if the environmental conditions are right. Babies are like seedlings because their physiological and psychological systems are unformed and very delicate. They are subject to stress responses that may be particularly prevalent where early experiences are problematic. These stress responses impact on brain development (Shore 2001). It is during the first months of life that the brain is at its most plastic and flexible, so that the baby can develop and fit into the world that he/she finds. This means that babies adapt to their environment in order to fit into their family, culture and community. The 100 billion brain cells with which a baby is born are not interconnected and most cannot function in isolation. They need to be organised into networks that require trillions of synapses between

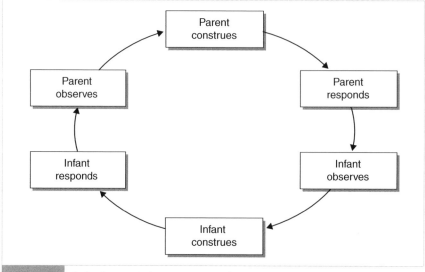

Figure 4.2 ● Cycle of parent–infant interaction (adapted from Davis et al 2002)

them. Although the development of these connections depends, to some extent, on genes, they also depend on early life events, particularly the early care and nurturing received from birth. Empathic care giving from an emotionally available caregiver, which is warm, affectionate, sensitive and attentive, providing patterned visual and auditory stimulation, particularly language, are critical if the baby is to achieve optimal brain development (Bee 2000). A serious lack of sensitive interaction in the early months will have long-lasting effects not only on infants' cognitive abilities, but on their ability to form lasting relationships. This sensitive interaction is as essential for growth as a diet that is rich in essential nutrients. The rapid growth that takes place in the first 3 years of life are a crucial time where social interaction and environmental predictability maximise development. It is during this time that children grow in their abilities to think and speak, learn and reason, setting patterns that will last a lifetime and lay the foundation for their values and social behaviour as adults. The quality and content of the baby's relationship with his/her parents or carers has an effect on the neurobiological structure of the child's brain that will be enduring. Once the brain is developed it is much harder to modify (Balbernie 2004).

Figure 4.2 illustrates the cycle of interaction between the baby and his/her parents or caregivers. Both parent and baby watch each other and then try to make sense of what they see and hear or experience and respond accordingly. This is a mutual process, with both the parent's and the baby's behaviour or response determined by the understanding that they are able to make of the other's actions. The experiences that the infant gains within this relationship then colours his/her anticipation of future relationships with others.

However, the difficult thing about this interaction is that the baby needs this care all the time. The baby needs a caregiver who is emotionally available, responsive and able to identify the baby's needs. Problems that interfere with the interaction and the ability to respond appropriately may trigger a spiral in a downward trend. For example, when a mother is depressed and unable to respond sensitively to her infant, the baby comes to accept that his/her needs will not be met and will also act in a depressed way (Field et al 1988). The baby's problems also seem to persist into later childhood (Murray 1992, Cooper & Murray 1998).

Gerhardt (2004) suggests that support for parents is crucial if they are to be 'good enough' caregivers. The tension that exists between the need to work and to be at home caring for the baby often leads women to make choices to do one or the other when, according to the evidence, they want to do both (Newell 1992). At home they may be isolated from social contact, leading to depression. At work they may be in a continual state of anxiety and guilt about the care of the baby. Neither choice seems beneficial. Both may lead to depression in either or both parents with consequences for their child's emotional and physical wellbeing both in infancy and, as we shall see, in later childhood through into adulthood.

Child mental health, physical wellbeing and development

In 1999 the Office for National Statistics (ONS) carried out its first national survey of child mental health in the UK (Meltzer et al 2000). It found that almost one in ten 5- to 15-year-olds were facing handicapping emotional or behavioural problems (Meltzer et al 2000). The latest ONS survey (Green et al 2005) makes depressing reading, showing no change at all in the prevalence of mental ill health in children in this age group. Longitudinal evidence shows that many child psychiatric disorders persist well into adult life, increasing the risks for mental health problems and difficulties in social functioning. More working days are lost due to mental ill health than physical conditions (World Health Organization (WHO) 1998). For young people and their families, as well as for society as a whole, the cost of child mental health problems is high. Preventing, identifying and treating psychological disorders, therefore, not only reduces misery for suffers and their families, but improves the functioning of the working population.

The ONS survey (1999) showed that in children with mental health problems, not only was there an increased risk of psychiatric disorder in later life, but also associated physical ill health. In mentally healthy children, 6% were rated as showing fair to very bad health generally, whilst 20% of those with a mental health disorder displayed associated individual physical complaints. Children with mental health problems were more likely to suffer with:

- bed wetting
- speech and language problems
- co-ordination difficulties and soiling
- increased risk of accidents
- increased risk of life-threatening illness during life.

Over one-third of children with neurological problems, such as epilepsy, were found to have mental health problems.

In older children those with a mental health problem had a higher prevalence of:

- smoking
- cannabis use
- alcohol abuse
- problems with literacy.

Other risk factors were also contributory factors to the prevalence of child mental health disorders. They were found to be more prevalent in lone families, reconstituted families where there were five or more children, where parents had no educational qualifications and where both partners were unemployed (see Table 4.1).

Worryingly, in an 18-month follow-up of the ONS survey children, it was found that many disorders and, in particular, conduct and hyperkinetic disorders, were persisting through childhood (Meltzer et al 2000). However, when a disorder-based approach is taken, as in the ONS study, the existence of problems that do not constitute a disorder may well be disguised. It was for this reason that a different approach was taken in Southwark, in London, where a random survey of 253 children 0–16 years in three GP practices was conducted to elicit problems and risk factors for mental health difficulties in one of the most deprived areas of

Table 4.1 ● Prevalence of child mental health disorders (after Meltzer et al 2000)

One parent	16%	Two parents	8%
Reconstituted families	15%	No stepchildren	9%
More than five children	18%	Two children	8%
No parental qualification	15%	Degree	6%
Both unemployed	20%	Both working	8%

the UK (Davis et al 2000). Semi-structured interviews were undertaken at home by psychologists trained in the methods to elicit problems and risk factors that were judged against predetermined criteria for severity. For children younger than 14 years, the interview was conducted with the main carer, who was mainly the mother. A list of 47 possible problems were identified, e.g. generalised anxiety, phobias, truancy, depressed mood, inattention, overactivity, eating problems, poor temper control, stealing.

At the same time, 28 risk factors were also identified, e.g. chronic child health problems, parental physical health problems, parental mental health problems, social isolation, trouble with police, marital problems. These risk factors interfere with personal social networks and, therefore, informal levels of support. Perhaps more importantly, they are factors that can jeopardise the attachment process and hence the parent–child interactions that provide the developing child with the opportunity to learn important social skills.

A similar study of 473 children aged 0–17 years recruited from seven GP practices in Lewisham, another London borough, found that between 20% and 37% of children had three or more significant problems (Attride-Stirling et al 2000). Approximately 48% had a least one psychosocial problem and 50% had three or more risk factors for child mental health problems. This indicated that every other child had a quite serious problem and one in five children had a group of severe problems. As many as one in two families were struggling with difficulties related to the development of psychosocial problems in their children. Whilst limited to one London borough, the Lewisham example is useful because it provides an insight into the most common problems. For 5- to 10-year-olds these included:

- tantrums in 16%
- generalised anxiety in 12%
- disruptive attention seeking in 11%
- inattention in 12%.

Similarly, the same survey highlighted risk factors, which included for parents or carers of 0- to 17-year-olds:

- adverse life events (trauma, family breakdown, abuse, accidents, etc.) 25%
- parent who had childhood learning difficulties 19%
- parents who had childhood emotional difficulties 23%
- parental postnatal depression 14%
- parents with mental health problems 23%
- parental physical health problems 17%.

All of the above may impact on the parent–child interaction cycle with consequences for child emotional and physical wellbeing. However, where risk factors are cumulative, the impact on health is all the more likely with consequences for adult mental and physical health.

Adult mental and physical health problems later in life

In the previous discussion of unhelpful parenting effects in childhood, it is self-evident that many of the consequences felt in childhood have the potential to also manifest as adult experiences. In particular, early impaired psychological functioning accumulates, triggering patterns of social dysfunction, an inability to cope with stress and a predisposition towards enduring mental illness as well as impaired physical functioning.

Russek and Schwartz (1997) showed, in a study obtained from undergraduates at Harvard University, that perceptions of parental caring predict the health status in mid-life. In the early 1950s, initial ratings of parental caring were obtained from a sample of healthy Harvard undergraduate men. During the 35-year follow-up investigation, detailed medical and psychological histories and medical records were obtained. The results showed that in mid-life those suffering from illnesses, such as coronary artery disease, hypertension, duodenal ulcers and alcoholism, had perceived their parents to have a significantly lower rate of parental caring items (i.e. loving, just, fair, hardworking, clever, strong) while they were in college. 'This effect was independent of the subject's age, family history of illness, smoking behaviour, the death and/or divorce of parents, and the marital history of subjects' (Russek & Schwartz 1997, p. 144). Furthermore, 87% of subjects who rated both their mothers and fathers as low in parental caring had diagnosed diseases in mid-life, whereas only 25% of subjects who rated both their mother and fathers high in parental caring had diagnosed diseases in mid-life. They concluded that:

> 'Since parents are usually the most meaningful source of social support for much of early life, the perception of parental caring, and parental loving itself, may have important regulatory and predictive effects on biological and psychological health and illness'.
>
> (Russek & Schwartz, 1997, p. 144)

Findings such as these suggest that parenting activities have implications for the costs to health, not just physically but also economically, as ill-health is costly to society in terms of time and resources.

Family and parenting support for a stronger economy

The economic importance of parenting can be understood at a number of levels. Within the plans laid out in the government's Child Poverty Review (HM Treasury 2004a), there is an explicit concern to move parents, and especially those separated from partners, into positions of employment where they can generate income for themselves and their children. This goal serves the political aspirations of delivering income directly into the households of materially deprived children, and reducing the number of children living in workless households. This later point could be of value for normalising the experience of working for an income especially in families where the decline of local industry has created a cycle of unemployment across generations. By working and generating income, parents will be contributing to the primary wealth-creating sector (Mustard 1996).

In situations where parents reject government efforts to get them into work and instead adopt homemaker roles that include child care, they become classified by the United Nations Economic Commission for Europe (UN/ECE) as economically inactive, but can at least be counted as providers of non-paid services (Hantrais 2004). Despite this classification it is argued that parents working effectively to improve family functioning do continue to contribute to a nation's economy even if indirectly, by supporting working partners or by nurturing children to grow into well-adjusted, socially competent adults. In these circumstances, parents will be contributing to what Mustard (1996) refers to as the secondary wealth-creating sector that affects the quality of the social environment within which the primary sector operates. The central importance of this role for the rest of society is often only appreciated when things go wrong and ineffectively parented children fail to develop the personal self-control necessary for avoiding a tendency towards anti-social behaviour and accident-prone risk-taking behaviour (Pulkkinen & Hamalainen 1995). Indeed, there is a need to recognise the potential bearing that positive parenting practices have on some of the externalities, namely anti-social costs and lost days from the workforce, that Wanless (2004) highlights as affecting health service provision.

The financial costs to health services from treating behaviourally disordered children are highlighted in research published by Guevara et al (2003). The evidence here indicated how children with behaviour disorders, like those with chronic physical conditions, made greater use of office-based consultations and accident and emergency services and even more use than children with physical disorders of prescribed medication. In a UK study, Scott et al (2001) also confirm these health service costs through their follow-up of children with anti-social behaviour, where the existence of conduct disorder was the greatest predictor of future costs. This research is referred to within the earlier *Every child matters*, government Green Paper (Department for Education & Skills 2003) and the pathway of consequences from not dealing with childhood oppositional and defiant disorders is clearly illustrated (Figure 4.3).

The financial burden to the National Health Service created by the treatment of behaviour disorders is a good reasoning to use preventive strategies. These need to include the offer of home visiting and parenting support groups in the ante- and postnatal periods, provided by health visitors working alongside midwives and other family community workers employed within Sure Start, children's centres, Children's Trusts and Primary Care Trusts. An American example of a home visiting scheme for adolescent mothers who were judged as high risk for child abuse and neglect, illustrated how child and maternal health outcomes could be improved and that the programme was a cheaper course of action than provision of county foster care (Sterling Honig 2001). It was thus a cost-effective means of boosting family mental health and preventing child abuse in high-risk families. A similar study in the UK has yet to be fully reported, but an initial report of the qualitative findings indicates positive outcomes on the practice of health visitors in enhancing parent–infant interaction (Brocklehurst et al 2004). Cunningham (1996) argues that the cost-effectiveness of parenting programmes

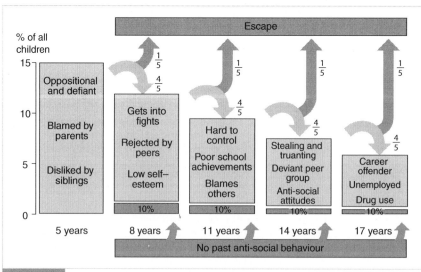

Figure 4.3 ● Continuity of anti-social behaviour 5–17 years from research conducted by Stephen Scott (reader in child health and behaviour and consultant child and adolescent psychiatrist) for the Home Office 2002

should be considered not just in terms of the money required to organise, administer and deliver parenting services, but also in terms of potential reductions in costs to public services created by anti-social behaviour. Certainly, in view of Guevara et al's (2003) findings, programme costs need to be compared to those incurred from ongoing A&E attendance, when behaviour disorders are not actively managed.

Positive parenting support should be taken seriously as a means of reducing financial burdens. Wanless (2004) explains costs as internal and external. Internal costs affect individuals and with parenting support they are experienced as psychosocial benefits with improved parental and child self-esteem and confidence (Barlow et al 2002, Olds et al 1997). These benefits have long-term consequences for child learning and later adult employment (Montgomery et al 1996) and for parents it may mean improved quality of life and better use of locally available resources. External costs by contrast affect society, because of the relationship between individual actions and social relations with others. The costs of financially investing in parenting support services are felt as benefits, as young people are better prepared for making a useful contribution to society. The external costs are therefore necessary for supporting growth of a healthy society (Stewart-Brown 2000), allowing civic activity and discouraging delinquency (Gatti et al 2003).

Alternatively, the external costs of not acting and failing to invest in parenting support will be felt by dealing with the ill-health and the 'havoc' that escalates from anti-social actions. Hughes et al (2000), in their report for Barnardo's, amply illustrate these through the cases of seven young people, who through early impoverished childhoods have become disconnected from society in adult life. They introduce Dean, who at 13 was frequently left unsupervised with his nine younger siblings. With limited social support from family and friends, and a partner who was often absent, Dean's mother felt overwhelmed. As Dean's behaviour became unmanageable he was excluded from school. Intervention through a Barnardo's family centre at the age of 13 offered some hope, but his tendency to bully and his anger meant that he was unable to function properly in a group. He had not developed the pre-requisite social skills many of us take for granted. He soon became involved in local crime activities and, at the time of the report had gone missing from police bail. At the age of 14 Dean was missing and, at that time, the failure to invest in his early childhood had cost £33 266. Yet an investment of £12 782 to cover the costs of additional support during his pre-school years and a further investment of £6000 during his primary school years would have saved £14 484. The early investment would have supported:

- additional home visiting from a health visitor
- the provision of parental support and education for his mother and any significant others
- support with drop-in attendance at a family centre
- educational support from age 9 at school.

Hughes et al (2000) also emphasise that by not acting earlier, Dean's rights under the UN Convention on the Rights of the Child 1989 had been infringed. It is fair to say that Dean's parents had let him down, but equally the State had done little better, letting both him and his mother down. What is also worrying is that children like Dean are more likely to repeat this cycle as they too take on parental responsibilities that are overwhelming and poorly resourced.

More heartening though is Joanne's story, also published in Hughes et al's report. Joanne, as a young mother of a 2-year-old, explained that she only felt able to attend a local mother and toddler group when a neighbour offered accompany her. This opportunity exposed her to the benefits of the group for her child and herself as she made increasing contact with the Barnardo's group facilitators. In a similar way, that Cochran et al (1990) explain, the social network accessed through the group broadened for her networking opportunities and sources of information about other community resources helpful to supporting child development. She became an active member of a reading with children project and started taking on secretarial responsibilities for the playgroup and women's group, culminating in her taking the lead on a drug awareness project and accepting a Whitbread Volunteer Action Award in June 2000. The investment that allowed Joanne to access community resources was estimated by Barnardo's as costing £2847, which is considerably cheaper than the costs they report for picking up the pieces evident in the other life histories told in the same report.

The examples above impress upon us the need to offer social support in the early years of children's lives, whilst being mindful of child *and parent* support needs. Failure to invest early will result in increasing health service expenditure and extra demands on other public services, such as schools and policing. CIVITAS, the Institute for the Study of Civil Society, would argue that existing fiscal policies are inadequately organised to support functional family life and instead promote lone parenthood (CIVITAS 2005b). In fact, the ONS (2004) survey shows that in 2001 23% of dependent children were living in lone parent households a rise of 5% since 1991. CIVITAS also believes that Britain's crime reduction policies are some of the most ineffective in Europe and suggest that an alternative strategy, offering social investment in the family, to encourage law-abiding lifestyles, would help to prevent young people from following anti-social pathways (CIVITAS 2005a). Other reports suggest that one in five children in the UK still lives in poverty and life chances remain very unequal for children from different backgrounds, and in many cases the gaps are not closing (Bamfield & Brooks 2006). However, the government remains optimistic and claims that child poverty, for instance, has already reduced in the last decade (HM Treasury and DfES 2005) and that the Every Child Matters programme of services represents considerable social investment in the family (HM Treasury 2004a). In monetary terms this is certainly true, but we cannot afford to assume that solutions will evolve because there is seemingly more financial investment. Community public health practitioners need to be proactive in ensuring that present government policy is translated into initiatives that support parents in their task of raising children. In order to do this effectively, practitioners need to be aware of the present policy initiatives that make family and parenting support imperative.

Policy initiatives that make family and parenting support imperative

In its preamble, the UN Convention on the Rights of the Child (UNICEF 1990) asserts that:

'The family, as the fundamental group in society and the natural environment for the growth and well-being of all its members, particularly children, should be afforded the necessary protection and assistance so that it can fully assume its responsibilities within the community.'

Article 18.2 goes on:

'For the purpose of guaranteeing and promoting the rights set forth in the present Convention, States Parties shall render appropriate assistance to parents and legal guardians in the performance of their child-rearing responsibilities and shall ensure the development of institutions, facilities and services for the care of children.'

'Wellbeing' as applied here is surely health in its widest sense. The idea that raising children is a joint venture between the State and parents recognises that all citizens bear a responsibility for children. The State, therefore, has a duty to provide assistance to parents, acknowledging the need for social support to enhance the opportunities for all children (Pugh et al 1994). Family support is necessary for family health and is, therefore, a public health issue and one which the government has a duty to encourage.

The death of Victoria Climbie in 2000 was a powerful force impelling the UK government to make its duty towards children a priority. This has led to a raft of policies and papers in response to the recognition that health, the police, social care and, in fact, all services had failed to prevent the abuse of Victoria that eventually led to her death. The centrality of the child has gained momentum since then and is set to underpin public health practice in this area. The UK government has taken a fresh look at how children can best be supported within society. We have seen the introduction of a new Children Act (2004) explained through the policy document 'Every Child Matters: next steps' and supported by the National Service Framework for Children, Young People and Maternity Services (DH 2004), all of which will have far-reaching consequences on parenting and family support provision. Table 4.2 summarises the abstracts and chronology of English government publications that have evolved into the programme that is now known collectively as 'Change for Children'.

The present government's vision for children as outlined in 'Every Child Matters: the next steps' (DfES 2004) sees parenting support embedded at each life stage. This is through universal services providing information advice and support, and through targeted and specialist services for parents of children who need them, and compulsory action through parenting orders as a last resort where parents condone anti-social behaviour or truancy (p. 6). The document is very clear on trying to shift away from associating parenting support with crisis intervention to a more consistent offer of parenting support throughout a child and young person's life. The vision is to provide a mixture of 'universal and targeted parenting approaches that include advice and information giving, home visiting and parenting classes' (p. 26). It states that support needs to be available at a variety of locations and focus on key transition stages in a child's, young person's or parent's life, and as such reflects a response to the knowledge base concerning childhood trajectories (Graham & Power 2004). Varieties of support include the involvement of schools in the commissioning of parenting programmes for children whose behaviour is causing problems or who are not attending (see http://www.teachernet.com). Parenting support is linked to the need for advice on employment and childcare, through Sure Start Children's Centres, and extended schools to enable parents to make the transition into work. This was the underpinning message of the Treasury review on child poverty (HM Treasury 2004a). The target is to halve child poverty by 2010 and eradicate it by 2020. Whilst this represents a refreshing outlook on the health of communities, a note of caution is to be had regarding the push towards encouraging parents to spend less time with their developing child, therefore lessening their ability to influence the child's direction.

The Children Act (2004) outlines, among other things, the arrangements under which Children's Trusts are to be set up. The primary purpose of these is to secure commissioning leading to more integrated service delivery and better outcomes for children and young people. Under the Act, services have a duty to co-operate to change the behaviour of those who work with children and families so that they experience not only more integrated services, but also universal services that are more responsive to need providing specialist support. It is envisaged that services will be co-located in extended schools or children's centres. Most areas should have a Children's Trust by 2006 and all areas by 2008.

The 'Every Child Matters: Changes for Children' document seeks to describe the outcomes sought, the shared approaches that need to be taken and the delivery mechanisms involved. Essentially it is about improving the five outcomes for children in partnership and making the changes involved in practice and organisation

Table 4.2 • Chronology of events and policy documents pertaining to parenting and family support

Publication/event	Date	Abstract	Available at
Death of Victoria Climbie	February 25th 2000	Health, Police, Social Care, etc., failed to realise and prevent the abuse that led to the death of Victoria Climbie.	
Public enquiry into events at Bristol Royal Infirmary	January 2002	The public enquiry into children's heart surgery at the Bristol Royal Infirmary from 1984 to 1995, led by Professor Sir Ian Kennedy. His report was published in January 2002. The DH's response included a commitment to improve children's health services, ensuring that children, like adults, are entitled to high-quality, safe services designed to meet their particular needs.	http://www.bristol-inquiry.org.uk/
Laming enquiry into death of Victoria Climbie	January 2003	Following Victoria's death a public enquiry was set up after the murder conviction of her carers, Marie-Therese Kouao and Carl Manning. This report sets out recommendations to address the root causes of the failure to prevent Victoria's death.	http://www.victoria-climbie-inquiry.org.uk/index.htm
National Service Framework (NSF) Hospital care standard for children	April 2003	The Standard for Hospital Services was the first module, published in advance of the full NSF, in response to the concerns raised in the Kennedy Report. It champions a central recommendation of the Report, and a principle of the NHS Plan, in advocating that services should be designed and delivered around the needs of users of services. This will be achieved through interagency partnerships and by empowering children and their families through full involvement in choices about their care.	http://www.dh.gov.uk/PublicationsAnd Statistics/Publications/Publications PolicyAndGuidance/Publications PolicyAndGuidanceArticle/fs/ en?CONTENT_ID=4006182&chk=oiSEI1

		The hospital standard, and later the full NSF, aims to ensure that there are seamless care pathways through services delivered for children and young people. As well as care delivered around their needs, the standard states that children and their families should be able to expect hospital services that provide effective and safe care in a child-friendly environment. This means clinical governance systems focusing on the particular needs of children and young people, that staff caring for them should have the appropriate training and skills to provide high-quality care, and that hospital environments should be safe, healthy and friendly places for children and young people.	
Emerging Findings document of Children's NSF	May 2003	The Emerging Findings consultation document was intended to make clear the direction the work on developing standards would take, with External Working Groups and with the engagement of key stakeholders. The document was also intended to identify key points for early consideration by service providers and commissioners. Overall the responses supported the proposals but stressed that significant challenges lie ahead. The terms of what it meant to have a comprehensive CAMHS service were defined. Summary outcome available at website.	http://www.dh.gov.uk/Consultations/ResponsesToConsultations/ResponsesToConsultationsDocumentSummary/fs/en?CONTENT_ID=4068486&chk=C5mHWB
Every Child Matters – consultation paper	8th September 2003	This paper set out the government's commitment to improving outcomes for all children and young people, including the most disadvantaged	http://www.everychildmatters.gov.uk
Every Child Matters: Next Steps	March 2004	Published on the same day as the Children Act was introduced to Parliament, this document set out the purpose of the Children Act and the next steps for bringing about change of children's services	http://www.everychildmatters.gov.uk

Table 4.2 ● (Continued)

Publication/event	Date	Abstract	Available at
NHS Improvement Plan	June 2004	Sets out the next stage of the government's plans for the modernisation of the health service. It signalled three big shifts: putting patients and service users first through more personalised care; a focus on the whole of health and wellbeing, not only illness; and further devolution of decision-making to local organisations. It required greater joint working and partnership between primary care trusts (PCTs), local authorities (LAS), NHS Foundation Trusts, NHS Trusts, independent sector and voluntary organisations.	http://www.dh.gov.uk/PolicyAnd Guidance/OrganisationPolicy/ Modernisation/fs/en
Treasury Child Poverty Review	12th July 2004	This examined the welfare reform and public service changes necessary to advance towards the long-term goal of halving child poverty by 2010 and eradicating it by 2020. The review set out the key measures to reduce child poverty in the medium to long term, in particular through improving poor children's life chances, where public services can make a huge contribution, as well as continued efforts to help people who can work into work, providing financial support to families and tackling material deprivation.	http://www.hm-treasury.gov./spending_ review/spend_sr04_childpoverty.cfm
Parental separation: Children's Needs and Parents' Responsibilities – consultation paper	21st July 2004	A Green Paper setting out proposals to help those undergoing parental separation to resolve disputes so that children's needs are better met. Recognises that the primary responsibility for caring for children rests with parents rather than with the State and focuses strongly on what children need and how parents can be assisted better to meet those needs during and after relationship breakdown.	http://www.dfes.gov.uk/childrensneeds/
The Chief Nursing Officer's review of the nursing,	3rd August 2004	This review was recommended in the Green Paper, Every Child Matters. It considered the needs of children with a wide	

midwifery and health visiting contribution to vulnerable children and young people		range of needs, recognising the vital role universal services have in early identification and prevention. It addressed all nurses, midwives and health visitors working in all settings and considered how they can be deployed to complement other services and to maximise benefits for children and young people. The findings and recommendations set the strategic direction for the professions. The review provided advice for service commissioners, managers and other agencies on how to develop and support an appropriately skilled nursing, midwifery and health visiting workforce to promote the wellbeing of children and young people.	http://www.dh.go.uk.PublicationsAnd Statistics/Publications/Publications PolicyAndGuidance/Publications PolicyAndGuidanceAricle/fs/ en?CONTENT_ID=4086949&chk=4JYgAb
NSF for children, young people and maternity services	15th September 2004	This set out national standards for the first time for children's health and social care, which promote high quality, women-and-child centred services and personalised care that meets the needs of parents, children and their families. It is a 10-year programme intended to stimulate long-term and sustained improvement in children's health. There is now a website, which gives examples of good practice for all the standards of the NSF.	http://www.dh.go.uk/PolicyAnd Guidance/HealthAndSocialCareTopics/ ChildrenServices/ChildrenServicesIn formation/ChildrenServicesInformation Article/fs/en?CONTENT_ID=4089111 &chk=U8Ecin http://www.info.dh.gov.uk/children/ nsfcasestudies.nsf
Children Act 2004	November 2004	Encourages integrated planning, commissioning and delivery of services: improved multi-disciplinary working, removing duplication, increasing accountability and improving the coordination of individual and joint inspections in local authorities. Made provision for a Children's Commissioner for England to act as an independent voice for children and young people, to champion their interests, concerns and views nationally. Children Trust arrangements set up through the Act, bringing together all services for children and young people in an area. A lead-professional model will be adopted where many disciplines are involved, and services will be co-located in extended schools or children's centres.	http://www.hmso.gov.uk/acts/ acts2004/20040031.htm

Table 4.2 (Continued)

Publication/event	Date	Abstract	Available at
		Trusts to be supported by integrated processes, like the common assessment framework. There will also be joint commissioning of services which entails: Shared decisions on priorities; identification of all available resources; joint plans to deploy them underpinned by pooled resources. Will ensure that those best able to provide the right packages of services can do so.	
Choosing Health – Making health choices easier.	16th November 2004	White Paper that set out how government will assist people in taking responsibility for their health by improving information and providing support in making healthy choices – including how we safeguard the health of children and young people.	http://www.dh.gov.uk/Publications AndStatistics/Publications/ PublicationsPolicyAndGuidance/ PublicationsPolicyAndGuidanceArticle/ fs/en?CONTENT_ID=4094508& chk=aNSCor
NSF for Children, Young People and Maternity Services – Supporting Local Delivery	December 2004	This performed two functions: 1. It sets out what the Every Child Matters: Change for Children programme means for health organisation in the same way as do other tailored documents for social services, criminal justice and schools and places the implementation of the NSF in the context of that wider programme. 2. It details the support the government will offer for implementation of the NSF to health organisations and their partners.	www.everychildmatters.gov.uk
Every Child Matters: Change for Children	December 2004	The Outcomes Framework provides a useful summary of Change for Children. It lays out the 26 public service agreement targets and 13 other key indicators for the implementation of Every Child Matters. See also,	http://www.everychildmatters.gov. uk/_files/8FDC0C06EA8CD5A77CCDA888 EED28FDF.pdf

	Common Assessment Framework Working together guidance Lead professional guidance Child Information Index.	
Sure Start Children's Centre Practice Guidance	December 2005	Lays down the good practice expected from Children's Centres especially in the areas of: Reaching the most disadvantaged families and children Increasing consistency in the level of support services offered Grounding children's centre practice in evidence Improving multi-agency working Raising the quality of early years provision Employing more highly trained and qualified staff.	http://www.surestart.gov.uk/ publications/?Document=1500
Support for parents: the best start for children	December 2005	A pre-budget report from the Treasury prior to the comprehensive spending review 2007. Encompasses: Economic and financial security for families as the foundation to improve children's lives Support for parents in managing the demands of parenthood and work/life balance Building stronger communities and regenerating deprived neighbourhoods Improving and reforming public services so they deliver for all children, young people and families in ways appropriate to their needs.	http://www.hm-treasury.gov.uk
Respect Action Plan	January 2006	The Respect Action Plan has six main strands: Supporting families, expanding parenting provision and establishing the National Parenting Academy for front-line staff A new approach to the most challenging families Improving behaviour and attendance in schools Activities for children and young people Strengthening communities Effective enforcement and community justice	http://www.respect.gov.uk

needed to make it happen. The five shared outcomes are: 1) being healthy, 2) staying safe, 3) enjoying and achieving, 4) making a positive contribution, and 5) achieving economic wellbeing. The shared approach is above all about putting the child at the centre of services and there is a major shift to prevention and early intervention. This means:

- dealing with complex problems (and people) in a joined-up way
- listening to children, young people and their families
- integrating services
- locating services in relation to need and convenience
- multi-agency working
- sharing skills
- sharing processes and language
- sharing and managing information
- joint commissioning and sharing resources
- performance management and inspection.

All these will be delivered through:

- Children's Trusts
- Extended schools
- Common Assessment Framework
- Child 'index'
- Local Safeguarding Children's Boards
- Healthy Schools Programme
- Child Health Promotion Programme
- Common Core Skills and Competencies
- Independent Inspectors.

The Chief Nursing Officer's review for the National Service Framework and Choosing Health focused on the being healthy and staying safe outcomes, but will impact and contribute to the outcomes that embody the 'Change for Children Approach', depending upon and informing shared projects.

Although parenting support is integral to achieving the five outcomes for children, it is yet to be seen whether interpretation of the policy at a local level, which clearly puts the child at the centre, will result in better support for parents and families. Community public health practitioners, including health visitors and school nurses may find themselves well placed to ensure that this happens.

Incorporating policy into practice: evidence of what works in parenting and family support

The challenge of the emotional wellbeing model comes with its translation into practice, when the modern world exposes parents and children to many competing social cues that may contradict efforts to behave in a manner that is both empathetic and respectful. Current government targets articulated through the Every Child Matters programme are perhaps naïve in the presumption that parents will know and understand how to act in a way with their child/children in order to support sound emotional development, and that wider communities are sufficiently equipped (emotionally healthy) to support such parenting actions. However, adults also need to understand themselves and the consequences of their own actions better before they can helpfully respond to those of their children, provoking further responses in the adult. The previously mentioned parent–child interaction cycle (Davis et al 2002) explains how a pattern of monitoring, construing and responding is repeated by parent and child as they observe and make sense of each other's actions and behaviours. Negative patterns of interaction that provoke distress in the other are to some extent in the hands of the parents, depending on their knowledge and understanding of the behaviours they observe not only in their child, but also in themselves. When taken in conjunction with what is now known about infant brain development, the centrality of parent–child interactions cannot be underestimated as the consequences are clearly more far reaching than might ordinarily be appreciated.

Service organisation

The manpower required to manage all these problems in society is vast and cannot be reasonably managed by specialists alone. It is clear anyway that highly specialist assessment and treatment may not be relevant in all cases. In practice, mental health promotion has to involve all people working in child and family services. If effective services are to be provided then education, social services and health need to take a broader view of their roles and to seriously consider the implications for their work of actively promoting the psychological wellbeing of everyone in their care.

Figure 4.1 (p. 71) illustrated the forms of support available in communities, but differing levels of support and, indeed, treatment will be necessary for differing complexity of needs. Studies have found that the likelihood of parents expressing a need for help increased with the number and severity of the problems experienced (Attride-Stirling et al 2001, Davis et al 2000). Quinton (2004) also reports that as many as 46% of families living in poor environments never use formal services.

Clearly then there has to be a non-stigmatising, accessible service for supporting parenting and families and identifying need offered at a universal level. Figure 4.4, based on the NHS Health Advisory Service (NHS Advisory Service 1995) recommended model for service delivery, identifies the role of tiers 1 and 1a, emphasising the close working relationship between the formal and informal systems of care. Workers at this level are confronted with parents and children with psychosocial issues on a daily basis and provide the first line of support. All those working at this level need to be trained to the National Occupational Standards (PESF 2005), to be able identify those who need help, offer advice and support and have sufficient knowledge of specialist services to be able to refer appropriately when necessary (DH 2003). Essentially they are providing a preventative and promotional service.

Tier 2 is the mental health professionals based in specific locations throughout the community. They may be nurses, health visitors, social workers, teachers or psychology graduates; however, they all have a mental health training and or experience of child mental health. Clearly they need to be working in close relationship with tiers 1 and 1a providing support, training, liaison and consultation. Tiers 1, 1a and 2 may collaborate to provide targeted parenting support either delivered in groups or through home visiting. Working at this level may be regarded as secondary prevention; tackling problems once they have arisen.

Tier 3 is the child mental health specialists working in generic multidisciplinary teams that serve several localities. These teams provide assessment and treatment services for the full range of problems and mental health disorders in conjunction with other agencies as appropriate. They will provide a mixture of short- and long-term interventions dependent on complexity of need. Here again tiers 2 and 3 need to be working together to provide one-to-one help for more complex problems within families.

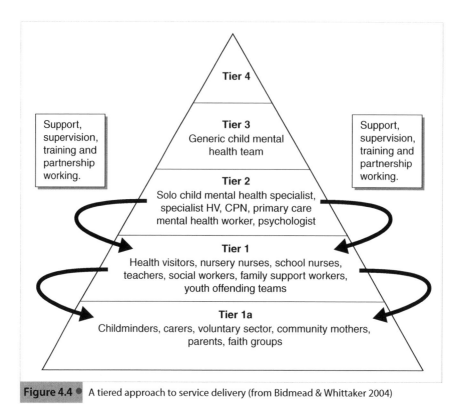

Figure 4.4 ● A tiered approach to service delivery (from Bidmead & Whittaker 2004)

Tier 4 comprises the highly specialist mental health teams serving several multi-disciplinary generic teams. Their services are commissioned at a regional or multi-district level and include in-patient services. Working together in partnership, these tiers of service can provide a comprehensive range of interventions appropriate to the complexity of need experienced by families within communities.

Specialist Community Public Health Nurses can be the leaders of teams that provide services at the preventative and promotional end of the needs spectrum. However, where they offer treatment for conduct disorder/behaviour problems, then the access to the group is typically by referral only. Most other parenting groups at tier 1 or 1a are open access, with self-referral being the most usual option (Bidmead & Whittaker 2004).

Service delivery

Nationally there is a huge variation in services that parents might be offered (Henricson et al 2001). Parents living in Sure Start areas may receive a very different service to others living in less needy areas. Sure Start services may be provided by a variety of professionals or volunteers according to local need, which, where there is best practice, has been defined in partnership with parents and children.

To meet this need for parenting support there has been a proliferation of various parenting programmes and interventions implemented by health visitors and school nurses and others. They have been at the forefront of developing parenting support and have been quick to recognise the need and to innovate, working in partnership with parents. Often this has been dependent on the enthusiasm of the few and has lacked strategic support, direction and co-ordination (Coren et al 2004). As various programmes have been developed, in the UK and elsewhere, resources have greatly multiplied to an array that may be confusing to parents and practitioners alike. To help to clarify the situation, consideration will now be given to some of the most popular and evidence-based interventions for parenting education and support programmes.

Home visiting

The universal provision of home visiting following the birth of a baby by a health visitor has been the envy of other countries, such as the USA, who have sought to replicate this provision (Olds et al 2002). Home visiting allows for an identification of need and then targeting of services as appropriate. However, research has also demonstrated that antenatal visiting is useful in helping to identify risk and resilience factors and establish the partnership relationship with the client so necessary for future service delivery (Puura et al 2002, Roberts et al 2002). Sadly this contribution of the parent–home-visitor relationship is rarely mentioned within the home-visiting literature when discussing effective outcomes. When carried out by trained health visitors, an antenatal visit that incorporates the parent's expectations of the infant and of themselves as mothers and fathers can be most effective in thinking about the transition to parenthood. It provides a forum to address psychosocial issues that may impinge on parenting ability, taking a problem-solving approach. It can build on the strengths and the resources that the parents-to-be have to enhance their parenting ability, and can be of considerable help to families and services alike in order to identify areas of need and concern (Puura et al 2005). A recent report from the Avon Longitudinal Study showed that women who were anxious at 32 weeks' gestation had a significantly increased risk of their children having behavioural problems at 4 years of age (O'Connor et al 2002). It was hypothesised that, in keeping with animal studies, maternal anxiety could affect fetal brain development. The study failed to take into account the effects of subsequent parenting practices on children's behaviour, but it is clear that this antenatal anxiety could be a contributory factor to childhood behaviour problems. Recent recommendations suggest that any preventative strategy needs to begin in the antenatal period (Bidmead & Whittaker 2004, Harker & Kendall 2003, North 2005).

The benefits of home visiting have been shown (Kendrick et al 2000) and incorporated into many Sure Start programmes so that those most in need can be identified, as it has been demonstrated that intensive home visiting to those in most need is most effective (Council on Child and Adolescent Health 1998). Research shows that effective home visiting needs to be carried out by nurses (Josten et al 2002, Olds et al 2002), and that more visits leads to better outcomes (Olds 2002). Nurses in the USA, where the studies were carried out, have additional training and carry out the functions that in the UK would be the responsibility of the community midwives and health visitors. The benefits of home visiting are shown in Table 4.3.

Transition to parenthood: Parents in Partnership Parent Infant Network (PIPPIN)

The focus of this programme, which begins in the antenatal period, is parent's relationships with each other and with the baby. It has a sound evidence base and has effective outcomes for mothers and fathers (Parr 1998). It is delivered by specially trained facilitators, who may be health visitors or midwives, and is a group-based intervention that aims to address the difficulties and joys of adapting to parenthood.

Traditional antenatal and postnatal classes/groups

These may be delivered by health visitors or midwives or together in a combined approach and are to be found in most areas of the UK. The quality of these classes remains patchy (Parr 1998). Pre- and postnatal support of this kind is also provided

Table 4.3 ● Outcomes of home visiting (after Bull et al 2004)

Evidence of effects of home visiting	Evidence unable to be determined	No evidence
Improved quality of home environment as measured by the Home Inventory Emotional and verbal responsivity of the mother Avoidance of restriction and punishment Organisation of the environment Provision of appropriate play materials Maternal involvement with the child Opportunities for variety in daily routine.	Prevention of abuse and neglect	Hospital admissions
Parent success in managing children's behaviour Sleep difficulties Feeding problems School behaviour problems in boys	Increased use of community resources	Uptake of immunisations and child health services
Improvements in child intellectual capacity (USA)	Impact on children's diet	Family size
Improvements in cognitive delay caused by prematurity, low birth weight, failure to thrive.	Take-up of welfare benefits	Maternal participation in the workforce
Reduced frequency of accidents in childhood	Client satisfaction	
Reduction of hazards in the home	Improvement in rates of breast feeding	
Changes in attitudes and beliefs, and improving parenting skills Management of postnatal depression (UK)		

by the National Childbirth Trust to parents who pay to attend. Many health visitors offer postnatal support groups to the new parents on their caseloads. These are not the same as parenting groups as they offer, for the most part, information about infant feeding, child development, childcare, toys, first aid and a variety of practical issues, and one of their aims is to reduce social isolation among women with babies. Groups that extend from the antenatal through to the postnatal period are thought to be most successful at achieving this particular outcome.

Brief encounters

Research has shown how distressing it is for children to experience the breakdown of their parents' relationship (Cockett & Tripp 1994). That parents too find this very distressing has been highlighted in research that looks at the impact on the ability of both parents to parent through the relationship difficulties (Walker 2005). Parental relationship difficulties are often implicated in a child's behavioural problem and there has been a considerable movement to encourage health visitors, midwives and community nurses to offer support for relationships when problems first start to occur (One Plus One 1998). That this contributes to the health of children and parents cannot now be disputed. The 'Brief Encounters' counselling offered by health visitors has proved highly effective and acceptable to new parents, and enabled one in five couples to be identified and given help, compared with one in twenty in the control clinics. The findings of the British Social Attitudes Survey (1992) reported by One plus One (1998) showed that only 2% of married people would turn to a marriage counsellor if they had a problem; they were much more likely to approach a family member or friend for support. they also turn to health care professionals with whom they have more contact at times of increased stress. This being so, One plus One, an organisation concerned to support relationships, who believe that 'Being a good partner is part of being a good parent' (One Plus One 2005) set up its 'Brief Encounters' training to help to enhance the skills and confidence of health visitors and other practitioners working in the community to detect the early signs of distress caused by relationship problems, so that they could respond constructively even when time was limited.

First parent home-visiting scheme

This scheme seeks to support first-time parents in the first year of their baby's life with an empowerment approach, which entails extra home visiting by specially trained health visitors (Barker & Anderson 1988).

Postnatal home visiting for postnatal depression

The provision of listening visits to mothers with postnatal depression has been shown to be an effective intervention for mothers and babies (Seeley et al 1996). Postnatal depression has been shown to have an adverse effect on the development of babies, particularly boys (Murray et al 1996), so it is particularly important that postnatal depression is identified as soon as possible and treated before damage occurs to the parent–child interaction cycle referred to earlier (see Figure 4.2.).

Volunteer and lay-visiting programmes

As noted by Whittaker and Cowley (2003) a number of these schemes have arisen, particularly in Sure Start areas. Examples of these include Community Mothers Schemes, Home Start and Newpin (Cox et al 1990, Oakley 1995). In a review of the effectiveness of volunteer schemes, Cox (1993) reported benefits of improved maternal confidence, self-esteem and coping skills. Similarly, Johnson et al (1993) identified maternal benefits in the form of reduced tiredness and depressive feelings and improved diet, following support from an Irish 'community mothering' scheme. These schemes all build on self-help ideals.

95

Educational/parenting programmes

These programmes have been fuelled by a desire in the UK to increase children's school readiness. However, parent–child interaction is enhanced by the parents being encouraged to help their children learn by enjoying early play together, sharing books and talking together from the earliest weeks. Examples of these education-based initiatives are Delta in Northern Ireland (Gillespie & McClean 2004), Parents as First Teachers in Berkshire (Farquhar 2002), PEEP in Oxfordshire (Evangelou & Syla 2003) and National Bookstart (Wade & Moore 2000). These programmes, which are gaining in popularity, have evidence of effectiveness with health visitors often taking the lead.

One-to-one approaches to children's behavioural problems by health visitors or school nurses

It is clear that not all parents want to attend groups for a number of different reasons (Austerberry et al 2004). However, there are a number of different approaches that health visitors and school nurses might use that do not involve the use of parent groups. Examples of these include the Solihull Approach (Douglas & Ginty 2001) and the Parent Adviser/Family Partnership Model (Davis & Spurr 1998, Davis et al 2002) (see Chapter 2), which are gaining in popularity. Group parenting programmes can often be used with good effect on a one-to-one basis in the home. According to Quinton (2004), health visitors have been seen as important sources of information and emotional support when children have behavioural problems.

Parenting groups

There are many parenting programmes offered in the community to help parents either relate more effectively to their children or manage their children's behaviour (Barlow & Stewart-Brown 2001). Examples include Family Caring Trust Programmes, which offers a range of courses from 0 to 6 years through the school years to parenting teenagers; Tameside and Glossop Positive Parenting, Family Links Programmes, which works with parents and with children in schools; NCH, handling children's behaviour, etc. Many of these programmes have been developed within the UK and are culturally acceptable to parents, who are very satisfied with the programmes. Typically, they report a better understanding of their children, less shouting, feeling calmer, more in control, enjoying their children more, less stress, realising the need to listen to their children, praising and encouraging them more, allowing their children to lead play, feeling less isolated, behaviour improvements in the children, using time-out, giving choices and using logical consequences, and less squabbling. They use a combination of video clips of parents in situations with children, discussion, role play and homework tasks where they try out various strategies at home with their own children. There are many unpublished evaluations of these programmes that show them to be acceptable to parents and practitioners alike. Very often parents will train to become parent leaders of the groups and work alongside the health professional, thus contributing to the building of social capital in the local area. There is some evidence to suggest that parent-training programmes also improve maternal psychosocial health in the short-term, although it is suggested that some caution should be exercised before the results are generalised to parents irrespective of the level of pathology present (Barlow et al 2002).

Infant massage groups

These have grown in popularity and recent empirical evidence suggests that there are benefits for parent–infant interaction and subsequent bonding process as well as child growth (Onazawa et al 2001, Zealey 2005) Many health visitors are trained to run these groups (see Resources section for details).

Referred parenting groups for conduct-disordered children (age 3–12)

Here a number of evidence-based approaches are suitable: The Incredible Years (Webster-Stratton & Hammond 1997), Triple P (Sanders 1999), Mellow Parenting for Vulnerable Families (Puckering et al 1994) (see Resources for information). These programmes emphasise the need for parents to ignore some behaviours that they do not like, praise what they do like, use encouragement, listen to their children, communicate clearly and effectively with children, use time-out, give choices and follow with logical consequences; they also highlight the importance of child-led play and spending quality time with the children. Mellow Parenting also works not only with the parent, but also with the parent and child. Parents in this programme also come to terms with their own experiences of being a child and possibly being at the receiving end of less than positive interaction with their own parents.

Parenting education in schools for young people

This may be provided by teachers or school nurses as part of the personal health and social skills curriculum. Some useful work in schools has been done by the Family Links programme (see Resources).

Support for fathers

Research shows that the involvement of fathers with their children is significantly related to positive outcomes for the child (Amato 1994, Flouri & Buchanan 2003) and that when the father is absent there are poorer outcomes (Amato 1993). It follows then that services need to engage fathers to support the parenting of their children. Research by Ghate et al (2000) showed that services were not very successful at engaging fathers for a variety of reasons. Examples included, female-dominated staff, no strategy for working with fathers, activities provided at family centres that were too female orientated, and that little was provided that catered to father's interests. The researchers concluded that fathers needed to be worked with as men, not just as child carers, a point also apparent in the findings of (Hendessi & Dodwell 2002) when reviewing 47 projects supporting younger parents. Services may be unused to thinking in this way and whilst some may have been successful in working with fathers in non-typical circumstances (e.g. lone fathers) they were less successful in engaging with other more 'ordinary' fathers. There are examples of good practice in work with fathers and training offered by Father's Direct (see Resources).

There are many other interventions and programmes that can be utilised to improve parenting support in the community. Moran et al (2004) provide a comprehensive review of the international literature and a searchable database of the effectiveness of these interventions.

Conclusions and implications for practice

In this chapter we have illustrated the centrality of family and parenting support for family health and wellbeing. Clearly, services need to plan to begin as early as possibly with preparation for relationships being taught within schools. Universal services need to be in place from the antenatal period onwards and at all the important transition stages of parenthood. These will include when parents are preparing to make the transition from being a couple to being mothers and fathers, support during the first year when babies are most vulnerable, when siblings are born, when toddlers begin nursery, when children begin school, when children pass from infants to junior school to secondary school, when children become adolescents and when adolescents become young adults. It is at these important transition stages that support needs to be available as necessary, which can be accessed easily with no stigma attached to asking for help appropriately. Not only will there be a saving in terms of human suffering and misery, but, as we have demonstrated in this chapter, investment in support services for parents will pay dividends in savings to the national health services, social services, education services and the criminal justice system.

Health visitors, specialist community public health nurses, school nurses, nursery nurses, midwives, early-years workers, children's centre staff, teachers, community mothers and others involved with families, all have a central role to play in providing this support. They are the people with whom parents come into contact on a daily basis and need to be able to provide a first line of support for parents, offering a listening ear and knowledge of local services that may be able to help the more complex problems. Effective universal parenting support programmes and intervention for more complex needs are available as we have demonstrated. There are implications for staff training and support, but it is an investment worth making.

The need to change the direction of service provision is now underpinned by a robust set of policies for putting the child and the family at the centre of service delivery. Areas of the country are now beginning to develop strategic plans for the implementation of children's centres, extended schools, children's trusts and local safeguarding children boards. Whether policy will be further translated into practice, so that with each of these new initiatives services are also implemented to support parents and families with sufficient numbers of well-trained and supported staff, remains to be seen.

DISCUSSION QUESTIONS

- How should health professionals resolve the difficulties of confidentiality of information within their extended role of partnership in care with other agencies and the voluntary sector?
- Can service providers break out of the narrow confines of their professionalism to work in true partnership with each other and with other agencies and community groups?
- How are the new extended roles of health visitors, school nurses, midwives and all who work with parents in the community to be fulfilled in the light of a resource shortfall?
- How can sufficient training for staff be funded so that parents are supported by well-trained, well-supported staff that have the requisite qualities and skills (see Chapter 2)?

References

Acheson D 1998 Independent inquiry into inequalities in health. The Stationery Office, London

Amato PR 1993 Children's adjustment to divorce: theories, hypotheses, and empirical support. Journal of Marriage and the Family 55: 23–38

Amato PR 1994 Father–child relations, mother–child relations, and offspring psychological well-being in early adulthood. Journal of Marriage and the Family 56:1031–1042

Attree P 2004 Growing up in disadvantage: a systematic review of the qualitative evidence. Child Care and Health Development 30(6): 679–689

Attree P 2005 Parenting support in the context of poverty: a meta–synthesis of the qualitative evidence. Health and Social Care in the Community 13(4): 330–337

Attride-Stirling J, Davis H, Day C et al 2000 An assessment of the psychosocial needs of children and families in Lewisham: final report. Lewisham Community Child and Family Service, London

Austerberry H, Wiggins M, Turner H et al 2004 Evaluating social support and health visiting. Community Practitioner 77(12): 460–464

Balbernie R 2004 An infant mental health service: the importance of the early years and evidence based practice. Online. Available: http://www.aimh.org.uk/the_importance_of_the_early_years.htm [18 June 2004]

Bamfield L, Brooks R 2006 Narrowing the gap: a manifesto to make Britain more equal. The Fabian Society, London

Bandura A 1995 Exercise of personal and collective efficacy in changing societies. In: Bandura A (eds) Self-efficacy in changing societies. Cambridge University Press, Cambridge, pp. 1–45

Barker D J P 1998 Mothers, babies and health in later life, 2nd edn. Churchill Livingstone, Edinburgh

Barker W, Anderson R 1988 The Child Development Programme: an evaluation of process and outcomes. University of Bristol, Child Development Unit, Bristol

Barlow J, Coren E, Stewart–Brown S 2002 Meta-analysis of the effectiveness of parenting programmes in improving maternal psychosocial health. British Journal of General Practice 52(476): 223–233

Barlow J, Stewart–Brown S 2001 Costs and effectiveness of community post-natal support workers. Researchers must now focus on effectiveness with specific groups of women. British Medical Journal 322(7281): 301

Bartley M J, Ferrie J, Montgomery S M 1999 Living in a high-unemployment economy: understanding the health consequences. In: Marmot M, Wilkinson R G (eds) Social determinants of health Oxford University Press, Oxford, pp. 81–104

Bee H 2000 The developing child. Allyn and Bacon, Needham Heights

Bidmead C, Whittaker K 2004 Positive parenting: a public health priority. CPHVA, London

Bifulco A, Moran P M, Ball C et al 2002 Childhood adversity, parental vulnerability and disorder: examining intergenerational transmission of risk. Journal of Child Psychology and Psychiatry (formerly Journal of Child Psychology and Psychiatry and Allied Disciplines) 43(8): 1075–1086

Brocklehurst N, Barlow J, Kirkpatrick S et al 2004 The contribution of health visitors to supporting vulnerable children and their families at home. Community Practitioner 77(5): 175–179

Bronfenbrenner U 2005 Making human beings human. Bioecological perspectives on human development. Sage, London

Brooks L 2005 Dr Spock on the naughty step. Online. Available: http://media.guardian.co.uk/site/story/0,14173,1418008,00.html [23 June 2005]

Brunner E 1997 Socioeconomic determinants of health: stress and the biology of inequality. British Medical Journal 314(7092): 1472

Buchanan A 2000 Present issues and concerns. In: Buchanan A, Hudson B (eds) Promoting children's emotional well-being. Oxford University Press, Oxford, pp. 1–27

Bull J, McCormick G, Swann C, Mulvihill C 2004 Ante-natal and post-natal home-visiting programmes, a review of reviews. Health Development Agency, London

Ceballo R, McLoyd V M 2002 Social support and parenting in poor, dangerous neighborhoods. Child Development 73(4): 1310–1321

Chandola T, Kuper H, Singh–Manoux A et al 2004 The effect of control at home on CHD events in the Whitehall II study: gender differences in psychosocial domestic pathways to social inequalities in CHD. Social Science & Medicine 58(8): 1501–1509

Children Act 1989 HMSO, London

Children Act 2004 HMSO, London

CIVITAS 2005a Fighting crime. Are public policies working? Online. Available: http://www.civitas.org.uk/pdf/crimeBriefingApr05.pdf [15 July 2005]

CIVITAS 2005b Tax credits favour lone parenthood. Online. Available: http://www.civitas.org.uk/pdf/taxCredits.pdf [14 July 2005]

Cochran M, Larner M, Riley D et al 1990 Extending families: the social networks of parents and their children. Cambridge University Press, Cambridge

Cockett M, Tripp J 1994 Children living in reordered families. Joseph Rowntree Foundation, York

Cooper P, Murray L 1998 Postnatal depression. British Medical Journal 316: 1884–1886

Coren E, Barlow J Individual and group-based parenting programmes for improving psychosocial outcomes for teenage parents and their children. (Cochrane Review). In: *The Cochrane Library*, Issue 2, 2004. John Wiley & Sons, Chichester, UK

Council on Child and Adolescent Health 1998 The role of home-visitation programs in improving health outcomes for children and families. Pediatrics 101(3): 486–489

Cowley S, Billings J R 1999 Resources revisited: salutogenesis from a lay perspective. Journal of Advanced Nursing 29 (4): 994–1004

Cox A 1993 Preventive aspects of child psychiatry. Archives of Disease in Childhood 68: 691–701

Cox A, Pound A, Mills M, Owen A L 1991 The evaluation of a home visiting and befriending scheme for young mothers: Newpin. Journal of the Royal Society of Medicine, Vol 84, (4) 217–220

Crawford A 2005 Parental guidance. Sunday Herald 6 March, 2005, p.13

Cunningham C E 1996 Improving availability, utilization, and cost efficacy of parent training programs for children with disruptive behavior disorders. In: Peters R D, McMahon R J (eds) Preventing childhood disorders, substance abuse, and delinquency. Sage, Thousand Oaks, CA pp. 144–160

Davey Smith G, Hart C, Blane D et al 1998 Adverse socioeconomic conditions in childhood and cause-specific adult mortality: prospective observational study. British Medical Journal 316(7145): 1631–1635

Davey Smith G, Lynch J 2004 Life course approaches to socioeconomic differentials in health. In: Kuh D, Ben–Schlomo Y (eds) A life course approach to chronic disease epidemiology, 2nd edn. Oxford University Press, Oxford, pp. 77–115

Davis H, Day C, Cox A et al 2000 Child and adolescent mental health needs assessment and service implications for an inner city area. Clinical Child Psychology and Psychiatry 5: 169–188

Davis H, Day C, Bidmead C 2002 Working in partnership with parents. Harcourt Assessment, London

Davis H, Spurr P 1998 Parent counselling: an evaluation of a community child mental health service. Journal of Child Psychology and Psychiatry 39: 365–376

Department for Education & Employment 1999 Making a difference for children and families: Sure Start. DfEE, London

Department for Education & Skills 2003 Every child matters. The Stationery Office, Norwich

Department for Education & Skills 2004a Every child matters: changes for children and young people. DfES Publications, Nottingham

Department for Education & Skills 2004b Every child matters: next steps. Department for Education and Skills, London

Department of Health (DH) 2001 The health visitor and school nurse development programme. Health Visitor Practice Development Resource Pack. DH, London

Department of Health (DH) 2003 Getting the right start: the National Service Framework for Children, Young People and Maternity Services – emerging findings. DH, London

Department of Health (DH) 2004 National Service Framework for Children, Young People and Maternity Services. DH, London

Douglas H, Ginty M 2001 The Solihull approach: changes in health visiting practice. Community Practitioner 74(6): 222–224

Evangelou M, Sylva K 2003 The effects of Peers Early Education Partnership (PEEP) on children's developmental progress. DfES, Nottingham

Farquhar S 2002 An evaluation of Parents as First Teachers Programme. Report 1. Online. Available: http://www.ecd.govt.nz/paft/EvaluationPAFT.pdf [14 July 2005]

Farrington D, Welsh B 1999 Delinquency prevention using family-based interventions. Children & Society 13(4): 287–303

Field T, Healy B, Goldstein S et al 1988 Infants of depressed mothers show "depressed" behaviour even with non–depressed adults. Child Development 59: 1569–1579

Flouri E, Buchanan A 2003 The role of father involvement and mother involvement in adolescents psycholgical well-being. British Journal of Social Work 33(3): 399–406

Galobardes B, Lynch J W, Davey Smith G 2004 Childhood socioeconomic circumstances and cause–specific mortality in adulthood: systematic review and interpretation. Epidemiologic Reviews 26(1): 7–21

Gatti U, Tremblay R E, Larocque D 2003 Civic community and juvenile delinquency. British Journal of Criminology 43(1): 22–40

Gerhardt S 2004 Why love matters: how affection shapes a baby's brain. Brunner-Routledge, Hove, UK

Ghate D, Hazel N 2002 Parenting in poor environments. Stress, support and coping, Jessica Kingsley Publishers, London

Ghate D, Shaw C, Hazel N 2000 Fathers and family centres: engaging fathers in preventative services. Joseph Rowntree Foundation, York

Gillespie N, McClean E 2004 An evaluation of the Delta Community Parenting Project. CENI, Northern Ireland

Graham H, Power C 2004 Childhood disadvantage and adult health: a life course framework. Online. Available: http://www.hda–online.org.uk/Documents/childhood_disadvantage.pdf [1 August 2004]

Green H, McGinnty A, Meltzer H, Ford T, Goodman R & Office of National Statistics 2005 Mental health of children and young people in Great Britain. Palgrave Macmillan, Basingstoke

Guevara J P, Mandell D S, Rostain A L et al 2003 National estimates of health services expenditures for children with behavioral disorders: an analysis of the medical expenditure panel survey. Pediatrics 112(6): e440–e446

Hantrais L 2004 Family policy matters. The Policy Press, Bristol

Harker L, Kendall L 2003 An equal start: improving support during pregnancy and the first 12 months. IPPR, London

Hendessi M, Dodwell C 2002 Supporting young parents: models of good practice. YWCA, Oxford

Henricson C, Katz I, Mesie J et al 2001 National mapping of family services in England and Wales: a consultation document. National Family and Parenting Institute, London

Hertzman C, Wiens M 1996 Child development and long-term outcomes: a population health perspective and summary of successful interventions. Social Science & Medicine 43(7): 1083–1095

HM Treasury 2004a Child poverty review. HMSO, London

HM Treasury 2004b Choice for parents, the best start for children: a ten year strategy for childcare. HMSO, London

HM Treasury, Department for Work and Pensions 2003 Full employment in every region. HMSO, London

HM Treasury, Department for Education and Skills 2005 Support for parents: the best start for children. HMSO, London

House J S, Landis K R, Umberson D 1988 Social relationships and health. Science 241: 540–545

Hughes M, Downie A, Sharma N 2000 Counting the cost of child poverty. Barnardo's, Ilford, UK

Johnson Z, Howell F, Molloy B 1993 Community mothers' programme: randomised controlled trial of non-professional intervention in parenting. British Medical Journal 306(6890): 1449–1452

Josten L, Savik K, Anderson M et al 2002 Dropping out of maternal and child health visits. Public Health Nursing 19(1): 3–10

Kendrick D, Elkan R, Hewitt M et al 2000 Does home visiting improve parenting and the quality of the home environment? A systematic review and meta analysis. Archives of Disease in Childhood 82(6): 443–451

Kirk R H 2003 Family support: the roles of early years' centres. Children & Society 17(2): 85–99

Kuh D, Ben–Schlomo Y 2004 A life course approach to chronic disease epidemiology, 2nd edn. Oxford University Press, Oxford

Kuh D, Hardy R, Langenberg C et al 2002 Mortality in adults aged 26–54 years related to socioeconomic conditions in childhood and adulthood: post war birth cohort study. British Medical Journal 325(7372): 1076–1080

Kuh D, Power C, Blane D et al 2004 Socioeconomic pathways between child-hood and adult health. In: Kuh D, Ben–Schlomo Y (eds) A life course approach to chronic disease epidemiology, 2nd edn. Oxford University Press, Oxford, pp. 371–395

Lerner R M 2005 Urie Bronfenbrenner: career contributions of the consummate developmental scientist. In: Bronfenbrenner U (eds) Making human beings human. Bioecological perspectives on human development, Sage, Thousand Oaks, CA, pp. ix–xxix

Llewellyn G, McConnell D 2002 Mothers with learning difficulties and their support networks. Journal of Intellectual Disability Research 46(1): 17–34

Lundberg O 1993 The impact of childhood living conditions on illness and mortality in adulthood. Social Science & Medicine 36(8): 1047–1052

Malone M 2000 A history of health visiting and parenting in the last 50 years. International History of Nursing Journal 5(3): 30–43

Meltzer H, Gatward R, Goodman R et al 2000 Mental health of children and adolescents in Great Britain. The Stationery Office, London

Montgomery S M, Bartley M J, Cook D G et al 1996 Health and social precursors of unemployment in young men in Great Britain. Journal of Epidemiology and Community Health 50(4): 415–422

Montgomery S M, Bartley M J, Wilkinson R G 1997 Family conflict and slow growth. Archives of Disease in Childhood 77(4): 326–330

Moran P, Ghate D, Merwe A 2004 What works in parenting support? A review of international evidence. Policy Research Bureau, DfES, London

Murray L, Hipwell A, Hooper R et al 1996 The cognitive development of 5 year-old children of postnatally depressed mothers. Journal of Child Psychology & Psychiatry & Allied Disciplines 37: 927–935

Murray L 1992 The impact of postnatal depression on infant development. Journal of Child Psychology and Psychiatry 33(3): 543–561

Mustard J M 1996 Health and social capital. In: Blane D, Brunner E, Wilkinson R (eds) Health and social organization towards a health policy for the 21st century. Routledge, London, pp. 303–313

NHS Advisory Service 1995 Together we stand: the commissioning, role and management of child and adolescent mental health services. HMSO, London

101

North J 2005 Support from the start: lessons from international early years policy. The Maternity Alliance, London

Nursing and Midwifery Council 2004 Standards of proficiency for specialist community public health nurses, NMC, London

O'Connor T G, Heron J, Golding J et al 2002 Maternal antenatal anxiety and children's behavioural/emotional problems at 4 years: report from the Avon Longitudinal Study of Parents and Children. The British Journal of Psychiatry 180(6): 502–508

Oakley A, Rigby A, Hickey D 1994 Life stress, support and class inequality. European Journal of Public Health 4: 81–91

Oakley A 1995 An evaluation of Newpin: a report by the Social Sciences Research Unit, Institute of Education, University of London. KKF Printing, London

Olds D L 2002 Prenatal and infancy home visiting by nurses: from randomized trials to community replication. Prevention Science 3(3): 153–172

Olds D L, Eckenrode J, Henderson C R, Jr. et al 1997 Long-term effects of home visitation on maternal life course and child abuse and neglect. Fifteen-year follow-up of a randomized trial. JAMA 278(8): 637–643

Olds D L, Robinson J, O'Brien R et al 2002 Home visiting by paraprofessionals and by nurses: a randomized, controlled trial. Pediatrics. 110(3): 486–496

Onazawa K, Glover V, Adams D et al 2001 Infant massage improves mother–infant interaction for mothers with postnatal depression. Journal of Affective Disorders 63: 201–207

One Plus One 1998 One Plus One family support project. Policy News. Bulletin Plus 2(4)

One Plus One 2005 Relationships today information sheets. Marital quality and parenting. Online. Available: http://www.opo.org.uk/springboard/index.asp [14 July 2005]

ONS 2004 http://www.statistics.gov.uk/cci/nugget.asp?id=716 accessed 2.08.06

Parr M 1998 A new approach to parent education. British Journal of Midwifery 6(3): 160–165

Parenting Education and Support Forum (PESF) 2005 National Occupational Standards. Online. Available: http://www.parenting–forum.org.uk/documents/NOS_March2005_Standards.pdf [15 July 2005]

Polansky N A, Chalmers M A, Buttenwieser E et al 1981 Damaged parents. An anatomy of child neglect. University of Chicago Press, Chicago

Power C, Bartley M, Davey-Smith G et al 1996 Transmission of social and biological risk across the life course. In: Blane D, Brunner E, Wilkinson R (eds) Health and social organization. Towards a health policy for the 21st century. Routledge, London, pp. 188–203

Puckering C, Mills M, Cox A et al 1994 Process and evaluation of a group intervention for mothers with parenting difficulties. Child Abuse Review 3: 299–310

Pugh G, De'Ath E, Smith C 1994 Confident parents, confident children: Policy and practice in parent education and support. National Children's Bureau, London

Pulkkinen L, Hamalainen M 1995 Low self-control as a precursor to crime and accidents in a Finnish longitudinal study. Criminal Behaviour and Mental Health 5(4): 424–438

Puura K, Davis H, Papadopoulou K et al 2002 The European Early Promotion Project: a new primary health care service to promote children's mental health. Infant Mental Health Journal 23: 606–624

Puura K, Davis H, Mantymaa M et al 2005 The outcome of the European Early Promotion Project: mother–child interaction. International Journal of Mental Health Promotion 7: 82–94

Quinton D 2004 Supporting parents: messages from research. Jessica Kingsley Publishers, London

Richards M, Hardy R, Kuh D et al 2001 Birth weight and cognitive function in the British 1946 birth cohort: longitudinal population based study. British Medical Journal 322(7280): 199–203

Roberts R, Loxton R, Campbell J et al 2002 European Early Promotion Project: transition to parenting. Community Practitioner 75: 464–468

Russek L G, Schwartz G E 1997 Perceptions of parental caring predicts health status in midlife: a 35-year follow-up of the Harvard Mastery of Stress Study. Psychosomatic Medicine 59(2): 144–149

Sanders M R 1999 Triple P-Positive Parenting Program: towards an empirically validated multilevel parenting and family support strategy for the prevention of behavior and emotional problems in children. Clinical Child & Family Psychology Review 2(2): 71–90

Scott S, Knapp M, Henderson J et al 2001 Financial cost of social exclusion: follow up study of antisocial children into adulthood. British Medical Journal 323(7306): 191–194

Seeley S, Murray L, Cooper P J 1996 Post-natal depression: the outcome for mothers and babies of health visitor intervention. Health Visitor 69: 135–138

Sheppard M, Gröhn M 2004 Prevention and coping in child and family care. Mothers in adversity coping with child care. Jessica Kingsley Publishers, London

Shore A N 2001 Effects of a secure attachment relationship on right brain development, affect regulation, and infant mental health. Infant Mental Health Journal 22: 6–77

Stattin H, Romelsjo A 1995 Adult mortality in the light of criminality, substance abuse, and behavioural and family-risk factors in adolescence. Criminal Behaviour and Mental Health 5(4): 279–311

Sterling Honig A 2001 When should programs for teen parents and babies begin? Longitudinal evaluation of a teen parents and babies program. The Journal of Primary Prevention 21(4): 447–454

Stewart-Brown S 2000 Parenting, well-being, health and disease. In: Buchanan A H B (eds) Promoting children's emotional wellbeing. Oxford University Press, Oxford, pp. 28–47

Sweeting M, West P 1995 Family life and health in adolescence: a role for culture in the health inequalities debate? Social Science and Medicine 40: 163–175

Turner H, Wiggins M, Austerberry H et al 2005 Use of postnatal community services: RCT evidence. Community Practitioner 78(1): 11–13

Wade B, Moore M 2000 A sure start with books. Early Years 20(2): 39–46

Wadsworth M 1996 Family and education determinants of health. In: Blane D, Brunner E, Wilkinson R (eds) Health and social organization towards a health policy for the 21st century. Routledge, London, pp. 152–170

Wadsworth M 1999 Early life. In: Marmot M, Wilkinson R (eds) Social determinants of health, Oxford University Press, Oxford, pp. 44–63

Walker J 2005 Relationships, quality of life and support for parents and families. Paper presented to Associate Parliamentary Group for Parents and Families, July 2005, London

Wanless D 2004 Public health policy in England: securing good health for the whole population (2). Online. Available: http://www.hm–treasury.gov.uk [28 June 2004].

Webster-Stratton C, Hammond M 1997 Treating children with early onset conduct problems: a comparison of child and parent training interventions. Journal of Consulting and Clinical Psychology 65: 93–109

Werner E E 1995 Resilience in development. Current Directions in Psychological Science 4(3): 81–85

West D J, Farrington D P 1973 Who becomes delinquent? Heinemann Educational Books, London

Whiteman M C, Deary I J, Fowkes F G 2000 Personality and social predictors of atherosclerotic progression: Edinburgh Artery Study. Psychosomatic Medicine 62(5): 703–714

Whittaker K, Cowley S 2003 Parenting support: where does it fit with public health roles? Community Practitioner 76(3): 100–103

Wilkinson R G (1999) Putting the picture together: prosperity, redistribution, health and welfare. In: Marmot M, Wilkinson R G (eds) Social determinants of health. Oxford University Press, Oxford, pp. 256–274

Woods J 2005 Who knows best – mother or TV? Online. Available: http://www.telegraph.co.uk/arts/main.jhtml [30 June 2005]

World Health Organization (WHO) 1998 World Health Report 1998. Life in the 21st century: a vision for all. WHO, Geneva

Zealey C 2005 The benefits of infant massage: a critical review. Community Practitioner 78(3): 98–101

Further reading

Bidmead C, Whittaker K 2004 Positive parenting: a public health priority. CPHVA, London

Gerhardt S 2004 Why love matters: how affection shapes a baby's brain. Brunner-Routledge, Hove

Ghate D, Hazel N 2002 Parenting in poor environments. Stress, support and coping. Jessica Kingsley Publishers, London

Moran P, Ghate D, Van der Merwe A 2004 What works in parenting support? A review of the international evidence. Policy Research Bureau, DfES. Nottingham http://www.prb.org.uk/wwiparenting/

Quinton D 2004 Supporting parents: messages from research. Jessica Kingsley Publishers, London

Stewart-Brown S 2000 Parenting, wellbeing, health and disease. In: Buchanan A, Hudson B (eds) Promoting children's emotional wellbeing. Oxford University Press, Oxford, pp. 28–47

Resources

Family and Parenting Institute

An organisation set up by the government in 1999 to support families in raising children. The Institute wants to make it easy for parents to find out what help is available and to ensure that parenting services provided by small and large organisations are more widely publicised. It will also lobby for better and more comprehensive services. The website has information for parents and professionals around managing difficulties in parenting. Some useful publications. Many free downloads.

430 Highgate Studios, 53–79 Highgate Road
London NW 5 1TL
Tel 020 7424 3460 Fax 020 7485 3590
Website: http://www.familyandparenting.org

Parenting UK

An umbrella organisation for all groups and agencies involved in parenting education and support. Very useful newsletters with summaries of research, resources available, training events and conferences. Worth becoming a member.
Website: http://www.parentinguk.org

Parenthood Education in Schools (PESF)

New website designed as a resource to promote best practice in parenthood education for children and young people in schools and is aimed at anyone involved in planning or delivering parenthood education. A guidance document, downloaded free, covers all key aspects of parenthood education and describes the links with the other parts of the PSHE curriculum and with citizenship education.

Unit 431 Highgate Studios, 53–79 Highgate Road
London NW5 1TL
Tel 020 7284 8370 Fax 020 7485 3587
E-mail: pesf@dial.pipex.com
Website: http://www.parenthood.org.uk

NCH

Works with children and young people offering diverse innovative services through local projects. Parenting Programme 'Handling Children's Behaviour'.

85 Highbury Park
London N5 1UD
Tel 020 7704 7000 Fax 020 7226 2537
Website: http://www.nch.org.uk

International Association of Infant Massage

Promotes nurturing touch and communication through training, education and research. In the UK, training and membership with regular newsletters and a support network of regional reps and instructors.
IAIM 56

Sparsholt Road
Barking
Essex IG11 7YQ
Tel 07816 289788, 0208 5911399 Fax 0208 5911399
E–mail: mail@iaim.org.uk
Website: http://www.iaim.org.uk; http://www.infantmassageinstitute.com

Family Links

Oxford-based charity established to encourage and teach nurturing and relationship skills. Pomotes public awareness of the need for emotional education. Offers training courses in the Nurturing Programme to professionals and to families. Foundation programme for PHSE in primary schools. Whole-school approach working with staff, pupils and parents.

Family Links
Peterley House, Peterley Road
Horspath Industrial Estate
Cowley, Oxford OX4 2TZ
Tel 01865 401800 Fax 01865 401820
E-mail: info@familylinks.org.uk
Website: http://www.familylinks.org.uk

Family Caring Trust (0–6 years, 5–15 years)

A Northern-Ireland-based charity concerned with the care of the family. Site summarises work of Trust and allows ordering of resources. Also contains information for parents who are having difficulties with parenting. Resources for parenting groups, all ages and family relationships.

East Berkshire Dept of Community Studies at the University of Reading report available from Elizabeth Hawkins, Head of Dept of Community Studies at the University of Reading, Bulmershe Court, Reading RG6 1HY.

Herts Social Services evaluation is also available from Family Caring Trust.

University of Ulster in co-operation with the Down–Lisburn NHS Trust, evaluation available from Family Caring Trust

Barnardo's South Lakeland Family Support Service evaluation by University of Leeds School of Continuing Education (July 2001).

Facilitator training available from Hallam Caring Services, Sheffield 0114 2554790.

8, Ashtree Enterprise Park
Newry Co. Down BT34 1BY
Tel 028 3026 4174 Fax 028 3026 9077
E-mail: office@familycaring.co.uk
Website: http://www.familycaring.co.uk

Mellow parenting

An evaluated, effective 13-week programme engaging hard-to-reach families with children under 5, and helping them make changes in their relationships with their children. One-year follow-up has shown lasting gains in maternal wellbeing, parent–child interaction, child behaviour and child development. The group explores parents, own upbringing and feelings about pregnancy plus video work in the home.

For training enquiries, contact: rmackenzie@acpp.org.uk
http://www.acpp.org.uk/events/displayDetail.asp?id=100160

The Incredible Years – Caroline Webster-Stratton

American site displaying range of programmes offered.

Contacts UK:
Dr Stephen Scott, Dept of Child and Adolescent Psychiatry
Institute of Psychiatry, King's College,
de Crespingny Park
London. SE5 8AF Tel 020 848 0467
E-mail: s.scott@iop.kcl.ac.uk
Website: http://www.incredibleyears.com
For training enquiries, contact:
Raija Kelly
Tel: 44 (0)20 7919 3810
E-mail: Raija.Kelly@slam.nhs.uk

Triple P

This Australian Positive Parenting Program is a multi-level, parenting and family support strategy aiming to prevent severe behavioural, emotional and developmental problems in children by enhancing the knowledge, skills and confidence of parents. It incorporates five levels of intervention of increasing strength for parents of children from birth to age 12. Now extended to parents of young people aged 12–16.

Trainers available Scotland, Stoke-on-Trent and Salisbury. See website for contact details.
http://www.triplep.net or email training@triplep.net

DELTA (Developing Early Learning and Thinking Abilities)

Offers support for parents through a series of between 4 and 6 consecutive sessions, which take place in the child's school. While the workshops involve issues, which are important to child development, it also aims to increase the self-esteem and confidence of the groups of parents. Useful site with resources that can be downloaded.

Antrim Board Centre
17 Lough Road
Antrim BT41 4DH
Northern Ireland
Tel: 028 9448 2222 Fax: 028 9446 0794
Website: http://www.neelb.org.uk/cass/earlyyears/contact/zy00014l.htm

PEEP (Peers Early Education Partnership)

An early-learning intervention aiming to improve the life chances of children in disadvantaged areas by raising educational attainment, by supporting parents and carers as first educators of their children.

The PEEP Centre
Peers School
Sandy Lane West
Littlemore
Oxford OX4 6JZ
Tel 01865 779779
E-mail: info@peep.org.uk
Resources can be downloaded: http://www.peep.org.uk

Parents as First Teachers

A universal programme for parents with children pre-birth to 5 years. Offers support to parents and children through home visiting, group support meetings, and a resource network with consideration of developmental milestones. Can be linked to a local school or community centre. USA developed but developing nationally in UK.

UK Head Office c/o Turners Court Youth Trust
9, Red Cross Rd.
Goring on Thames
Reading RG8 9HG
Tel 01491 874234 Fax 01491 875370
E-mail: turnerscourt@turnerscourt.f9.co.uk
Website: http://www.paft.org.uk

Fathers Direct

Provide a range of resources, research, and training for working with fathers. Summary of research on Fatherhood available to download. Also 'Dad Magazine'.

Herald House
15 Lamb's Passage, Bunhill Row
London EC1Y 8TQ
Tel 020 7920 9491 Fax 020 7374 2966
E-mail: mail@fathersdirect.com
Website: http://www.fathersdirect.com

Midwives, health visitors, prison workers or Youth Offending Teams
Duncan Fisher
Tel 01873 858010

Community development as a public health function

Yvonne Dalziel

Key issues

- **The origins and influences on community development**
- **Exploration of the key concepts of community development in health**
- **Refocusing public health practice to a model of community development**
- **The development of methods appropriate to a community development ethos**
- **Application of community development process to key areas of public health practice**

Introduction

It is generally agreed that poor health and poverty are inextricably linked and that ill health will not be solved by medicine alone, but by more effective public health measures and socio-economic change. Access to a sustainable income, an equitable and accessible food supply, tackling crime, responding differently to mental health issues, housing and environmental needs and the building of social capacity are some of the issues which, it is suggested, if addressed would have a long-term impact on community health. That poverty is the key indicator in poor health is now indisputable (Marmot & Wilkinson 1999, The Black Report, Townsend & Davidson 1982), but the historical relationship between the NHS and medical/clinical model of health has arguably compounded the problem of inequality in health. Until recently the sole focus of the NHS has been primarily on treatment and disease and, although these are undeniably important, there has been a tendency to view health as only treatment and cure. The preventive aspect and the impact of poverty on health have traditionally been believed to have been outside the scope of medicine, and health promotion/improvement, when it occurred, has been regarded mainly as relating to individual behaviour change based on an information giving process.

The NHS value system has encouraged ways of working to address health needs that are, arguably, more comfortable culturally for higher socio-economic groups. Little or no focus has been placed on how the people with the poorest health might perceive a system that seems to ignore their needs. People struggling with stress and financial difficulties, or who feel themselves outwith societal norms, need different, more creative ways of allowing their legitimate voice in the decision-making process. Much of the profound inequity in peoples' health is socially determined and arises from the circumstances in which people live and work. Poverty is more than low income, a lack of education and poor health. It is also an experience of feeling powerless to influence the social and economic factors that determine wellbeing. Poor health exacerbates existing poverty and poverty is most often a political problem, i.e. people are poor because of structural, man-made situations.

Failure to recognise and address the issue that much of our ill-health lies out-with what the NHS currently offers results in the NHS treating poverty and the impact of poverty as a medical condition. This only serves to increase the health inequalities gap and ultimately leads to the medicalisation of poverty and an increase in health inequality.

The adoption of the ideology and methods of community development offer workers involved in public health work an approach to address the inequalities in health that underpin many of the health problems in our communities. This chapter will briefly explore the historical context of community development and the radical influences on the community health movement in the 1960s and 1970s that are arguably still pertinent to the implementation of a public health strategy today.

This chapter suggests that it is the approach to health and a change in the underlying values in relation to health that will create new ways of working and so make a difference. The difference will come from a model of public health that gives the individual and community the tools and knowledge to make the changes for themselves and their families. The outline of a model of community development that focuses on child health will suggest how the application of the methods to one area of health activity can have an impact on the health of the wider community. Finally, the chapter suggests that if a new way of thinking about health is to develop, one that focuses on addressing inequalities and using community development as a mainstream approach, then health workers will need strong leadership, changes in the education curriculum, and the development of structures and policies to support them in thinking and doing differently.

Community development: origins and influences

Although community development is now gaining recognition as an approach to health, the methods and thinking that constitute community development are not new. Jones (1990) suggests that it was used by colonial governments to 'ensure the governability and modernisation of their empires' (p. 32). It was more recent events, however, that nurtured its growth and its value as an approach to addressing health issues.

According to Jones (1990), community development and health work had evolved over the previous 10 years, incorporating a number of different influences that had built onto a basic community development model. The growing movement in health occurring in the last few decades has used community development as an ideological and practical framework to bring about change in how health as a concept is regarded. Previously used as a method in community work to address housing and social policy needs, the first health projects using community development principles did not appear in the UK until the late 1970s. The emergence, in the late 1960s and 1970s, of social movements like the women's movement, civil rights, black power and the self-help movement, was a key influence in supporting the growth of the approach.

A social movement is defined as: 'collectively acting with some continuity to promote change in the society or group to which it is a part' (Turner & Killian, quoted in Schiller & Levin 1983, p. 1344). The social movements of this time grew from the disaffection of people who felt marginal to and excluded from decision-making processes. It was a reaction to the dominant male, white, middle-class systems and the attitudes that discriminated against women, black people and the poor. The movements demanded justice, freedom, democracy and the end of discrimination. Underpinning their emergence was a belief system that held the primacy of individual experience as the basis of knowledge and expertise.

The primary challenge of both the women's health movement (which grew out of the women's liberation movement) and the self-help movement was to demystify health knowledge and retake its ownership from the male-dominated medical profession, which so jealously guarded it as its own. As a consequence, they developed an anti-professional view of health and the causes of ill health and encouraged individuals to become experts in their own bodies. They encouraged people to view what they knew, derived from their own experiences, as being as important as the theoretical knowledge that had evolved conceptually and been filtered through a dominant male medical ideology. In consciousness-raising and self-help health groups, women began to see how this latter view of themselves was reinforced by their contact with the medical profession and that it adversely affected their health and their access to health services.

The Black Report (Townsend & Davidson 1982) indicated that the groups for whom the social movements had, potentially, the greatest impact, that is, those who are socially and economically disadvantaged, who are more likely to experience poorer health and have shorter lives than more affluent people. The community development ethos will bring into the awareness of public health workers that these groups of people, and others who feel socially excluded from mainstream society, e.g. homeless, disabled, have knowledge and experience about their own lives that, when harnessed, can strengthen and sustain their communities.

The right of people to participate in health decisions is enshrined in the Alma Ata Declaration of 1977 (World Health Organization (WHO) 1978). It states that 'the people have a right and a duty to participate individually and collectively in the planning and implementation of their care'. The desire for a public health movement to tackle health problems resulted, in 1981, in the WHO policy Health For All by the year 2000. Central to the attainment of its targets is the development of primary care and the concepts of participation, collaboration and equity that were central to the Alma Ata Declaration.

The dominance of the medical model in public health thinking, and its focus on epidemiology and medicine, has left an ontological deficit in what health workers working in public health know about the poorest communities; what they need to promote health and to build the social capacity of their neighbourhoods and communities. Involvement in public health work, through activities like community-based needs assessment, public involvement in primary care planning and delivery of services, would legitimate the community development approach and support the move away from the clinical model based on individual, transactions to a social contract with entire communities (Ashton & Seymour 1988). To fit the new agenda of addressing social, as well as individual, change in health, health workers require a change in their approach to health as a concept, and to the methods and the activities of its daily practice.

Poor people define their poverty in terms of lack of opportunities, lack of power and lack of security so this broader definition of poverty will require a broader set of actions to fight it. The impact of providing social services to the poor has been less than expected, mainly because interventions do not respond to poor people's real needs.

The key tenets of a community development approach, collective action, self-determination, democracy and promotion of self-confidence are central to any policy to tackle inequalities in health and to address poverty. Community development as a concept is now high on the health agenda, however it is defined; but the way in which it fits into public health work and whatever activities health workers might engage in to bring about change are still not mainstream.

Elements of community development

A community development approach is a useful way to move from exclusion to inclusion in the decision-making process for marginal groups and the principles of the approach could form an essential ideology for groups of health workers. The approach is concerned with the notion of shared power between health professionals and lay people and the move from dependency to involvement. The concepts which underpin this approach are about equal access to resources, promoting democracy and involvement in decision making about health, taking action to bring about change, sharing power and working in partnership with communities.

Underlying each is the concept of shared authority. This means that each person takes equal responsibility for the decision making and each is accountable for the outcomes. Although conceptually different, each element of community development is related to, and has an impact on, the others. For example, when individuals are involved as equal partners and their knowledge affirmed, skills used and opinions heard, then they feel more in control and, in turn, are more able to begin to form alliances with others to bring about the changes they desire. A brief outline of each of the different elements will demonstrate this.

Equity

Although very closely connected and often confused as one concept, equity and equality are not the same thing. People all have the right to equal access to available health services for the maintenance and promotion of health but, to be fair, people do not all need to be treated in the same way. Instead, those who stand to benefit the most and whose needs are the greatest are given priority: this is 'equity'. In a culture of scarce resources, this may mean unequal distribution, even taking away from the most well off to give extra services to the most needy. All too often, what happens is the opposite; those most in need have the worst access to services. Inequalities in health care are not only about the provision of services but also how services are delivered. Addressing inequalities means challenging practices that discriminate against individuals on whatever basis – poverty, race, disability, language, sexuality or age – in the provision of essentials for health. It also involves examining the provision, quality, uptake, accessibility and availability to those who have the greatest need.

Empowerment

This is also discussed at length in Chapter 6. Rappaport defines empowerment as 'the process by which people, organisations and communities gain mastery over their lives' (1984, p. 3). The empowerment process involves building individual and collective confidence and raising the esteem of individuals and communities through valuing their knowledge and experience and supporting them to be part of the decision-making process. Kiefer (1983) views empowerment as attainment of what he calls 'participatory competence'. Beigal (1984) views empowerment as both capacity and equity: capacity being use of power to solve problems and equity referring to getting one's fair share of resources. Empowerment skills include problem-solving, assertiveness and confidence-building strategies.

Participation

The concept of participation is about supporting people who are affected by decisions, to have some influence over their outcome, and for nurses it is an

---

Box 5.1

Levels of participation or involvement

1. **Information giving** – details of services, decision-making structures, helplines, media slots, etc.
2. **Gathering information** – views on existing services, needs assessment, concerns about services, focus groups, community meetings
3. **Consultation** – asking for comment on formulated plans or proposals
4. **Involvement in policy development and decision making** – getting users directly involved with management to develop training and quality standards for professional staff
5. **Joint working** – equal basis to develop projects, services, information packs, local forum, community health projects
6. **Community or user control** – involvement in planning and delivering services

(Adapted from Taylor et al 1988)

---

important approach to the attainment of health. Perceptions of power affect participation. Steve Lukes (1974) suggests that there are different levels of power: the visible manifestations of power, the unseen but tangible manifestations of power and internalised powerlessness. People on the margins of society experiencing this third level of powerlessness become passive and dependent. Believing themselves unable to influence events and decisions affecting their lives, they consciously exclude themselves from opportunities to be part of the process of decision making. People who experience internal powerlessness are often those who do not attend for clinic appointments, come to parentcraft classes or attend their children's school evenings. They don't believe their involvement can make a difference to their lives.

Keifer suggests that participatory competence is a life-long achievement and includes three aspects:

1. Development of a more positive self-concept or sense of self-competence.
2. Construction of more critical or analytical understanding of surrounding social and political environment.
3. Cultivation of individual and collective resources for social and political action.

Consultation, rather than participation, happens when decisions have already been made and there is little likelihood of any change but the public is still asked to comment about a proposal. This is a poor substitute for real participation and being part of the planning process. There are six different levels of participation or involvement from information giving to user control (Box 5.1).

Health workers can support their communities to be involved in any of these different levels. Involving people as part of the decision-making process is beneficial not only to the people living in communities but to the service providers. Giving users a voice in what they need avoids the mismatch of services and may be, in the long run, more economical. However, for community development it is the spin-off from involvement, as much as the development of relevant services, that is important. Involvement as a process is in itself health improving. As people begin to feel connected and valued their self-esteem rises, along with their levels of confidence. They feel more in control of their lives and so better able to take up health messages.

Box 5.2

Features of alliance building

- Commitment to the shared goals of the alliance
- Community involvement in all alliance activities. Community representatives must have the necessary training and skills to participate equally
- Communication where partners share relevant information and commit to simplicity, openness and honesty
- Joint working with equal ownership and appropriate input from each partner
- Accountability
- Evaluation is built into alliance work and results used constructively

(From Funnell et al 1995)

Partnership and alliances

A key concept in the community development process is partnership and the building of alliances. Alliance is defined as partnership for action; a virtual organisation that is created by the interaction between partner agencies and sectors (Duffy 1996). The purpose of agencies working together and with local people is to develop common priorities and strategies on issues and policies that affect health. Partnerships for health work involve a wider spectrum than that usually associated with the health sector. For example, a health alliance would involve nurses working in partnership with agencies such as environmental health, education, social work, voluntary organisations, health projects, work places and local industries. Funnell et al (1995) identify six key features of alliance building (Box 5.2).

There has been some shift in the movement within primary care towards supporting partnership and alliances with other practitioners rather than just other health professionals. This new thinking about health and public involvement, and the benefits of community partnerships to health workers in relation to pooling information, knowledge, experience, skills and resources, is an important part of new ways of working. Joint working can be more efficient, effective and can widen and deepen the impact of health initiatives. In return, health workers must be willing to share knowledge and power with each other, other agencies and, importantly, the community and to be involved in supporting community involvement.

Collective action

The author's and other experienced community development workers' experiences suggest that the knowledge of what constitutes community development in primary care is very incomplete. Many health visitors maintain that they have been working in community development for years and need learn nothing new. They believe that running groups, giving input into a women's group or working with mother and toddler groups is community development. Small-group work is an important method in community development and is to be encouraged but it is not the whole story. What is missing from primary care is the action part of community development. Concepts like partnership or equity are very palatable, empowerment is what many feel they are doing already, but collective action is more frightening because it is about the transfer of power and control. When health workers talk about doing community development what they more rightly mean is that they are working with a community-based approach.

The difference between community development and community-based work is not well understood and the use of the term 'community development' to describe what is essentially community based can lead to confusion. Essentially the differences are quite profound and adoption of one set of activities without the right mindset will lead to different outcomes. There is nothing wrong with community-based work and many argue that it will eventually lead to community development (Labonte 1998). However, the author's experience is that it can be difficult to shift from initial dependency into shared authority and if that is the final aim then why not start off that way? The use of community based rather than community development denotes a failure to let go of power (Table 5.1).

It can be seen from this matrix that the level of involvement of the participants in community-based activity is on the passive dependent continuum, whereas when a community development approach is used the user involvement is at a more active involving level. When challenged about where the power lies in a community-based activity, many workers will say that the users decide what the agenda or programme is so that makes it community development. However, if the knowledge imparted comes from a professional perspective and is located within a professional context with professional boundaries, there is a chance that, in terms of cultural competence, the information may not relate to the lives of individuals living in different social, cultural or financial circumstances. More empowering is for one of the group to seek out the information on behalf of the rest of the group. For example, if a group member collects information about healthy eating or parenting and then shares this knowledge with others, it is not

Table 5.1 ● Community-based vs. community development work

Community-based work	Community-development work
Professional control – health worker manages budget, finds funding, controls use of venue , opens up and closes building, etc. Worker sets and manages the agenda	User/community control – shared authority between users and workers, e.g. management committee where members have equal rights Share equal responsibility for success of activities
Professional knowledge and experience used and valued	Members may chair steering group and are involved in decision making Members control own budget and are part of making applications for funding
Focus of the group is to impart knowledge. Group facilitated by professional	Members set the agenda Local and individual knowledge and experience valued as much as professional knowledge
Invited speaker gives a talk from professional perspective and invites questions	Members of the group seek out and present their own information on a topic Members have responsibility for negotiating outside support Members lead sessions
Often professional venue/location, e.g. health centre	Usually community location, e.g. village hall, health project

only more empowering for members, but more likely that the information is better understood, given that it relates to the cultural context of the members. It will then have more impact. The worker's role is one of facilitating a different kind of process.

The author is involved in a project to recruit local people and then train them to work with their peers in poorer areas. This programme has had an impact on reducing the mystique of professional medical and health knowledge and of engaging the community in tackling its own issues, not in a victim-blaming way, but in a way that builds individual and community capacity and leaves something behind when the activity finishes.

Collective action is when people act together to bring about change in circumstances that they identify need to be changed. The women's health movement and radical groups of the 1960s and 1970s are examples of collective action. Today, self-help groups formed around a variety of issues and pressure groups, like disability coalitions or environmental groups, use collective action to bring about policy and structural change. When community development is working well it is evidenced by visible collective action. Health workers working with groups where they make the tea or put away the toys because that is what they perceive the participants want or need should question what kind of role they are undertaking with the group and what the consequences of their actions are likely to be. Rather than supporting dependency and passivity they could instead help initiate social action within their neighbourhood to bring about changes in individual and community confidence and self-esteem.

Working with and for communities to improve health and wellbeing

Community nurses, especially health visitors, have been supporting a range of families, not just vulnerable families, for years and are increasingly being viewed, with other community nurses and school nurses, as an untapped resource for promoting wider community health. They are the ideal practitioners to take forward the new agendas in health described in the recent government documents *Towards a healthier Scotland* (Scottish Office 1999) (and others). They are in the community, have easy access to large numbers of families and individuals, develop the kind of relationships that engenders trust and, importantly, the principles of health visiting support them to work for policy change and to support collective action for health.

Labonte (1998) maintains that community development offers the best means by which health authorities can begin to tackle the determinants of health. The model he offers would provide public health workers with a methodological and philosophical framework. It involves:

- the adoption of a model of positive health
- an analytical model of health determinants
- community development as a theory of social change
- a model of community development practice
- an accountability framework
- development of methods appropriate to community development ethics.

A model of positive health

The World Health Organization's (WHO) definition of health is well used but, arguably, its concern with promoting health rather than dealing with illness is rarely fully understood or operationalised within a health context. A change in how health as a concept is viewed would switch health workers' primary focus from an illness- and disease-prevention focus to an emphasis on promoting health and wellbeing. Labonte's model of positive health views health as being more about the quality of our emotional and social situations than about our experience of disease or disability. This model includes elements like:

- feeling vital and full of energy
- having a sense of purpose in life
- experiencing a connectedness to 'community'
- being able to do things one enjoys
- have good social relationships
- experiencing a sense of control over one's life and living conditions.

A model of positive health would move the focus primarily away from a disease- and illness-prevention model to one that supports the development of building individual and community capacity. In child health, the switch would be from screening activities, such as hearing tests and vision testing, to focusing on the life circumstances in which children live. With this approach, a sense of meaning, promoting self-confidence and the family's relationship to the wider community would be viewed as being as important as an individual child's development.

An analytical model of health determinants

It is thought that inequality in health has psychological as well as physical effects. An understanding of how unequal access to resources may adversely affect health is not clearly understood, but Wilkinson argues that the psychological effects of poverty and limited access to resources can create chronic anxiety. He suggests that the deep divisions in our society both reflect and are a cause of unaffordable financial and human waste that is significant. He maintains that there is evidence to suggest that national infant mortality rises if the rich get richer while the real incomes of the poor remain constant (1996). An analytical model would view housing, a clean and nourishing environment, access to food and appropriate services as essentials for health and determinants that needs assessment would incorporate as standard.

Community development as a theory of social change

Community development is an idea that 'encompasses a commitment to a holistic approach to health; one which recognises the central importance of social support and social networks'. A community way of working attempts to 'facilitate individual and collective action around common needs and concerns identified by the community itself and not imposed from outside' (Adams 1989). The emphasis is on working collaboratively to address equity, support democracy and the participation of the community in issues that affect their lives, and taking collective action to offer a more empowering and positive health promotion message. Principles and values of community development involve:

- combating social exclusion, poverty and disadvantage
- anti-discriminatory action in relation to race, age disability, gender, sexual orientation
- commitment to community-led, collective, democratic processes of action empowerment and participation
- preventive action

- commitment to partnerships between common interest groups governments and citizens
- public issue and public policy focus
- range of activities from self-help services to campaigning action.
  (From: Voluntary Activity Unit 1996)

A model of community development practice

Labonte's model of community development outlines a range of social organisations and relationships necessary for the promotion of health. The activities associated with the development of these relationships could form the core activities for health workers to engage in tackling the key determinants of health, e.g. housing, poverty and environment. Labonte describes them as 'strategic spheres' that rely on their interrelatedness and dependency on one another for change to occur.

Support of individuals

Community nurses are one group of workers already engaged in the support of individuals, but community development emphasises individual support as an essential component of the strategic approach to social change. Personal support would include basic support, empathy and affirming trust, advocacy, counselling, education and crisis intervention, as well as referral to other agencies or community groups. Where this approach deviates from mainstream community nursing or social work is in the belief that promoting confidence by enabling the development of new skills and opportunities is not enough on its own. Support must take place within a framework that views personal support as an important component of social or collective action to bring about social change.

Development of support groups

Concepts of democracy, participation and empowerment are central to a community development approach. Local democracy means everyone having a say in what is right for them and for their community, creating structures to encourage participation and involvement, working together to improve the community and influence local policy and enabling people to take effective action. Here the individual support, which is an essential part of health work, is extended to encourage people to come together to improve social support and increase social networks. It is believed that this process builds support for personal change, overcomes 'learned helplessness', and creates the ground for social action to occur.

The process of involvement is an empowering action in itself. The author's experience of helping a women's group set up a food co-op in their neighbourhood demonstrated that health gain for the volunteers was not limited only to an increased intake of fruit and vegetables, but to the increase in self-esteem resulting from their involvement. Being part of the project supported the concept of health outlined by Labonte in that women felt an increased sense of purpose and of being connected to their community. Involvement in activities that facilitate participation, like joining a food co-op or taking part in a management group, can often be difficult for groups that feel themselves marginalised. It could be part of mainstream public health practice to encourage involvement by supporting engagement with educational programmes that build confidence or to develop access to information through making documents and literature more available.

Community organising

Community development is about bringing people together to deal with the issues and needs in their area that they define as problematic. It is about working from expressed needs, helping create structures where individuals are not powerless and where there is a commitment to include people who feel excluded because of poverty, disadvantage and isolation. Public health activity would help communities to organise to take effective action through developing support groups, working with people to plan things and to identify issues for action. One of the difficulties of the community development approach is the involvement of individuals who are under-represented in the democratic process. Community nurses and others, using their contacts and the nature of the relationships they develop, could play an important part in reaching such individuals and encouraging them to become involved in local action on community defined needs.

They also have an important role in strengthening communities and helping them develop resources. Social capital is often referred to as 'social glue' and is claimed to impact on health in a number of ways, e.g. by increasing life expectancy and decreasing infant mortality. Loosely, it means developing social trust, reciprocity and mutual support between neighbours and creating services in the community that are relevant and support empowerment amongst their users. Social capital is also demonstrated by involvement in civic activities, e.g. voting, going to church, participation in local events.

Alliance building, political action

Community development methods and concepts support a view that empowered communities should work in partnership with local authorities, local businesses and health professionals to bring about change. They are all key stakeholders in the promotion of health. As argued earlier, improvements in public health are more dependent on changes in social and economic policy than on medicine, and so the involvement of agencies like housing, police and education working collaboratively with local communities in the promotion of health is essential.

An accountability framework

Accountability is similar to evaluation, although it is broader in meaning. Labonte makes the point that accountability is often more of an ethical or moral nature than a legal matter. Public health workers would have what he calls a 'dual accountability tension' in that health authorities employ them and so they have accountability to their employers; but in working alongside the community as equal partners they would also have accountability to them. The conflict that can arise for workers when local people are challenging their employing authority about services they want is not the problem that Labonte suggests it might be, if current policy about involvement and working from needs of local people is adhered to.

Development of methods appropriate to community development ethics

In order to enhance and support community development ways of working it is essential that public health workers be aware of and can use methods of working and evaluating community development that uphold the values of the approach. The Voluntary Activity Unit (1996) offers these suggestions in relation to evaluation that are equally valid for undertaking other community development initiatives:

- Work with communities must be negotiated to ensure that the criteria and methods used are sanctioned by the constituencies on whose behalf they act.
- Communities are encouraged to ask a series of questions about evaluation such as:
  - what will be evaluated and by whom?

- what perspective will be used to identify success or failure?
- what methods will be used?
- what happens to the products of evaluation, who will have access to it and for what purposes?

- Evaluation should be regarded as a learning process for communities and the other agencies involved and so there must be a commitment to involvement of them as evaluators. The process then is always based on partnership and collaboration rather than on a lone researcher.
- Evaluation should be regarded an empowering process that increases community and personal knowledge, raises self-esteem and confidence and allows for community control.
- Recognition is needed that qualitative data are as valid as quantitative information. As motivation for action often springs from the quality of personal and community life indicators and measures must reflect lived experience and give commitment to the voice of people not usually asked for their views.
- Resources need to be made available to allow real participation, e.g. training, crèche or sitter support or translation facilities.
- Value to be given to the process as well as to task goals, e.g. getting people together or involved is acknowledged as an outcome of a piece of community work.

Working with a community development approach will not only involve a change in practice for the public health workforce, and the need to enhance skills such as group work, but will also radically change the relationships health workers have with the people with whom they are involved. They will no longer be working *for* patients or clients, but working *with* them, acknowledging the value of local expertise and knowledge, and being able to support the emergence of leaders from within the community to take things forward.

Community development activity

Underpinning the community development approach are a set of activities designed to mobilise neighbourhoods or communities of interest to harness their own skills and resources to provide action for change. These activities are encompassed within the community development process. In many ways the community development process parallels Labonte's (1998) model of community development practice discussed earlier. There are four distinct elements in the process: reflection, analysis, developing strategies and taking action. One element has an impact on the other, which leads onto the next and so on in a continuous cycle. Several discrete stages of activities support the elements; some may overlap or happen simultaneously, like Labonte's model, but they are all, nevertheless, integral to the process.

Craig (2000) offers a model of public health practice for nurses that this section builds on to outlines the community development process and its accompanying activities.

Networking or 'just hanging about'

This involves visiting mother and toddler groups, women's groups, the local cafe and talking to people to find out who the key individuals are in a community. The purpose is to build up a picture of the neighbourhood, the culture and the values of the local people, what their needs are and where their interests and energy lie in addressing them. Nurses are very attached to the notion of doing something and find the idea of 'hanging about' very challenging. They may feel guilty about

Community development as a public health function

119

doing nothing when in fact 'hanging about' is doing something different. It is a complex process in which one tries to shed the professional uniform and be open to whatever is happening without judgement. It means watching and listening and absorbing what goes on while building relationships, making current and future contacts, and deciding whom to involve further. It is a process of seeing and being seen, being accepted as part of the community without being in the community and hopefully, if it is being done properly, being trusted.

Identifying supports in the community

Developing from 'hanging about' and still part of networking is the next stage. Here public health workers move onto encouraging people to become involved in addressing local health needs. They may need support to do this, e.g. awareness-raising sessions to help them focus on issues of health and to clarify what health means to them. They may also need help to organise themselves to progress to the action stage. This may mean the group becoming constituted and seeking charitable status. Groups often need to be formalised in this way to obtain funding and, although often initially resisted, it can be a very good process for a group. It helps members clarify their aims and objectives and begin to learn about how organisations operate, even one as small as theirs, and that there are different roles and tasks to be undertaken.

Needs assessment and identifying issues

It will be important for the public health worker to be working closely with local people to identify main concerns, identifying what needs to be done and developing support to do it. This can be achieved by running a health day in the community centre or doing community profiles or needs assessment. It was discussed earlier how people who perceive themselves as excluded from society due to poverty, colour, class or homelessness find it difficult to participate due to feelings of powerlessness – often called apathy or indifference by professionals. The public health workforce could help communities perceived to be on the margins, like people who are homeless or vulnerable families with children on the 'at risk' register, to be part of activities like community profiling and needs assessment by involving them in the process. That involvement could, according to Burton and Harrison (1997), produce benefits:

- Providing information from people's lived experience. This may produce the impetus for action in the community.
- Enabling new structures to develop as a framework evolves for allocation of tasks. Groups of people getting together to undertake pieces of work can together create new opportunities for further action.
- Enabling people to increase their knowledge about their community. The process of asking questions of neighbours and others creates a wider knowledge of what is in their neighbourhood for those involved in the process.
- Facilitating personal development and the acquisition of new skills. Training is usually necessary for those involved in asking the questions and analysing and disseminating the data.
- Creation of more effective services by feeding the information back up through the system. This helps health authorities commission services that are more meaningful to community need.
- More democratic health service through public involvement at all levels.

Often at this stage it is not possible to undertake a formal needs assessment, due to lack of resources, funding and personnel, or it may not be appropriate because the needs are apparent.

Testing ideas on informal networks

Instead of formal needs assessment, groups may decide to take action on what they perceive to be their immediate health difficulties and then through a variety of methods check this out with the larger community. These can include:

- informal contact
- holding training days
- small surveys
- discussion groups
- running a seminar or conference in the community.

Workers at this stage in the process will be shaping, collecting and getting support for ideas, setting up support groups, offering opportunities for volunteering, training and supporting participation.

Bringing together key individuals to develop strategies

This next stage in the process is clarifying opportunities for change and developing strategies. One group the author worked with identified a lack of trained crèche workers to care for their children while they were engaged in committee meetings as an issue. With key workers, locally, they decided to seek funding and to offer a training course for local people wanting to work in crèches. Another area identified for action was the lack of shops, locally, selling quality affordable fruit and vegetables. After holding a public seminar and asking other projects involved in food work to speak about setting up a fruit and vegetable co-op, the group decided to take action collectively and set up its own fruit and vegetable co-op.

Taking action with the community

This next stage supporting the action of the community around its defined needs is a key one for a public health worker working with a community development approach. Activities at this time will focus on supporting communities in seeking funding to initiate new ventures, or to develop existing projects and build alliances between the community and people who can help them. This may mean setting up evaluation or monitoring systems for projects and community activities and to support their growth and development. These activities will be underpinned by sharing information, joint working and networking.

One of the outcomes of the community development process must be to influence policy. However, policy change need not be huge change. The creation of new structures, however small, can impact on policy. The courses for crèche workers referred to earlier were so successful that other agencies asked to employ the workers and soon the availability of training began to alter crèche policy in the area. Community education workers eventually undertook to organise and fund the training, and to compile a register of trained workers. After the establishment of the food co-op, volunteers started working with other agencies and eventually community centres locally began to reduce the sales of sweets and to offer fruit instead to youth and children's groups. The community cafe widened the variety of food for sale and tried to reduce the amount of fried food it offered. Playgroups and nursery schools implemented healthy eating policies and local primary schools supplied fruit in tuck shops. The local GP practice even provided core funding to sustain the food co-op.

To bring about major change that will impact on the lives of the most discriminated people in our society requires that local people have access to the existing decision-making structures like health boards, city councils and government so that their voices can be heard. Influencing policy is a key principle of health visiting but is one that nurses have shied away from in the past. There may be several reasons for this; the structures for nurses to feed into policy have not existed, it is regarded as 'too political', but it may be also that nursing, as a low-status profession, is implicated in the lack of action by nurses. Like the low-status groups they work with (women and children, the poor and older people), nurses do not readily avail themselves of the active participation in the democratic process that may bring about change. Like these groups, this may also be a manifestation of their internalised powerlessness (Lukes 1978). If nurses are to be involved in other people's empowering process, there may need to be a place in nurse training to focus on the 'participatory competence' of nurses to prepare them to be able to engage in this.

The impact of community development work can be considerable. The crèche training provided employment for local women, offered new skills and knowledge, and improved childcare in crèches. The establishment of the food co-op impacted on food costs, created a new community focus, and led onto new training courses. It also initiated the development of new groups and community activities. It is clear from these brief examples of food work and child care that working alongside local people in this way can have a considerable impact on public health issues through influencing policy, locally, to bring about structural changes. However, in the future the public health workforce will not only be about undertaking different activities, but also applying different methods to existing practice.

Health workers' workloads are defined by caseloads in many cases. A caseload of under-5's will by definition restrict public health nurses to spending time developing a relationship with individuals, primarily, being available when they have a crisis, visiting them at home, seeing them in the clinic, giving advice and counsel, and generally overseeing the development of their children. This individualistic model of care undertaken by many health workers feeds the ego and the sense of being important and vital to others. It encourages health workers to know the answers and creates dependence on the part of the patients/clients for their knowledge and skills. The current individualistic culture and medical model structures in the workforce, coupled with the statutory obligation to fulfil certain responsibilities for individual families, further supports this dependence and renders casework as a core activity very powerful. A small study of health visitors trained in community development methods (Dalziel 1997) showed that, given a choice between community development work or responding to caseload demands, the caseload was made priority every time. This was because of external client demand and pressure from GPs and nurse managers to maintain the status quo.

Recent research carried out for Lothian Health (Dalziel & McLachlan 2000) in relation to community development training in primary care found that primary care staff liked this way of working and wanted to do more, but felt constrained by caseloads and lack of support within the structures. The research suggests that in order for community development to be integrated into mainstream working, it needs:

- Recognition within NHS structures and at all levels of management of the value of this kind of training and the community development way of working.
- Consideration of practical support for the training including how practice-based health professionals can be released to attend training.
- Funding of posts for dedicated workers to provide ongong advice and support to implement the approach.
- Further research to assess the health gains of such activities.

Applying the community development process to key areas of child public health

The introduction of new government papers on public health has created a change in attitudes to a community development way of working. Perhaps the days of an individual health visitor working in isolation in community development activities, which is in conflict, philosophically, with mainstream colleagues with whom the person is meant to be working, is changing. The benefits of having all public health workers with a caseload working in a community development way as opposed to a lone community development worker are substantial:

- Ready access to an existing communities of interest, i.e. women with young children, older people, antenatal, or to other groups with which public health workers are involved.
- General acceptance by other professionals of their role in community health.
- Existing knowledge of the area and available services.

Child health and community development

Although most areas of current health activity are amenable to a community development approach, child health is good place to start. Child health is at the core of public health activity and has a potential effect on community health that may be as yet untapped. Individual family work is valuable and can be retained within a community development framework, but, arguably, this focus on individual care and individual contact also prevents any possible social action to solve community or population problems from being discovered. What individual visiting reveals are individual symptoms of a wider community stress: bits of a jigsaw that all look the same, but are in fact unique and only make sense when fitted together with the other pieces. The individual approach, on its own, can do little to change the life circumstances that contribute to unhealthy lifestyles and illness. Without a population approach, work with families sits outside the new public health agenda.

The changing focus on positive health that values being connected, having a sense of purpose, and a focus on strengthening communities makes many traditional child health activities insufficient for the new agenda. The current activities are located within a personal care strategy and so have a remit for child health that focuses on surveillance, screening and advice to mothers about feeding, weaning, sleeping behaviour, etc. Focus on a positive model of health as opposed to illness prevention would create different priorities for action. Although immunisation, weighing, hearing and vision testing and developmental testing are important activities, without locating the causes and solutions to what is found by surveillance within a bigger community picture, they are of little value and need to be replaced by an emphasis on different criteria for health. Instead of the questions child health workers traditionally ask about weight, hearing and developmental progress they might ask questions that more properly focus on a wider public health agenda like:

- Has this child access to good food, adequate shelter, and a safe environment?
- Is there the potential in this family/community for him/her to develop supportive, nourishing relationships and a sense of belonging?
- Is there the opportunity for him/her to be educated and do fulfilling work when he/she is older?

- Is there freedom from discrimination and harassment?
- Are there accessible relevant health and social welfare services in the area?

In this agenda, good housing, abolition of poverty, opportunity for nourishing social relationships, for fulfilling work in the future and a pleasant environment are viewed as essentials for the promotion of health and of equal status as immunisation and child development.

A community development public health approach would move the emphasis away from an exclusive focus on individual behaviour to participation, collaboration with the local community and some understanding of the social circumstances that create ill-health. Key areas of child health that are amenable to this change include:

- well baby clinics
- child development
- child protection.

Well baby clinics

It could be argued that traditional child health clinics encourage and support a dependency culture, where young parents feel pressurised into taking their child to the baby clinic 'to be checked'. This might have overtones of the policing role of public health nurses but also, perhaps, professional input encourages them to feel that what they know about their child is not enough on its own and needs to be confirmed or supported by health workers. This can be disempowering and deskilling for parents. Clinics also operate very much on an individualistic model of care with individual advice and support being offered, often in a cultural and social vacuum. Advice and help that lies outwith this prevailing culture will be largely ignored. Child rearing is an activity embedded in cultural norms and women from the same culture can and do offer advice and help as part of their natural interaction with young mothers. They are then likely to be more acceptable purveyors of guidance and support than health workers. Health professionals often demonstrate unconscious contempt for the input of lay women by calling their knowledge 'old wives tales' to diminish its value. A community development approach to public health would use this valuable community resource and incorporate it into a new structure for young parents. The Patchwork community clinic in Edinburgh is a good example of this approach in action.

The Patchwork experience

A group of health visitors in an area of high deprivation in the city were aware that the traditional service they offered to parents was often inadequate and not meeting the complex myriad of needs resulting from economic and social disadvantage. After completing the *Community Development in Primary Care* (Dalziel 1999) training programme run by the author, they decided to work differently.

Following the community development process they ran a series of focus groups to find out what local parents wanted and then worked with them to achieve action for change. They formed a steering group composed of parents, health visitors and representatives from community education and from the local health project. They then moved the baby clinic from the general practice building to the community centre. This shift from buildings that are medically orientated into community centres, where the environment fosters social and community activities, immediately created a more equal partnership and reduced the perceived authority of the health visitor. In this model of shared authority, child rearing is returned to the community where it rightly belongs. Health visiting activities then centre on working with the child-rearing constituency, lay workers and parents, to find out what needs they have, not necessarily by formal needs assessment but by talking to them, forming support groups or organising child-rearing seminars or exchanges in which they are equal participants. Parents are part of the decision-making progress and can dictate what happens in Patchwork.

The Patchwork experience encourages new friendships amongst the women and reduces the isolation that can lead to postnatal depression. It acts as a source of information about what is happening in the community, encourages breastfeeding support groups, and runs parenting groups around issues defined by the parents. These events promote good practice, help parents learn about social relationships, and allow them to get support and help for difficulties from each other. Community education workers involved in the initiative encourage parents to produce their own local leaflets on best child health practice and on sources of support and help locally. The social action resulting from this new structure is currently around antenatal education and breastfeeding. The uptake of traditional parentcraft classes run by health visitors and midwives is very poor. One of the Patchwork volunteers was interested in addressing this issue and is working with a local midwife finding out what women who live in this area want from antenatal education and how they can be involved as peer educators. She has also started, with some other women, a breastfeeding support network. Arguably, this will make as much or more impact on local women as the breastfeeding strategies currently devised within cultural and social vacuums by professionals.

Valuing local expertise and knowledge around something as seminal as child rearing is part of building social capital. The acceptance of lay knowledge and experience alongside professional expertise strengthens partnerships with communities and will ultimately shift patterns of dependency from health professionals and diminish community helplessness.

Child development

Working alongside parents and lay workers in a community-based child-rearing 'clinic' with local parents it would be possible to organise or facilitate a range of child development activities to help parents be the expert in their child's development. It may take several forms, e.g. booklets, seminar-type activities or fun events but local parents would be actively involved in developing information on stages in child development for themselves and other parents. In this paradigm, new parents are encouraged to monitor their child's progression, reporting when something seems not OK, rather than being dependent on the health worker to be the judge of what is normal. Arguably this is what parents, relatives and friends do anyway in their day-to-day contact with a child. Parents could also have open access to other services, child psychology, speech therapy or vision and hearing testing if they decide that they need it. Shifting the responsibility to the parents to judge child progression and changing structures to support this reduces dependency, increases knowledge and confidence, and promotes self esteem.

Child protection

In the preface to her book *The case of Mary Bell* (who was convicted of murder when a child of 10 years old), Gita Sereny says 'The reason such tragedies happen is that there is still too much ignorance within families about how to live and how to love.' It is no accident that vulnerable families living in poverty in poor social circumstances are more often involved in child protection issues. Due to the stress of living with multiple difficulties, children of such families are usually exposed to more harm than more affluent families. Overburdened with debt and lack of money, often experiencing psychological and relationship difficulties, drug or alcohol addiction or mental health problems, many families cannot sustain the support and nourishment necessary for their children's health because of their own needs. The public health agenda would view the development of resources, services and relevant support to respond to such parental need as the way forward. The work of public health nurses mobilising communities, and supporting the development of local resources like credit unions and welfare advice may prevent some of these family relationships breaking down irreparably. Community development concepts applied to child protection issues would view equity in resources and a collective and democratic approach as being more likely to offer the support individuals and communities need than individual home visiting on its own.

Public health workers need to be part of the movement to encourage a shift away from an individual blaming and punishment agenda to one of looking at what communities have and what families in difficult circumstances need to support them. It would offer an opportunity for perpetrators and suspected abusers to be involved in support and training programmes to help them look at their violence and the correct use of their power, and also to harness that knowledge and experience to help others. This is part of building social capital.

Conclusion

The chapter is being written at a time when Hall 4 (Hall and Elliman 2003, Scottish Executive 2004) is being implemented and there is a drive to encourage nurses and other health workers to engage in public health work. Community development training has been undertaken throughout most of the country and, although nurses are keen to work in this way and view the community development approach as an attractive way to engage with communities and address the inequalities within disadvantaged neighbourhoods, it hasn't, to date, quite happened. Health inequalities are quite rightly now high on the agenda of public health but new styles of working, although developing, are also not quite there yet. The use of community development concepts, like joint working and partnership with the community, public involvement in primary care services, addressing equity and inequality issues, collective action and an empowering agenda, will provide primary care staff with the thinking and the methods to work differently.

In time, a community development approach could dismantle the current health care culture and do much to help public health workers undo some of the learning imbued by nurse and other professional training that encourages a separation from the needs of poorer communities. It could challenge the notion that health professionals are the only experts in health and suggest that housing, education or development workers are equally engaged in health improvement. If this way of working became more commonplace, the dominant culture of professionally held power and expertise in health would hopefully give way to a culture of shared authority between health workers and the communities that they serve. It would bring with it the recognition that individuals can be active partners rather than passive recipients in the process of engagement in health improvement. Core work for health staff would shift to involvement and joint working with the community in primary care planning and delivery, a targeted emphasis on resources to address inequalities in health and a reduction in surveillance and policing.

The adoption of this approach is far reaching and offers public health workers a set of principles that will move the profession into a new era in its development. It may be the beginning of the separation of nursing from the shadow of medicine and the emergence of community nurses as autonomous practitioners divorced largely from the medical model and working as public health promoters building social capacity.

This new paradigm for health could see workers no longer constrained by the hierarchical nature of health care but working across professional boundaries to shift the energy and resources from medicine and illness to issues that concern the community at large; accountable for their work and its outcomes to the communities they serve.

Paradigmatic shifts in public health cannot happen in isolation, but need to be supported by major structural change within health organisations. Integration will only happen when the appropriate culture and structures are in place to support the approach. If the community development approach to public health is to be allowed to have the impact it could, it needs to stop being marginal and viewed as an 'add on' to what is perceived as core work. It has been less favoured in the past as a way of working by health workers because it is slow and for a while what is going into it will be largely invisible. It also involves workers shedding the dependent, relatively distant, professional relationship fostered by caseload as core activity and adopting a relationship where working alongside people rather than for them is preferred. It may be that health workers are drawn to fulfilling the caseload remit because it is clearer, more highly valued and, initially, emotionally more rewarding.

Public health workers will need leadership at all levels if it is to achieve this major cultural and organisational change. It needs strong informed leadership at a government level, in health boards and authorities, trusts and at a local level. It will require changes in the professional education curriculum, post registration training, a rethink about student placements and an allocation of resources to make the transition. It needs brave management to gather the lone community development health or project workers in from the margins of health to the centre of public health work. To use their innovation, radical ideas, skills and knowledge and to make their activities central and not an 'extra' that health workers have no time to do. The experience and contacts gained by these workers will form the core of the new curriculum of the future and their skills used to train and support others.

Community development, properly funded and supported with relevant training, offers a way of working for the public health workforce that could have a profound influence on the health improvement agenda and on the shape of nursing and other professions. It can help support the changing relationship between health workers and other agencies, create opportunities to work in partnership with a range of new partners and welcome their support in tackling the health inequalities agenda.

DISCUSSION QUESTIONS

- Does the training of health professionals help or hinder practitioners in developing the public health agenda?
- Should the social determinants of health set the agenda for community health practitioners?
- Is surveillance a relevant component of public health/health visiting?
- Who cares for the children – community or professional relationship?
- Can community health practitioners risk an analysis of existing power?

References

Adams L 1989 Health Cities, healthy participation. Health Education Journal in Community Development and Involvement in Primary Care. Freeman R et al King's Fund 1997

Ashton J, Seymour H 1988 The new public health. Open University Press, Buckingham, UK

Beigal DE 1984 Help seeking and receiving in urban ethnic neighbourhoods: strategies for empowerment. In: Rappaport J, Swift C, Hess R (eds) Studies in empowerment: steps towards understanding and action. Hawthorn Press, New York

Burton P, Harrison L 1997 Identifying local health needs. Policy Press, University of Bristol

Craig P, Lindsay G 2000 Nursing for public health: population-based care. Churchill Livingstone, London

Dalziel Y 1997 Community development in primary care. Unpublished report Edinburgh Health Care NHS Trust, Edinburgh

Dalziel Y 1999 Community development in primary care. Lothian Health, Edinburgh

Dalziel Y, McLachlan S 2000 Preliminary Report of the CHART project. Lothian Health, Edinburgh

Duffy S 1996 Partnerships in action. Health Education Board for Scotland, Edinburgh

Funnel R, Oldfield K, Speller V 1995 Towards healthier alliances. London Health Education Authority

Hall D, Elliman D (eds) 2003 Health for all children, 4th edn. Oxford University Press, Oxford

Jones J 1990 Community Development and Health Education: Concepts and Philosophy, from Roots and Branches Papers from OU/HEA 1990 Winter School on Community Development and Health. Open University Press, Buckingham, UK

Kiefer CH 1983–4 Citizen empowerment: a developmental perspective. Prevention in Human Services 3(23): 9–37

Labonte R 1998 A community development approach to health promotion. Health Education Board for Scotland, Edinburgh

Lukes S 1974 Power; a radical view. Macmillan, London

Marmot M, Wilkinson R (eds) 1999 Social determinants of health Oxford University Press, Oxford

Rappaport J, Swift C, Hess R (eds) 1984 Studies in empowerment: steps towards understanding and action. Hawthorn Press, New York

Schiller PL, Levin JS 1983 Is self-care a social movement? Social Science and Medicine 17: 1343–1352

Sereny G 1998 Cries unheard. The case of Mary Bell. Macmillan, London

Scottish Executive, Women and Children's Health Unit 2004 Health for all children, 4th edn. Guidance on implementation in Scotland, Edinburgh, Scottish Executive. http://www.scotland.gov.uk/consultations/health/hfac.pdf

Scottish Office 1999 Towards a healthier Scotland. HMSO, Edinburgh

Taylor P, Peckham S, Turton P 1988 A public health model of primary care – from concept to reality. Birmingham: Public Health Alliance. Family Practice Vol 16, No. 2, 209–210. © Oxford University Press 1999

Townsend P, Davidson N 1982 Inequalities in health. Penguin, Harmondsworth

Voluntary Activity Unit 1997 Monitoring and evaluation of community development in Northern Ireland. Department of Health and Social Services, Belfort

Wilkinson R 1994 Divided we fall. British Medical Journal 304: 1113–1114

Wilkinson R 1996 Unhealthy societies: the afflictions of inequality. Routledge, New York

World Health Organization (WHO) 1978 Alma Ata 1977. Primary health care. WHO, UNICEF, Geneva

Further reading

Marmot M, Wilkinson RG (eds) 1999 Social determinants of health. Oxford University Press, Oxford

Mackereth C 2006 Community development. New challenges, new opportunities. CPHVA, London

Complex community-based initiatives

6

Anna Houston

Key issues

- The development of complex community-based initiatives (CCIs) in the UK
- Explanation of why the CCI approach is complex
- The components of a CCI approach
- Practice examples from CCIs in the UK
- Lessons from CCIs that community professionals can apply to practice

Introduction

In recent years much has been made of new ways of working in the community to deal with the issues of social exclusion, particularly in isolated, under-resourced areas of the UK. Improving health and t-ackling inequalities by narrowing the gap between social groups has been regarded as a key aspect of New Labour policy (Hunter 2004). One method of achieving this has been to develop community-based initiatives supported by substantial government funding (Hills 2004).

These complex community-based initiatives (CCIs) have been defined as: neighbourhood-based agencies, for local people, employing both lay and professional workers with the aim of providing sustained goal-oriented home (outreach) and centre-based services that offer 'information, guidance and feedback, joint-problem-solving, help with securing entitlements and services, encouragement, and psychological support' (Halpern 1990, p. 470).

Beyond this it was also acknowledged that CCIs varied in size, shape and aims. However, they all had one main goal and that was to promote positive change in the 'individual, family and community circumstances in disadvantaged neighbourhoods by improving physical, economic and social conditions' (Kubisch et al (1995, p. 1). These various elements within a CCI were supposed to be delivered in a devolved way, synergistically offered by different agencies working together across a variety of spheres. This could be: youth development, centre and home-based family support, community planning, housing and benefit support, job training, adult education, mental health care, economic development and employment readiness, life opportunity activities and child-care with many programmes using cross-agency funding to extend these elements inventively.

Policy

Inequality has been described in the literature as 'two, three or even fourfold differences in death rates between social classes' (Wilkinson 1996). Between 1979 and

1997 health inequalities were not raised at all at policy level (Neuberger 2003). Proactive community-based prevention work was a low priority area for government policy development. The Acheson Independent Inquiry (Department of Health (DH) 1998) acted as a kick-start to the incoming Labour administration regarding the inequality debate. The ideal of prevention was resurrected and some importance given to implementation through the role of community-based workers, such as health visitors. The 39 recommendations from the report gave the New Labour administration three priority areas regarded as crucial to improve the health of the less well-off:

1. Evaluate government policies for their impact on health inequalities.
2. A high priority should be given to the health of families with children.
3. Steps should be taken to reduce income inequalities and improve the living standards of poor households.

Government had recognised that improving the nations' health and narrowing the widening gap between social groups provided a challenge in policy making that exceeded any single government department's responsibilities (Hunter 2004). However, there continued to be a focus on 'downstream' issues that gave priority to secondary and acute care rather than the more 'upstream' public health focused, determinants of health issues.

Public health has had a low profile in the UK because of: 1) the power of the medical profession to drive forward a focus on the curative role; 2) the creation of an NHS resolute on the priority of resourcing the acute hospitals; and 3) a scarcity of evidence demonstrating the benefits of public health interventions (Neuberger 2003).

Following the Acheson Inquiry (DH 1998), four types of cross-government initiatives (Neuberger 2003) were developed:

1. *Treasury*: to tackle the underlying inequalities in wealth, such as children's tax credit, working families tax credit, increased child benefit provision, minimum wage and a new childcare strategy.
2. *Complex community-based initiatives:* to give heavily financed and focused help to disadvantaged areas: Sure Start, Healthy Living Centres, New Deal for Communities and Health Action Zones.
3. *NHS:* target-driven programmes associated with policy, such as Saving Lives (DH 1999), addressing mortality and morbidity reduction associated with coronary heart disease, cancer, suicide and accidents; or Choosing Health (DH 2005), focusing on issues such as obesity, substance misuse and the offer of a more personalised service, but crucially, personal responsibility for health was also key. Inequalities targets were developed to address infant mortality and geographical variation in life expectancy.
4. *Better access to health care*: additional monies for NHS in areas with poor health, new personal medical services that would provide primary care in under-resourced areas as well as a new public health role for Primary Care Trusts (PCT) to involve them in health improvement and prevention service provision and planning.

Why bother developing a public health approach or initiating a CCI? Part of the impetus from the government perspective was economic because safer, healthier communities are good for the economy and this prevents a continuing rise in demand for illness services as well as higher rates of absenteeism from work (Neuberger 2003). From an economic perspective, healthy communities attract investment, venture capital and speculation while unhealthy areas don't (Hunter 2004). Wanless (HM Treasury 2004b) added impetus to the process by stating that better public health initiatives significantly impact on the demand for health services. He was concerned that too much emphasis went into 'downstream' NHS acute care provision rather than focusing on 'upstream' initiatives that would improve and sustain health. The population, Wanless suggested, had to be health literate with availability of more useful advice and education so that they could be enabled to make informed choices about their life and their health. A public health approach had the capacity to save the government £30 billion by 2022 (Hunter 2004) because it would keep the focus on a proactive preventive approach to service delivery encouraging wellness maintenance rather than illness support. However, this issue is complex and it has been suggested that it is inadequate to take some of the worst off out of poverty and then assume that inequalities in health will be reduced (Shaw et al 2005).

Sure Start: a CCI

Sure Start (Department of Education and Employment 1999) was a national programme, initially available in England, then rolled out later to Northern Ireland, Scotland and Wales. Information on the slightly different expectations in the four parts of the UK can be accessed via the Sure Start website (see resources list for further information on Sure Start). Like many other CCIs it was designed to tackle the roots of disadvantage and inequity, by addressing policy to prevent social exclusion (Roberts 2000). Sure Start centred its resources and support at the start of life and followed government monitoring, target and evaluation mechanisms (Houston 2003a, 2003b). A special policy team (The Sure Start Unit) managed the new community system, both policy and strategy.

Before any programme is set up to be preventive it is necessary to have an understanding of the phenomena that are to be prevented, and to understand the political elements and the unintended consequences of managing the prevention strategy (Sinclair et al 1997). Early childhood complex community-based initiatives were developed in 1964 in the USA specifically to enrich the pre-school environment and to enhance the development of infants and toddlers with the aim of 'closing the gap between disadvantaged children and their more advantaged peers by raising poor children's levels of social and educational competence' (Brookes-Gunn et al 1994, p. 924).

Sure Start was regarded as a 'two-generation' programme because an important part of its focus was parental involvement as well as child services. Sure Start was developed alongside a raft of different community-based measures, such as Health Action Zones, Healthy Living Centres, New Deal for Communities, the National Strategy for Neighbourhood Renewal and Local Strategic Partnerships, with Connexions, The Children's Fund and, currently, the development and roll-out of Children's Centres (see additional resources) all part of the Labour administration's 'community' drive and commitment to reducing inequalities when it came to power in 1997.

Many of these new community-based organisations brought with them new management systems that existing community structures, both statutory and voluntary, had to somehow plug into. For example, Sure Start and Local Strategic Partnerships (LSP) had many elements in common in their neighbourhood approach. The community-based intervention process for LSP and Sure Start involved developing: a management board structure, often with an executive; a community or parent forum and task-based groupings for topic areas, for example, a Family Support Team (Sure Start) or community safety task group in the LSP structure (Office of the Deputy Prime Minister 2004).

Sure Start as a CCI was based in post-code bounded areas defined as deprived (Department of Education and Employment 1999). Parents who had a child in the 0–4 age group and who were resident in the defined area could access the local programme. Socially impoverished neighbourhoods tend to operate on a scarcity economy, there may be fear of exploitation, or of being beholden to others (Garbarino & Ganzel 2000). Those on the very edge of the margins are socially excluded from the community, reciprocity is distrusted, and neighbourliness fails to flourish. Countering this, with a remit of social inclusion, the Sure Start CCI focus was to be on four main over-arching aspects:

1. Improving social and emotional development.
2. Improving health.
3. Improving the ability to learn.
4. Strengthening families and communities.
   (DH 2002) (see Tables 6.1 and 6.2).

Against a backdrop of international commitment to early years development, UK government planning from 1997 onwards, particularly in the wake of the Acheson Report (DH 1998), involved: children's services, remediation of child poverty and family support (HM Treasury 2004a, Lloyd 2000, Wainwright 1999). Additionally there was a focus on equality of opportunity to paid employment, education and training (Wainwright 1999). In poor neighbourhoods the type of support from family, friends and services is more likely to be fragmented, narrow

Table 6.1 ● Sure Start aims at government level

Aim	Provision
Better access to early education and play	Two generational (involve parents as well as children)
Use of evidence-based practice	Non-stigmatising (avoid the label 'problem families')
Better health services for children	Multi-faceted in approach (education as well as health)
Increased support and advice on family issues	Persistent (last long enough to make a difference)
Empowered communities where change is locally led (by parents)	Locally driven: based on consultation and involvement of parents and local communities
	Culturally appropriate and sensitive to the needs of parents and children

Table 6.2 ● Sure Start at government level (from DH 2002)

Objectives	Themed areas
Improving social and emotional development	Outreach and home visiting
Strengthening families and communities	Support for families and parents
Improving health	Play, learning and children
Improving the ability to learn	Primary and community health care
	Special needs support
	Building community involvement
	Management and evaluation
	Smoking cessation and community participation scheme
	Employability link
	Promoting a learning environment (DH 2002)

and difficult to access (Hanson & Carta 1995). Sure Start would counter this by providing care that was:

- two generational (involving parents as well as children, centre-based and outreach)
- non-stigmatising (avoiding the label 'problem families')
- multi-faceted in approach (education as well as health)
- persistent (lasting long enough to make a difference)
- locally driven: based on consultation and involvement of parents and local communities
- culturally appropriate and sensitive to the needs of parents and children.

A substantial amount of research existed, including a 'review of reviews' demonstrating that early intervention benefited disadvantaged and 'at-risk' children, improving cognitive, language, motor and socio-emotional development as well as improving family functioning (Casto & Mastropeiri 1986). Results from the methodologically strongest studies also demonstrated substantial positive long-term effects from early childhood intervention support that were able to go beyond baseline measurement techniques (Gomby et al 1995).

A key feature of the UK government's approach was that 'joined-up' social problems demanded 'joined-up' solutions (Hunter 2004). Sure Start would have the support of the:

- *Treasury*: income transfer policies such as tax credits, and the Sure Start maternity grant
- *Department for Education and Skills*: developing a strategy for childcare, and also the Neighbourhood Nursery Initiative (NNI) (the Sure Start programme was facilitated by the Department for Education and Skills through the Sure Start Unit)
- *Social Exclusion Unit* with neighbourhood renewal (Cabinet Office 2000)
- *Home Office:* focusing on family policies (Glass 2001, Home Office 1998).

The government promoted public health through a proactive interventionist approach aimed at helping families and communities, particularly in deprived areas. The role of Sure Start (Table 6.1 and 6.2) within the existing pre-school UK structure was to enhance, develop and support organisations in the community already offering pre-school activity. Sure Start was also charged with developing more and better childcare facilities, e.g. crèche support, to allow parents to train and to return to the workforce as part of an employability anti-poverty drive. Good-quality, out-of-home day care for children has been shown to have a positive impact on the cognitive development of the child (Campbell & Ramey 1994, Schweinhart 2003, Schweinhart et al 1993).

Stress and social support are ecological influences that impact on parenting and child development, particularly in high-risk populations. Informal professional support was positively linked to increased maternal satisfaction with parenting (Crnic et al 1986) and the level of support offered to parents during the first 2 years of life was a predictor of the child's increased cognitive functioning at aged 5 years (Crnic & Stormshak 1997).

Ongoing policy commitment to a child-centred approach

In the late 1990s, government policy demonstrated strong commitment to community, family and child-focused policy initiatives. Documents such as *Every child*

133

matters (Department for Education and Skills 2004) supported early intervention to support parents alongside professional integration and 'joined-up' services. The policy aim was:

- supporting parents and carers
- early intervention and effective protection
- accountability and integration – locally, regionally and nationally
- workforce reform.

There were five key outcomes for children and young people in *Every child matters*: be healthy, stay safe, enjoy and achieve, make a positive contribution and achieve economic well-being. The report stated that:

'The government has built the foundations for improving these outcomes through Sure Start'

(Department for Education and Skill 2004: section 11).

The aim of improving the lives and health of children and pregnant women was part of the recent policy strategy; this would be done by setting standards for health and local authority service provision (DH 2004). In the new standard-setting – National Service Framework for Children Young People and Maternity Services (DH 2004) (see additional resources list), there were to be a number of elements aimed at better integration and co-ordination between agencies:

'The Children Act 2004 provides the legislative foundation for whole-system reform to support this long-term and ambitious programme. It outlines new statutory duties and clarifies accountabilities for children's services. But legislation by itself is not enough: it needs to be part of a wider process of change.'

(*Every child matters: change for children* 2004).

Explaining the complexity of CCIs

Part of the complexity within these community systems is 'vertical': attempting to make change at individual, family and community levels and pre-supposing that interaction between these three levels already exists (Kubisch et al 1995). Community-based interventions are 'heterogeneous and complex' and are, therefore, about creating a shift of rationale from a top-down professional agenda to a bottom-up community involvement approach (Hills 2004). Additionally, a 'horizontal' complexity can be created by bringing statutory and voluntary organisations into the new structure, along with their own management systems (e.g. in Sure Start) where each partner organisation manages workers that they 'second' into the new system:

'...most of the government's attempts to address inequality and disadvantage...have involved complex cross-sectoral long-term initiatives that rely on action by local partnerships to put national policies into practice.'

(Coote 2003, p. 16)

This complexity within CCIs has been examined to reveal a number of important issues such as:

- a macro-economic climate that militates against community capacity building
- a dynamic and constantly changing intervention highly responsive to neighbourhood voices

- broad outcomes that are difficult to measure and operationalise, such as 'empowerment' and 'community capacity building'
- absence of a comparator area leading to the question: Is the change the result of the intervention or would it have occurred anyway (Kubisch et al 1995)?

The complexity of the many-levelled, multi-layered structure leads to lack of clarity about what is being evaluated and, therefore, difficulty in establishing any link between the input and output (Hills 2004).

Seven further degrees of complexity (from the findings of Health Action Zones) have been highlighted (Barnes et al 2003):

- *Levels:* the complexity of input and management at different levels involving different local organisations.
- *Time:* measurable improvements in health status can take 10 years or more to achieve. Initial acceptance of a long-term process can give way to short-term political imperatives requiring achievement of government targets rather than locally determined strategies.
- *Scope:* overlaying intervention on existing mechanisms can mean blurring of the boundaries of where the intervention begins and ends.
- *Players:* the breadth of the intervention can involve a wide range of players with different levels of power and interest in the intervention affecting the eventual outcomes.
- *Strategies and models*: when the intervention is wide-reaching the use of different and sometimes competing models or theories can lead to difficulty in concluding exactly 'what works'.
- *Rules and conditions*: governing bodies can promise flexibility and freedom at the outset that can fail to be realised coupled with the imperative of targets and working with partners who have varying degrees of formal and informal governance systems.
- *The problem context*: (the example of Health Action Zones) there can be limitations associated with the ways in which different theoretical frameworks (e.g. social constructionist, complexity theory, new institutional theory) can assist in understanding both the processes and outcomes associated with complex initiatives.

Finally, Judge and Bauld (2001, p. 24), from the viewpoint of evaluating Health Action Zones, stated that complex community-based initiatives have multiple broad goals:

- They are highly complex learning enterprises with multiple strands of activity operating at many different levels.
- Objectives are defined and strategies chosen to achieve goals that change over time.
- Many activities and intended outcomes are difficult to measure.
- In open systems it is virtually impossible to control all the variables that may influence the conduct and outcome of the evaluation.

This complexity of the system results in a process that is 'more value driven than evidence based' (Coote 2003, p. 16). Experience (from US-based CCIs) identified that agreeing upon long-term outcomes was straightforward because they are often broad and uncontroversial. The interim outcomes pose more difficulty because both scientific and experiential knowledge about the links between early, intermediate and long-term outcomes is undeveloped in the area of complex interventions. The hardest part of the process is in defining interim activities and outcomes and then being able to link those aspects to the longer-term outcomes (Connell & Kubisch 1998). Table 6.3 demonstrated this issue by showing some of the unexpected long-term outcomes in the longitudinal follow-up of US CCIs, and additionally

Table 6.3 ● US major experimental studies reporting pre-school early intervention programme outcomes

Study	Type	Interveners	Participants	Measures	Outcomes	Extended outcomes/ issues
1. The Perry Preschool Study (Schweinhart et al 1993) five cohorts between 1962 and 1965 High Scope Research Foundation Longitudinal study	Curriculum-based preschool 5 days per week, For 2.5 hours per day For 2 years before school entry Plus supportive teacher home visits	Teaching staff Piagetian approach where children are regarded as active learners	123 black youths, from low-income families with IQs below 90	Emphasis on child-initiated learning: i) scholastic success ii) socio-economic success iii) social responsibility Participant review at 19 and again at 27 years of age	Attendees were more likely: 1. to attend school 2. to graduate 3. to gain employment 4. to go to college 5. to be self-supporting 6. to be socially responsible in adulthood There was less: 1. teenage pregnancy 2. crime 3. welfare dependence (Schweinhart et al 1985)	Cost benefit analysis results: savings on the initial investment = three and a half times the cost of 2 years of preschool and seven times the cost of 1 year of preschool (Schweinhart et al 1985) Follow-up at 19 years and 27 years of age
2. Chicago Child and Parent Centers (Fuerst & Fuerst 1993) Six centres, 12-year follow-up Federal funding through	High quality preschool education, parent involvement, and support, smaller class sizes and an intensely structured	Teaching staff	680 inner city children A high proportion received 4 years of early intervention	i) Scholastic success ii) Facilitate parent involvement in children's education	Attendees showed 1. improvement in both reading and math scores by the 8th grade 2. more likelihood	The cost of maintaining children in this type of intervention was twice that of regular school placement.

Programme / study	Intervention	Participants	Aims	Findings	Follow-up
education Longitudinal study	preschool learning programme, for 3 year olds to first grade in school			of graduating through a higher rate of school completion 3. lower rates of school drop-out 4. lower use of special education services (Reynolds et al 2001)	Follow-up at 12 years Significant improvement in the educational results of young black girls with the 4-year programme
3. Syracuse University Family Research Programme (Honig & Lally 1982) University experiment (5 years) Longitudinal study	Child development trainers (paraprofessionals trained to work with families) Extensive home visiting, child care, health, nutrition and social services programme prenatally until school entry	108 families: participants were single parents with a mean age of 18 years, the majority of families were very deprived and Black	i) Cognitive development and intellectual ability ii) 'Maximise family functioning'	1. No scholastic difference on school entry 2. Improved socio-emotional functioning 3. Significant difference in reduced delinquency rates, seriousness of offences and cost of crime 4. Little impact on income and career advancement of families	Reduction of delinquency was an unexpected successful by-product of the other achievements (Zigler et al 1992) Participants expressed more positive feelings about themselves, took an active part in solving problems and saw schooling as a vital part of life (Lally et al 1988) 10 year follow-up: 1. long-term positive impact of school functioning of girls 2. improved family unity 3. increased pride in their children

(Continued)

Table 6.3 ● (Continued)

Study	Type	Interveners	Participants	Measures	Outcomes	Extended outcomes/issues
4. Houston Parent Child Development Center (PCDC) (Johnson 1990) There were matched studies in two other Development Centres: Birmingham Alabama serving black and white families and New Orleans serving black families (Halpern & Larner 1988). University experiment (2 years)	Parent child education programme Included children aged 1–3 years 550 hours of participation from the families involved: twice-monthly home visits, from 12 months, for the first year Attendance at the centre in the second year for parent classes Centre sessions: three 1-hour sessions 4 days per week Twice-monthly evening meetings for both parents	Multi-disciplinary approach	97 mother–child pairs Low-income Mexican American families	Aim: foster the development of competence in young children by helping parents become effective teachers of their young children: i) scholastic success ii) foster intellectual and social competence	1. Little initial difference 2. Later primary education scores were significantly higher on reading, language and vocabulary scales 3. Significant reductions in child behaviour problems 4. Lower rate of disruptive behaviour at age 8–11 (Johnson 1990)	Improvements in mothers' use of affection, praise, criticism and restrictive control Less use of critical language 53% level of attrition in the experimental group

Programme	Description	Approach	Sample	Aims	Outcomes	
5. The Carolina Abecedarian Project (Campbell & Ramey 1994) University experiment (from infancy to age 8 years) Longitudinal study	(Halpern & Larner 1988) Family weekend activities; Nutritional supplements; Social services support and a curriculum-based preschool programme with an emphasis on language development	Multi-disciplinary approach; Low child–teacher ratio; Year-round programme, with transportation from 7.30 am to 5.30pm each weekday for 5 years; Four cohorts of children in centre-based study	57 infants from low-income families	i) Cognitive and fine motor development ii) Social, adaptive and language skills iii) Gross motor skills	1. Significantly higher scores on cognitive development 2. Significantly higher at age 8 years in math and reading 3. Less grade retention (less likely to be held back a year)	Follow-up at 12 and 15, 21 years Maintained academic achievements and enhanced performance in adulthood Delayed parenthood Maternal further education
6. Project CARE (a second-generation Abecedarian project) 54-month study	Centre and home-based comparison study of early intervention. (family education component in the home setting – weekly home visits)	Multi-disciplinary approach	Low-income families 25 families in home only group 16 families in the centre plus home group	Foster positive child development and encourage parents to meet their own needs for information, support and resources	Centre plus home visits showed significant positive result No effects for the home-only group It has been suggested (Farran 2000) that the family education home visiting component had a negative effect on the progress of the child	

(Continued)

Table 6.3 ● (Continued)

Study	Type	Interveners	Participants	Measures	Outcomes	Extended outcomes/issues
7. Yale Welfare Research Programme Pregnancy until infant is 30 months	Home visits Paediatric care and house-calls when necessary High-quality day care Regular child development assessments	Multi-disciplinary approach	High-risk minority families, low-income, deprived area Mothers of first-born infants	To improve the bonds between parents and their offspring Better social and school adjustment for children	Project children had less absenteeism Greater maternal involvement in child's education	10-year follow-up Mothers continued their education Families were self-supporting Intervention boys were better socially adjusted and displayed positive classroom behaviour Project children had better academic achievement Smaller family size Siblings also demonstrated better school attendance, progress and less remedial help

some of the failures of high early input with poor longer-term outcomes; both features examined in depth elsewhere (Karoly et al 1998).

However, the problem is compounded by a lack of explanation of how the intended and unintended consequences occurred. It has been established that most CCIs do not easily lend themselves to scientific measurement:

> '...they are messy and indeterminate, their impact on illness and mortality rates is often indirect, and they may not show any clear results within the lifetime of a single parliament.'
>
> (Neuberger 2003, p. 9)

Re-orienting community-based services was about developing collaboration between the statutory, voluntary and community sectors (Heenan 2004). Providing multi-faceted services in UK CCIs was also about targeting the wider determinants of health at a local level by providing new mechanisms to reach out to the excluded or marginalised in the community, such as HAZ, Sure Start or Healthy Living Centres. Additionally, the focus was on altering access to services for those most in need to assist their health improvement. These structures provided opportunities for: 1) local consultation processes; 2) improved gateways to information and advice on benefits, welfare and employment; and 3) re-designing local health services to enable people to engage in building and sustaining the capacity of their own local community.

It was thought that formal non-CCI services were less responsive or able to fulfil the task of reaching out and offering the consultative, sustained, non-stigmatising, multi-faceted support needed to encourage the wellbeing of young families in particular. The argument was that informal systems like CCIs could encourage and involve people at the grass-roots level to give opportunities to and to develop local potential in community members, who would then be enabled to sustain their community in the long term.

As inequalities endured, with a growing gap between rich and poor, the disparity between those with different amounts of 'potential' for good health was highlighted (Bartley 2004). Without help, some were destined to lead a less privileged, socially excluded life. Could CCI programmes developed within the informal local system in the community (such as Sure Start or HAZ) help and somehow confer on people an 'ability to manage their consumption, leisure and use of health services in a more health-promoting manner' (Bartley 2004, p. 10).

Examples from practice Sure Start: 1

This study example from practice addressed quantitative measurement and qualitative approaches to access local information from consumers about changed service provision. The 'traditional' community midwifery service was changed to a Sure Start Service (with some supportive local midwifery service NHS Trust funding) to a new 24-hour, 7 days a week midwifery service provided by five dedicated Sure Start midwives who were also involved in running a breastfeeding Baby Café and providing proactive advice, support and information (Houston & Bennett 2004).

Tables 6.4 and 6.5 illustrate the difference made to the community by the impact of Sure Start team midwifery in one area. The national and regional statistics show a consistently high caesarean section and instrumental delivery rate in comparison with the team midwifery approach. Comparison of pre-Sure-Start area statistics with post-Sure-Start data showed a trend towards lower rates in caesarean section, instrumental delivery and episiotomy with a corresponding positive increase in the level of normal delivery.

Additionally, qualitative responses were examined in detail in order to make further changes to the new system after it had been running for the first year. One

Table 6.4 ● Comparison of national local and Sure Start Statistics 2002–2003

Type of intervention	National statistics 2002–2003	London region statistics 2002–2003	Local statistics hospital 2002–2003	Sure Start team midwifery June 2002–May 2003
Normal delivery	67% (20% inductions)	65%	67%	75%
Caesarean section	22% (10% elective)	23.3%	20%	13.5%
Instrumental deliveries	11%	11.3%	12%	11%
Episiotomy (in normal deliveries)	13%	12%	11%	6%
Epidural	21%	–	–	5.3%

(DH 2004) NHS Maternity Statistics, England: 2002–2003 published March 2004 & Local Sure Start Team Midwifery Statistics (data subject to rounding and totals may not agree)

Table 6.5 ● Comparison of local Sure Start area statistics

Type of intervention	Sure Start area/ pre-Sure Start June 2001–May 2002	Sure Start team midwifery June 2002–May 2003
Normal delivery	69.5%	75%
Caesarean section	16.5%	13.5%
Instrumental deliveries	14%	11%
Episiotomy (in normal deliveries)	9.2%	6%
Epidural	18.2%	5.3%

client summed up the meaning of the change echoed by many on the new Sure Start system:

> 'I just feel that the care was so good I felt it was like BUPA or something like that. It was so good you thought you would have to pay extra for it.'

With some adjustments, the service is still running, and continues to be very well regarded by local women. This type of service provision meets the policy aim of a more personalised, choice-driven service. Mainstreaming this particular Sure Start example, to a wider area beyond the Sure Start patch, is complex because of issues associated with: continued funding when the Sure Start funding stops, staffing and recruitment issues within the midwifery profession, and recent hospital access boundary re-drawing where the main midwifery service unit will be further away from the local community.

Examples from practice in Sure Start: 2

A Sure Start programme wanted to find out if it had improved the quality of speech and language provision through working in a more multi-agency way, and at the same time altered access to service provision at community level.

The Sure Start Speech and Language Therapy Team aimed to impact on *access* and *speed of referral* using as their tools *flexibility* and *home-visiting*. The shift to a proactive preventive model meant that children were seen by the Sure Start speech therapist at an earlier point in time.

The documentary analysis (Houston & Parker 2005) addressed specific factors that could be used as a comparator in some ways between what had existed before and the new CCI Sure Start system. The factors highlighted were:

- Total number of children who failed to attend for initial assessment at the speech and language clinic.
- Total number of children appointed for initial speech and language assessment.
- Total number of children assessed at the speech and language clinic and placed on a further waiting list for implementation of their care plan.
- Total number of children assessed and discharged from the service.
- Total number of children not yet assessed where the parent contacted to say they were unable to attend the assessment.

Although the data sets available were not an exact comparative match, there was enough information to examine trends that could help the Sure Start programme to look at quality and review provision and access. It also allowed the Sure Start programme to look at the pre- and post-Sure-Start speech and language service delivery locally. Additionally, the speech and language management system wanted to know what elements (in the new system) 'worked' prior to mainstreaming decisions regarding absorption of innovative practice into the forthcoming Children's Centre system.

Table 6.6 showed that following referral into the system, 56.2% ($n = 296$) of children offered initial speech and language assessment appointments did not attend for initial assessment. Of this initial 56.2% of children, 28.52% ($n = 150$) of parents simply didn't turn up. A further 27.76% ($n = 146$) of those in this 'not yet assessed' category, contacted the service to say they were unable to attend the appointment given and, although re-appointed, a portion of this same 27.76% never returned to the service for any attention (specific numbers 'never returning' to the service were not available).

Aside from the initial assessment waiting list (3 months), there were 36.88% ($n = 194$) of children on the second waiting list (around 6–9 months wait for implementation of their care plan following initial assessment). Only 6.8% ($n = 36$) of children were discharged from the service following the initial assessment. This last figure is in some ways a tribute to the quality of the initial screening system (carried out predominantly by the health visitor). This demonstrated that following referral from another professional (the health visitor) the majority of cases could be deemed 'true' appropriate cases requiring remedial support and care from the speech and language therapist.

These data demonstrated that based on the overall quality of 'true' referrals present, a high number who needed help never came back. Failure to access the service early means that:

- the child will enter the treatment system later (probably at school entry)
- the child will need remedial help requiring time away from lessons
- late-stage diagnosis of the problem may mean it is more difficult to treat
- more speech therapy input increases the cost of late-stage treatment
- speech and language delay impacts on literacy and future learning.

Table 6.6 ● Waiting list and DNA data for one speech and language clinic-based service in the local area (22-month period) 2002–2004 (from North 2005)

Month	Total appointed	Did not arrive	Through to 2nd waiting list	Discharged	Unable to attend
Sep-04	16	4	9	2	1
Aug-04	8	5	2	1	0
Jul-04	25	6	11	2	6
Jun-04	25	10	8	2	5
May-04	27	6	12	4	5
Apr-04	26	6	17	3	0
Mar-04	35	7	19	1	8
Feb-04	29	7	13	0	9
Jan-04	17	4	9	0	4
Dec-03	25	7	10	1	7
Nov-03	28	7	7	4	10
Oct-03	27	6	12	3	6
Sep-03	20	3	7	0	10
Aug-03	25	6	11	0	8
Jul-03	16	3	8	1	4
Jun-03	11	4	3	0	4
May-03	34	15	7	2	10
Apr-03	14	6	4	0	4
Mar-03	28	8	7	0	13
Feb-03	34	15	2	4	13
Dec-02	16	6	6	0	4
Nov-02	40	9	10	6	15
Total	526	150	194	36	146
Percentage		28.52%	36.88%	6.84%	27.76%

Included in these data were a small number of children above 4 years, time constraints precluded extrapolation of this small but additional constituency

One speech therapist spoke about making the change to the new Sure Start system:

'…it was really scary coming from clinic [caseload based] where you are literally running chasing your tail, 60 in that school 40 in that school, into Sure Start where there was no-one to see at first because it was a shift to preventive work. It was a very different situation to be in. Right from the start we decided that prevention was the way to go.'

Respondent G. FG2 (Houston & Parker 2005)

Table 6.7 shows the Sure Start totals of 124 children who were seen by the Sure Start Speech and Language team (just over 1 whole-time equivalent in staffing hours). Assessment on the community waiting list (non-Sure-Start) was driven by the 'target to be seen': within 13 weeks (but this is often longer). In the non-Sure-Start system the delay between assessment and introduction of the therapy (the time on the second waiting list) was 9 months. This made the entire process a 12-month experience for the family, in the (non-Sure-Start) clinic-based traditional system, if they were able to stay the course.

Table 6.7 ● Sure Start speech and language therapy services statistics (25-month period) 2003–2005 (from North 2005)

Date	Ref	Seen 1 week	Seen 2 weeks	Seen 4 weeks	Therapy offered	Contact: continued attempts	Advice & discharge	Other
Feb-05	2	2			1		1	
Jan-05	4	4			1		3	
Dec-04	1	1						1MOA
Nov-04	8	6	2		3	3	1	1 drop-in given
Oct-04	6	3	2	1	4		1	1
Sept-04	3	2	1		2			1 R&A
Aug-04	5	4	1		2	1	2	2 R&A
Jul-04	3	3			2			
Jun-04	4	2	1	1	2		1	1A&R
May-04	7	4	3		5		1	1A&R
Apr-04	5	1	2	2	5			
Mar-04	7	5	1	1	1	2	2	2A&R
Feb-04	5	5			2			1 joint visit P&E 2A&R
Jan-04	5	5			3	1		1 A&R
Dec-03	5	2	3		1		1	3A&R
Nov-03	8	5	3		3		1	4 A&R
Oct-03	5		2	3	3			2A&R
Sep-03	6	5		1	3		3	
Aug-03	4	2	2		1	1	1	1A&R
Jul-03	4	4			1			2A&R
Jun-03	2	2					1	1A&R
May-03	5		5		2		2	1A&R
Apr-03	11	6	4	1	7		2	
Mar-03	4	3	1		3		1	
Feb-03	5	3	2		2	2	1	2 followed up: community stammering team
Total	124	79	35	10	60	9	26	30
Percentage		63.7	28.2	8	46.5	7.2	20.9	24

MOA: moved out of area; A&R: advice and review; R&A: review and advice; P&E: play and education

The difference, or the impact of the Sure Start service was illustrated by the 124 children referred into the Sure Start Speech and Language system where:

- 63.7% of children were seen for assessment within *1 week* with an immediate instigation of remediation work offered, if required
- a further 28.2% were seen *within 2 weeks*
- the remaining 8% were seen *within 4 weeks* of referral.

In the Sure Start system it was found that there was no initial wait for assessment and no second waiting list between assessment and remediation. In practice this meant that 92% of children were seen within 2 weeks of referral into the Sure Start system. A very high number of those same children began their remediation support programme straight away. This change was made possible because, at the outset, the Sure Start Speech and Language team made a conscious decision to develop a personal, flexible service within a multi-agency frame. This focused on reducing the level of circulating paper, such as appointment letters and forms, and instead increased telephone and face-to-face personal contact (Houston & Parker 2005).

Box 6.1

A note on data collection at grass-roots level

Very often, practitioners are paralysed into inertia because of the 'not good enough' data or the 'can't get data' debate. Both of these examples presented here, with their flaws, are data sets of 'what was available' offered by two sets of very busy practitioners who were able to say 'this is what I have already in the local system, what can we do with it, what does it show?' Both 'real world' data examples are useful in providing very local situational evidence of the meaning of the change and they show trends that can guide practitioners and managers in taking important next steps. However, if as a practitioner you do not collect any data, then even useful trends can be difficult to discern.

Health Action Zones (HAZ) CCIs

Health Action Zones were established in 1998. They were to be trailblazers for modernisation based on a number of principles (McKinnon et al 2001) these were:

1. *Achieving equity:* reduce health inequalities, promote equality of access to services and improve equity in resource allocation.
2. *Engaging communities:* involve the public in planning services, empower service users and patients to take responsibility for their own health and decisions about their care.
3. *Working in partnership:* recognise that people receive services from a range of different agencies and that these services need to be co-ordinated to achieve the maximum benefit.
4. *Engaging front-line staff:* involve staff in developing and implementing strategy, develop flexible and responsive organisations, encourage and support innovation in service delivery.
5. *Taking an evidence-based approach:* develop a more structured, evidence-based approach for service planning and delivery as well as application of effective procedures and interventions.
6. *Developing a person-centred approach:* develop services around the needs of people and deliver them as close to people as appropriate.

7. *Taking a whole-systems approach:* recognise that health, social and other services are interdependent and need to be planned and organised on a whole system basis to deliver seamless care and tackle the wider determinants of health.

Service provision has gone through various stages: *separatism* where each agency delivers their own contribution in isolation, *competition* where separate purchasing providers are in competition with each other and *partnership* where collaborative working is the ideal (Hudson 2005). Most recent CCIs have been driven by the need for professionals to work together and to integrate towards a 'whole' systems approach and to include, in some way, the members of the local community.

The Health Action Zone initiative (another type of CCI) was one of the first to be set up when the Blair administration came to power in 1997. A total of 26 HAZ were set up between 1998 and 2001. This covered a population of 13 million people in 34 health authorities and 73 local authority areas. They were aimed at delivering services through innovation and collaboration. They were focused in areas of high deprivation, serving populations that ranged in size from 180 000 to nearly 1.5 m people. A Health Action Zone was a partnership between the NHS, local authorities and the voluntary and private sector. Key to this new innovative process (similar to the ideals in Sure Start) was the involvement of local community members. The aim was to improve the health of the community and reduce persistent health inequalities by delivering appropriate interventions at a local level (Barnes et al 2003).

This was a new approach to public health work. The aim was to provide resources to link health, employment, regeneration, housing, education, and anti-poverty initiatives in an effort to respond to the needs of vulnerable groups in under-resourced communities. HAZ were to be the key 'catalyst' towards encouraging existing organisations to innovate, work together, and remove barriers to community development.

Examples from practice HAZ: 3

Many HAZ projects developed local plans designed to improve health and modernise local services within a health authority area. They addressed areas of focus within the seven HAZ principles and were able to develop cross-sectoral partnership-based plans. All of the initial HAZ plans were strong on problem identification and also on formulation of long-term aims. Some HAZ CCIs were able to identify routinely available statistical indicators that could be used to monitor progress (Judge & Bauld 2001).

The Merseyside example of St Helens and Knowsley HAZ is an example of cross-sectoral partnership planning. Its aim was to 'reduce health inequalities across the region; narrowing the gap between the least and most healthy, as well as improving the well-being and quality of life for all people'. The web-based information for local people showed the 'Health Plan for: physical activity, employment, housing, healthy eating, teenage pregnancy and rehabilitation'. The website (see additional resources information) had a variety of local authority, local area and health-related links for community members, such as this example, 'Sleepnet – everything you wanted to know about sleeping disorders, but were too tired to ask: http://www.sleepnet.com'.

The Merseyside HAZ received annual funding and had four goals that were to address specific challenges. The partners in the five districts had targets, outcomes and indicators to measure progress and success (see Table 6.8). It seemed, with the development of HAZ and other CCIs, that 'population-based, system level interventions that focus on competency building and the promotion of protective factors' were now considered to be 'suitable alternatives to the deficit-oriented medical model' (Nelson et al 2001, p. 654).

Table 6.8 ● An example of Health Action Zone goal planning

Goal 1	Reducing levels of poor health, preventable death, impairment and disability	NHS focused: promote increased access to quality services, assist people in management of common illness, expand the role of health care professionals, such as health visitors, pharmacists engage in dealing with ill health, violence and accidents caused by alcohol
Goal 2	Promoting healthy employment opportunities	Regeneration and employment focused: support measures that can increase employability Improve the employment and training prospects of young people and marginalised groups Promote healthier workplaces
Goal 3	Increasing the proportion of people who have an active independent life	Provide better services to prevent loss of independence and opportunity for older people and other excluded groups Support individuals following major illness Promote local community transport initiatives to reduce isolation felt by excluded groups in the community
Goal 4	Enhancing quality of life	Address the concerns of local communities through transport, environmental improvements, housing and community safety initiatives Promote community development through projects that befriend focus on healthy living and self-help initiatives Encourage access to affordable healthy food and support healthy eating for all age-groups

Based on Merseyside Health Action Zone

Criticisms of the CCI approach

Complex community-based initiatives are not without critics, who believe that the empirical case for intensive family preservation services has yet to be made because of failure in evaluative rigour (Gelles 2001). CCIs are 'hard to evaluate because of their size and the speed with which they are being rolled out, and because they are trying to address multiple problems within shifting political environments' (Coote et al 2004, p. 48). They are not operationalised in a consistent way, making comparison of 'like with like' problematic (Ritchie et al 2004, p. 52). They have all 'been inspired by ideas of what should happen rather than any certainty about what would happen' (Coote 2003, p. 16).

Also, in a climate of research contention, it takes political will to redirect scarce resource into intensive services, even if they prove later to be a cost-effective use of money (Utting et al 1993). The intervention itself is often evolving alongside any evaluation being undertaken. Within this complex system the potential exists for interventions to do 'harm as well as good' (Judge & Bauld 2001, p. 19), as shown in Table 6.3 (page 136). Mindick (1988) cautioned against CCIs that were poor in quality and resulted in disempowering individuals instead of giving people a sense of self worth in their lives.

Sure Start was offered to communities with a 10-year funding stream that, although designed to gradually diminish by 2008, offered some stability, and time for some element of change to occur as the roll-over into Children's Centres was anticipated. For other examples, such as the Healthy Living Centres (HLC) (funded through the Big Lottery Fund) there was little contingency funding to carry them beyond a 2007/8 cut-off from their funding stream and with financial uncertainty in Primary Care Trusts, many HLC programmes, however worthwhile, have experienced great difficulty in mainstreaming their proactive preventive work into the PCT or local authority agendas.

Alongside this problem, because this type of intervention is without precedent, it is often the case that the people who commission and contribute to the evaluation process 'lack appropriate experience' (Coote et al 2004, p. 48) or 'knowledge, skills and other resources to document the unfolding intervention or interpret findings in a political context' (Fawcett et al 2003, p. 32). HAZ programmes, for example, have been criticised for lack of clear, logical pathways linking problems, strategies, milestones or targets that were associated with long-term outcomes or goals; they were not good at 'filling in the gap between problems and goals' (Judge & Bauld 2001, p. 21).

What are the components of intensive community-based work?

Short-term benefits of CCIs, particularly those with a preschool focus, tend to be developmental in nature, such as increased cognitive ability, whereas long-term benefits of early childhood interventions have been shown to be social in nature (Karoly et al 1998), for example, economic independence in adulthood (Schweinhart & Weikart 1993). Children need:

- appropriate environmental nutrients at each and every stage
- support services that are present for a significant part of the growing years
- an intervention that targets the ecology in which children are raised as well as offering educational tasks in a preschool setting (Zigler & Styco 2001).

It is important that services are family centred and matched to the needs of local people, and there needs to be a better understanding of the use of high-quality services (Oberklaid et al 2003). Olds et al (1997) demonstrated that high levels of home visiting support resulted in fewer subsequent children, families spent less time on government welfare and there was less maternal arrest and conviction. Early intervention models must be more flexible and able to cope with a wider diversity of need and of service delivery system (Richmond & Ayoub 1993).

Therefore the key messages from successful CCIs are:

- partnership with users is important
- the initiative should be sited within the neighbourhood
- there should be respect and understanding for issues of race and culture
- interagency/interdisciplinary co-operation is important
- creative and responsive services attending to outreach and engagement
- clarity about child protection issues (Pinkerton & Katz 2003).

Predictors of delinquency reviewed by Farringdon (1996) were poor parenting, childhood anti-social behaviour, parental and sibling offending, low educational attainment, low intelligence and separation from parents. For children most at risk in society, interventions that reduce isolation and nurture interpersonal relationships can have a positive effect on child wellbeing (Runyan et al 1998). Dunst et al (1986), in their work with families who have children with special needs, demonstrated that social support and social networks were a mediating factor in personal wellbeing for families, additionally supportive connections for mothers, predicted less perceived difficulty in helping their child to develop social skills (Melson et al 1993). A number of positive components of good-quality early childhood CCIs (Schweinhart et al 1993) involved:

- active learning curricula for children
- staff trained in early childhood education
- effective management with systems for in-service training of staff and supervisory support
- partnership working between staff and parents with extensive outreach to parents at least monthly.

Community involvement and family support are integral to the optimal development of the child (Blackman 2002). At least two competing models of intervention exist for children. The traditional model aims to remediate the pathological deficits in the individual child, whereas the ecological one concentrates on mediating the effects of poor environment by strengthening the protective factors in the child's world (Quiery et al 2003). It has been shown, in a population-based study, that social and environmental factors play an important role in the social, physical and cognitive development of children (To et al 2001). An effective preschool programme, therefore, must involve the family as a whole and not just the child, because parental participation is crucial (Zigler & Styco 2001).

Lessons learned in CCIs suggest that parents like:

- services that are easy to understand and use
- flexible staff who are able to respond to unexpected demands
- staff who have time to build a trusting relationship with community members
- the child being seen as a member of the family and the family as a member of the community
- enthusiastic leadership with clear aims for the CCI
- continuity of service staff and provision in the CCI.
  (Sinclair et al 1997).

Is there a public health role for community practitioners in a CCI?

What is to become of 'traditional' community services in this new world of CCIs, particularly with the arrival of Children's Centres as a one-stop shop, next step to Sure Start programmes? Available to a wider population this 'new' service means more integration and cross-agency working with continued complexity of targets and impact measurement. An example of this integration is the use of the Common Assessment Framework (CAF), a tool designed by government to encourage integrated assessment processes and better multi-agency working. It was developed as a result of poor working practices and assessment issues associated with child protection failures, in cases such as Victoria Climbié (Laming 2003) (see Chapters 4 and 11).

Growing the integrated Children's Centres model from a Sure Start beginning out into the wider population is a challenge that has created anxiety in professionals currently involved in Sure Start. The tension is associated with fearing that the 'jam' will be spread too thinly and the intensive in-depth nature of the work will be lost.

However, perhaps there is an opportunity for community professionals to learn from and adapt some of the messages from CCI practice and research into their own system. Sullivan and Skelcher (2002 p. 50) highlighted the role, the skills and attributes of practitioners working across boundaries in collaborative enterprises that are public service based:

'…these individuals are often referred to as reticulists, people who are able to bring networks together and help others identify relevant linkages between them and other actors'.

Reticulate means to form into a network and Sullivan and Skelcher (2002) identified a number of different roles that reticulists might undertake as 'boundary spanners' with the ability to gather a network together: convenor, capacity builder, catalyst, network relationship operator (see also, Chapter 3). These seemed very appropriate to a number of community-based professionals, both in and outside of the CCI system, but most particularly of relevance to the role of the health visitor, who has the training and the potential to undertake the elements described. Reticulists are self-managers who possess sound organisational skills. They are:

'…skilled communicators, able to "talk the right language" in whatever forum they find themselves. They have excellent networking skills giving them the ability to gain entry to a variety of settings and to seek out and "connect up" others who may have common interests or goals. Their capacity to empathise enables them to see a situation from a variety of points of view which, combined with their communication skills makes them effective negotiators, they are people who can see the "bigger picture" and understand how different partners can contribute to achieve shared goals. They are able to understand the constraints and opportunities provided by different organisational contexts and how this might affect behaviour. They are individuals who are able to think laterally and think creatively and to use these capacities to problem solve and to take risks to achieve their goals'.
(Sullivan & Skelcher 2002, p. 100)

The arrival of Children's Centres means a government commitment to more integration, not less, and possible continued complexity of targets and impact measurement. Reticulists will be very important in helping to develop and maintain an integrated, inter-linked structure. We need to improve how practitioners learn from each other (Coote 2003) in a linked system and also within CCIs how they can be supported and enabled to contribute to the evidence as shown by the practice examples highlighted here.

Policy has dictated that whatever the approach that is implemented, the aim should be for community professionals both in the statutory and voluntary sector to:

'…communicate and agree policies and protocols that ensure there is a "seamless" service'.
(Department for Education and Skills 2001).

What lessons can community professionals learn from a CCI approach?

Even though there has been a government drive towards absolute interest in outcomes, it is important to understand the different processes that may be involved in generating appropriate knowledge: it is then imperative to link this understanding to learning and changing (Coote 2003). In many of the Health Action Zone programmes, professionals found it difficult to identify exactly how they might intervene to address problems; further, they were unsure of what

151

Box 6.2

Checking service provision

Does the service address client needs?

Place

- Is the service sited in the neighbourhood, providing easy access to clients?

Access

- Is the service easy to understand and use?
- Is the service flexible and able to respond to unexpected demands?
- Is information provided to allow clients to make informed decisions about their needs?
- Is it possible to work with other agencies to develop intellectual development for children through play (e.g. offer high-quality toys and games at well baby/child health clinics for older siblings)?

Two generational

- Does the service address family as well as child issues?
- Is the service broad based or single focus?
- Is it possible to work with other agency partners to offer socialisation where under-5s have an opportunity to mix with other children (e.g. development checks in an informal 'tea-party' setting where parents and children can meet and share)?
- Is it possible to work with other agency partners to develop a networks approach for other age groups, such as the elderly to reduce isolation?

Support

- Does the service allow the building of a trusting, non-stigmatising relationship?
- Is there respect and understanding of race and culture issues (internally within the organisation and outwardly with clients)?
- For preschoolers, does the service offer positive parenting programmes that are cross-sectoral and multi-agency utilising the skill of partner agencies?

Outreach

- Is the service centre based or does it have a home-visiting/outreach component (is there openness to partnership working with other agencies to deliver different sorts of services in non-health service premises – both centre-based and home visiting)?
- Is the service driven by the consumer or the professional (how well does the service consult with consumers)?
- Is the client allowed to be a collaborator in the decision-making process with the service providers (e.g. is the service wedded to a relationship-diminishing, checklist approach (Houston & Cowley 2002, Cowley & Houston 2003, 2004) to assessing client needs)?
- Does the service work with other agencies to offer support/respite assistance to families (e.g. drop-in clubs to alleviate stress, or offer mechanisms for support of isolated parents who can meet and share)?

Empowerment

- Does the service seek to build on family strengths? Or is the focus on family problems and weakness?
- Is the help and support offered to clients paternalistic or empowering?
- Is there evidence of multi-agency working to ensure that all parents are offered appropriate access to benefit advice?
- Is there evidence of work with other agencies to develop programmes and support structures that empower and protect at-risk groups such as teen parents?

Box 6.3

Checking service provision

Does the service meet professional aims/aspirations?

Articulating aims

- In project work, are professionals able to communicate their starting hypothesis and how this might be related to critical aspects of the social, economic and political environments?
- In project work, can the professionals identify in a credible and evidence-based way, why the planned expenditure might lead in the direction of the long-term outcomes that they seek to realise?
- In project work, can the professionals identify at the outset ways in which the planned process can be monitored and evaluated?

Commitment to learning

- Does the system allow professionals to innovate in a supported environment, aware but supportive of risk?
- Do the professionals commit themselves to a continuous process of learning from feedback? Starting with i) their own reflective practice, ii) management supervision, iii) client consultation, and iv) project evaluation.
- Does the system, and the professionals within it, have the ability to modify their position on the basis of new knowledge?

Management

- Does the service have enthusiastic leadership with clear aims?
- Is there continuity of staff?
- Is there real partnership with users (e.g. parent/professional board with representative meetings on a regular basis)?
- Is there interagency/interdisciplinary co-operation with good communication?
- Is there clarity about child protection and elder abuse issues?

Dissemination

- Does the professional and the organisation take time to value and disseminate, discuss and learn from project work and share outcomes both positive and negative with other agencies (as an example from practice in two Sure Start programmes linked by evaluation, there were, over a period of 3 years, at least 6 separate days dedicated to dissemination of completed work, more than 650 reports printed for distribution, covering seven topic areas, and six conference presentations given on the separate work of the two programmes).

advantage or disadvantage they expected would flow from such interventions and how exactly this would relate to their strategic goal (Judge & Bauld 2001).

Questions for all professionals to ask when reflecting on their own service provision in light of the CCI findings are presented in Box 6.2 and 6.3. The first addresses the client 'needs' in positive service provision and the second the professional imperatives in developing positive forward-looking service provision.

Conclusion

In addressing the level of success of CCIs, the long-term as well as the short-term advantages must be considered. Politically there is desperation to grasp proof of short-term gains in light of the resource and funding that has been put into community-based interventions in recent years. Latent effects have been highlighted in the literature from the USA through long-term follow-up studies (see Table 6.3). These have shown such things as avoidance of delinquency, decreased need for remedial help in school as well as the emergence of individuals who are economically independent from state support.

However, in respect of Sure Start for instance, the most recent national evaluation report at the time of writing (NESS 2005, Report 13) has been widely discussed because of its critical findings into Sure Start the CCI. The report suggested that not all families were helped by Sure Start and that, for some, the presence of Sure Start in an area made their lives worse (Belsky et al 2006).

The report failed to chime with some local Sure Start programme evaluations where a positive impact was identified (de Jager & Houston 2006, Houston & Parker 2005, Turner et al 2004). The NESS (2005) report itself received critical reviews because, although the study was based on a cross-section of children, it was claimed that 'it did not ask participants if they had actually used Sure Start services' (Community Practitioner 2006).

The National Evaluation process had produced a series of implementation and local context findings prior to NESS report 13, which is readily available on its website alongside other early impact findings. Results demonstrate short-term and intermediate effects, but will not be able to speak of the long-term outcomes for fam-ilies and communities assisted by additional neighbourhood-based resources.

However, in spite of the many difficulties highlighted here in making a CCI work and providing evidence of effectiveness, commitment remains for this type of approach:

> 'In the UK there is still a strong political will to intervene for social change, backed up by vast resources. There is a stronger commitment than ever before to preventing illness and reducing health inequalities'.
>
> (Coote et al 2004, p. 51).

The government is continuing with its agenda on anti-social behaviour, tackling such issues as nutritionally based problems in society and developing the anti-poverty strategy. There is a real opportunity for community professionals, such as health visitors, to let go of previously hampering 'medical model' practices to seize the chance of returning to proactive preventive work (as seen in the examples presented here). Prevention is currently very suited to this present political interventionist community-focused agenda.

Government is asking for a greater level of integration of services in a climate of mainstreaming where the agenda is about moving away from predetermined bounded provision of CCIs. There is the potential to develop a universal delivery system in Children's Centres that has the ability within it to target those in the community with additional needs using the lessons learned from all the CCI systems. This offers a golden opportunity for all community-based reticulists to seize the day and help to develop and build on the evidence of the public-health-focused CCIs, towards maintaining integrated, upstream services for the community.

DISCUSSION QUESTIONS

- Can complex community initiatives be mainstreamed into statutory services?
- How do you use evidence-based practice to extract the innovation from an area-based initiative and make sure that it gets mainstreamed?

- How do area-based services fit with professional health services, which are used to intervening with individual clients?
- How can complex community initiatives best be evaluated?
- What skills do professionals need to evaluate area-based activity?

References

Barnes M, Sullivan H, Matka E 2003 The development of collaborative capacity in Health Action Zones: a final report from the national evaluation. Online. Available: http://www.haznet.org.uk/hazs/evidence/HAZ_collc_cap.pdf [accessed 26 July 2005]

Bartley M 2004 Health inequality: an introduction to theories, concepts and methods. Blackwell, Malden, MA

Belsky J, Melhuish E, Barnes J, Leyland AH, Romainiuk H and the National Evaluation Team 2006 Effects of Sure Start local programmes on children and families from quasi-experimental, cross sectional study. British Medical Journal 332(7556): 1476

Blackman J 2002 Infants and Young Children.Early intervention: a global perspective 15(2): 11–19

Brookes-Gunn J, McCormack MC, Shapiro S, Benasich AA, Black GW 1994 The effects of early education intervention on maternal employment, public assistance, and health insurance: the Infant Health and Development Program. American Journal Public Health 84: 924–931

Cabinet Office 2000 National strategy for neighbourhood renewal: a framework for consultation. The Social Exclusion Unit, London

Campbell FA, Ramey CT 1994 Effects of early intervention on intellectual and academic achievement: a follow-up study of children from low-income families. Child Development 65(2): 684–698

Casto G, Mastropieri MA 1986 The efficacy of early intervention programs: a meta-analysis. Exceptional Children 52: 417–424

Community Practitioner 2005 Sure Start Review 79(1): 2

Connell JP, Kubisch AC 1998 Applying a theory of change approach to the evaluation of comprehensive community initiatives: progress, prospects and problems. In: Fulbright-Anderson K, Kubisch AC, Connell JP (eds) New approaches to evaluating community initiatives, vol 2. Theory measurement and analysis. The Aspen Institute, Washington DC

Coote A 2003 Mist opportunity. Health Service Journal 113(5884): 16–17

Coote A, Allen J, Woodhead D 2004 Finding out what works: understanding complex community-based initiatives. Kings Fund Publications, London

Cowley S, Houston AM 2003 A structured health needs assessment tool: acceptability and effectiveness for health visiting. Journal of Advanced Nursing 43(1): 82–92

Cowley S, Houston A.M 2004 Contradictory agendas in health visitor needs assessment. A discussion paper of its use for prioritizing, targeting and promoting health. Primary Health Care Research and Development 5: 240–254

Crnic KA, Greenberg MT, Slough N 1986 Early stress and social support influences on mothers and high risk infants' functioning in late infancy. Infant Mental Health Journal 7(1): 19–33

Crnic KA, Stormshak E 1997 The effect-iveness of providing social support for families of children at risk. In: Guralnick MJ (ed.) The effectiveness of early intervention. Paul Brookes Publishing, Baltimore, pp. 209–225

Department of Education and Employment 1999 Making a difference for children and families: SureStart. Department of Education and Employment, London

Department for Education and Skills 2001 SEN Code of Practice Section 10.1 Online. Available: http://www.teachernet.gov.uk/_doc/3724/SENCodeOfPractice.pdf [accessed 28 February 2005]

Department for Education and Skills 2004 Every child matters: next steps Department of Education and Skills Publications Nottingham Online. Available: http://www.everychildmatters.gov.uk/_files/A39928055378AF27E9122D734BF1F74.pdf [accessed 2nd March 2005]

Department of Health (DH), Acheson D (ed.) 1998 Independent inquiry into inequalities in health: The Acheson Report. London Stationary Office. Online. Available: http://www.archive.official–documents.co.uk?documents/doh/ih/ih.htm [accessed 26 July 2005]

Department of Health 1999 Saving lives: our healthier nation (Cm: 4386). The Stationery Office, London. Online.

155

Available: http://www.archiveofficial–documents.co.uk/document/cm43/4386/4386.htm; Executive sumary: http://www.dh.gov.uk/asset-Root/04/0493/29/04049329.pdf [accessed 26 July 2005]

Department of Health (DH) 2002 Sure Start Information Bank. Sure Start, London. Online. Available: http://www.SureStart.gov.uk [accessed 5 January 2005]

Department of Health (DH) 2004 National Service Framework for Children, Young People and Maternity Services: Executive Summary. Online. Available: http://www.dh.gov.uk/Publications-AndStatistics/Publications/Publications PolicyAndGuidance/PublicationsPolicy-AndGuidanceArticle/fs/en?CONTENT_ ID=4089100&chk=Egpznc [accessed 4th March 2005]

Department of Health (DH) 2005 Choosing health: making healthier choices easier. The Stationery Office, London

de Jager M, Houston AM 2006 Main-streaming Sure Start speech and language therapy services. Community Practitioner 79(3): 80–83

Dunst CJ, Trivette CM, Cross AH, 1986 Mediating influences of social support: personal, family and child outcomes. American Journal of Mental Deficiency 90(4): 403–417

Farran DC 2000 Another decade of interven-tion for children who are low income or disabled: what do we know now? Cambridge University Press, Cambridge, pp. 510–548

Farringdon DP 1996 Understanding and preventing youth crime. Joseph Rowntree Foundation, York

Fawcett SB, Boothroyd R, Schultz JA, Francisco VT, Carson V, Bremby R 2003 Building capacity for participatory evaluation within community initiatives. Journal of Prevention and Intervention in the Community (Special Issue: Empowerment) 26(2): 2136

Fuerst JS, Fuerst D 1993 Chicago experi-ence with an early childhood program: the special case of the child parent center program. Urban Education 28(1): 69–96

Garbarino J, Ganzel B 2000 The human ecology of early risk. In: Shonkoff JP, Meisels SJ (eds) Handbook of early childhood intervention, 2nd edn. Cambridge University Press, Cambridge, pp. 76–93

Gelles RJ 2001 Family preservation and reunification: how effective a social policy? In: White SO (ed.) Handbook of youth

and justice. Kluwer, New York Academic/Plenum Publishers. Online. Available: http://www.ssw.upenn.edu?CCPPR?pdf/family_preservation.pdf [accessed 6 May 2004]

Glass N 2001 What works for children – the political issues? Children and Society 15: 14–20

Gomby DS, Larner MB, Stevenson CS, Lewit EM, Behrman RE 1995 Long-term outcomes of early childhood programs: analysis and recommendations. The Future of Children 5(3): 6–24

Halpern R, Larner M 1988 The design of family support programs in high-risk communities: lessons from the child survival/fair start initiatives. In: Powell D (ed.) Parent education as early childhood intervention: emerging directions in theory research and practice. Ablex Publishing, Norwood, NJ, pp. 181– 207

Halpern R 1990 Community-based early intervention. In: Meisels SJ, Shonkoff JP (eds) Handbook of early childhood intervention, 1st edn. Cambridge University Press, Cambridge, pp. 469–498

Hanson MC, Carta JJ 1995 Addressing the challenges of families with multiple risks. Exceptional Children 62(3): 201–212

Heenan D 2004 A partnership approach to health promotion: a case study from Northern Ireland. Health Promotion International 19(1): 105–113

Hills D 2004 Evaluation of community-level interventions for health improvement: a review of experience in the UK. Health Development Agency. Online. Available: http://www.had.nhs.uk [Accessed 16 June 2005]

HM Treasury 2004a Spending review: child poverty review. Online. Available: http://www.hm–treasury.gov.uk/spending_review/spend_sr04/associated_docu-ments/spending_sr04_childpoverty.cfm [accessed 7 June 2005]

HM Treasury 2004b Wanless D (ed) Securing good health for the whole population: final report. The Wanless Report. HM Treasury, London

Home Office 1998 Supporting families: a consultation document. The Stationery Office, London

Honig AS, Lally JR 1982 The Family Development Research Program: retro-spective review. Early Child Development and Care 10: 41–62

Houston AM 2003a Sure Start: s complex community initiative. Community Practitioner 76(7): 257–260

Houston AM 2003b Sure Start: the example of one approach to evaluation. Community Practitioner 76(8): 294–298

Houston AM, Bennett F 2004 Examining the impact of Sure start team midwifery from a client and a professional perspective. Sure Start, Romford, UK

Houston AM, Cowley S 2002 An empowerment approach to needs assessment in health visiting practice. Journal of Clinical Nursing 11(5): 640–650

Houston AM, Parker L 2005 North Leyton Sure Start: The impact of inter-professional working on service delivery for Sure Start and the Children's Centre. Sure Start London

Hudson B 2005 Partnership working and the children's services agenda: is it feasible? Journal of Integrated Care 13(2): 7–12

Hunter DJ 2004 The future is public health: is public health finally rising to the top of the agenda? New Economy 11(4): 201–206

Johnson DL 1990 The Houston Parent-Child Development Center Project: Disseminating a viable program for enhancing at-risk families. Prevention in Human Services 7(1): 89–108

Judge K, Bauld L 2001 Strong theory, flexible methods: evaluating complex community-based initiatives. Critical Public Health 11(1): 19–38

Karoly LA, Greenwood PW, Everingham SS, Hoube J, Kilburn MR, Rydell CP, Sanders M, Chiesa J 1998 Investing in our children: what we know and don't know about the costs and benefits of early childhood interventions. The Rand Corporation, Santa Monica, California

Kubisch AC, Weiss CH, Schorr LB, Connell JP 1995 Introduction. In: Connell JP, Kubisch AC, Schorr LB, Weiss CH (eds) New approaches to evaluating community initiatives: concepts, methods and contexts. The Aspen Institute, Washington DC

Lally JR, Mangione PL, Honig AS 1988 The Syracuse University Family Development Research Program: long-range impact of an early intervention with low income children and the families. In: Powell DR, Sigel IE (eds) Parent education as early childhood intervention: emerging directions in theory, research and practice. Ablex Publishing, Norwood, NJ, pp. 79–104

Laming 2003 The Victoria Climbié Inquiry: report of an inquiry by Lord Laming. Online. Available: http://www.victoria–climbie–inquiry.org.uk/finreport/finreport.htm [accessed 2 August 2006]

Lloyd E 2000 Changing policy in early years provision and family support. NCVCCO Annual Review. Journal No. 2 NCVCCO, London, pp. 65–80

McKinnon J, Bauld L, Judge K, Lawson L 2001 Monitoring Interviews: Autumn 2001 Summary Report University of Glasgow. Online. Available: http://www.haznet.org.uk/hazs/evidence/nat_monitor–pm–intvws–aut01.doc [accessed 7 June 2005]

Melson GF, Ladd GW, Hsu HC 1993 Maternal support networks, maternal cognitions, and young children's social and cognitive development. Child Development 64: 1401–1417

Mindick 1988 Lessons still to be learned in parent empowerment programs: a response to Cochrane. In: Powell D (ed.) Parent education as early childhood intervention: emerging directions in theory research and practice. Ablex Publishing, Norwood, NJ pp. 51–65

North J 2005 Support from the start: lessons from International Early Years Policy. The Maternity Alliance, London

Nelson G, Prilleltensky I, MacGillivary H 2001 Building value-based partnerships: toward solidarity with oppressed groups. American Journal of Community Psychology 29(5): 649–677

NESS (National Evaluation of Sure Start) 2005 Early impacts of Sure Start local programmes on children and families (Report 13) HMSO, DfES Publications, London

Neuberger J 2003 Tackling inequalities in health: the local dimension. Public Management and Policy Association, London

Oberklaid F, Goldfeld S, Moore T 2003 Community based services and the needs of families is there a mismatch? Journal of Paediatrics and Child Health 39(2): 93–94

Office of the Deputy Prime Minister 2004 LSP evaluation and action research programme, HMSO, London. Online. Available: http://www.odpm.gov.uk [accessed 26 July 2005]

Olds DL, EckenrodeJ, Henderson CR, Kitzman H, Powers J, Cole R, Sidora K, Morris P, Pettitt LM, Dennis L 1997 Long-term effects of home visitation on maternal life course and child abuse and neglect: fifteen-year follow-up of a randomised trial. The Journal of the American Medical Association 278(8): 637–643

Pinkerton J, Katz I 2003 Perspective through international comparison in the evaluation of family support. In: Katz I, Pinkerton J (eds) Evaluating family support: thinking internationally, thinking critically. John Wiley, Chichester, pp. 3–21

Quiery N, McElhinnery S, Rafferty H, Sheehey N, Trew K 2003 Empowering parents: a two-generation intervention in a community context in Northern Ireland. In: Katz I, Pinkerton J (eds) Evaluating family support: thinking internationally, thinking critically. John Wiley, Chichester, pp. 207–225

Reynolds AJ, Temple J, Robertson DL, Mann EA 2001 Long term effects of an early childhood intervention on educational achievement and juvenile arrest: a 15-year follow-up of low income children in public schools. Journal of the American Medical Association 285(18): 2339–2346

Richmond J, Ayoub CC 1993 Evolution of early intervention philosophy. In: Bryant DM, Graham MA (eds) Implementing early intervention: from research to effective practice. The Guildford Press, New York, pp. 1–17

Ritchie D, Parry O, Gnich W, Platt S 2004 Issues of participation, ownership and empowerment in a community development programme: tackling smoking in a low-income area in Scotland. Health Promotion International 19(1): 51–59

Roberts H 2000 What is Sure Start? Archives of Disease in Childhood 82(6): 435–437

Runyan DK, Hunter WM, Socolar RS et al 1998 Children who prosper in unfavourable environments: the relationship to social capital. Pediatrics 101: 1

Schweinhart LJ 2003 Benefits, costs and explanations of the High Scope Perry Pre-school Program. Paper presented at the Meeting of the Society for Research in Child Development Florida. Online. Available: http://www.highscope.org/Research/PerryProject/Perry–SRCD–2003.pdf [accessed 2 April 2004]

Schweinhart LJ, Barnes HV, Weikart DP, Barnett WS, Epstein AS 1993 Significant benefits: the High/Scope Perry Preschool Study Through Age 27. Monographs of the High Scope Educational Research Foundation, No. 10. High Scope Press, Ypsilanti, MI

Schweinhart LJ, Berrueta-Clement JR, Barnett WS, Epstein AS Weikart DP 1985 Effects of the Perry Preschool Program on youths through age 19: a summary topics in early childhood. Special Education 5(2): 26–35

Schweinhart LJ, Weikart DP 1993 A summary of significant benefits: the High Scope Perry Pre-School Study through age 27. High Scope Press, Ypsilanti, MI

Shaw M, Davey Smith G, Dorling D 2005 Health inequalities and New Labour: how the promises compare with real progress. British Medical Journal 330: 1016–1021

Sinclair R, Hearn B, Pugh G 1997 Preventive work with families: the role of mainstream services. National Children Bureau, London

Sullivan H, Skelcher C 2002 Working across boundaries: collaboration in public services. Palgrave, Basingstoke

To T, Cadarette SM, Liu Y 2001 Biological social and environmental correlates of preschool development child. Care Health and Development 27(2): 187–200

Turner E, Houston AM, Mears P 2004 Implementation of the Sure Start language. Measure Community Practitioner 77(5): 185–189

Utting D, Bright J Henricson C 1993 Crime and the family: improving child rearing and preventing delinquency. Occasional Paper 16, Family Policy Studies Centre, London

Wainwright S 1999 Anti-poverty strategies: work with children and families. British Journal of Social Work 29: 477–483

Wilkinson RG 1996 Unhealthy societies: the afflictions of inequality. Routledge, London

Zigler E, Styco S 2001 Extended childhood intervention prepares children for school and beyond. The Journal of the American Medical Association 285(18): 2378–2380

Zigler E, Taussig C, Black K 1992 Early childhood intervention: a promising preventive for juvenile delinquency. American Psychologist 47(8): 997–1006

Further reading

Bartley M 2004 Health inequality: an introduction to theories, concepts and methods. Blackwell, Malden, MA

This book sets out to provide a road map through the bigger issues emanating from inequality research and offers signposts to the most important elements such as socio-economic position, models of aetiological pathways, social ecology, gender inequality, ethnic inequality and the part played by social policy. It is a helpful and easy to read text.

Reason P, Bradbury H 2001 Handbook of action research: participative inquiry & practice. Sage Publications, London

This book challenges the idea that research or inquiry can only be done from an ivory tower perspective. Part Three: 'Exemplars' has some inspiring examples that community practitioners may find encouraging to their practice.

Shonkoff JP, Meisels SJ (eds) 2000 Handbook of early childhood intervention, 2nd edn. Cambridge University Press, Cambridge

This is the definitive text on current thinking on the subject of 'Early' as in preschool 'Intervention' and 'Complex Community Initiatives'. This book offers a link to a wealth of other writers on this topic and highlights the many important aspects of development of this model of service delivery.

Tones K, Green J 2004 Health promotion planning and strategies. Sage Publications, London

This is a positive revision of preventive health promotion models alongside information on how to systematically address strategy development. The settings and methods chapter is of particular interest to practitioners who might feel bereft of ideas on where to start with strategy development.

Resources

Health Action Zones

'Engaging the organisations, partners and communities that make up the 26 Health Action Zones': more information can be found on the Department of Health website.

HAZ information is now mainly available through HAZ at the Department of Health or more likely through the HAZ area-specific websites; HAZnet is now closed off as a repository.

Merseyside: St Helens and Knowsley Health Action Zone Health Partnership: http://www.sthhaz.org.uk/sthhaz/sthhaz.nsf/links/main?opendocument

New Deal for Communities (NDC)

NDC helps some of the most deprived neighbourhoods in the country by giving grants to community-based partnerships for neighbourhood renewal. Online. Available: http://www.neighbourhood.gov.uk/page.asp?id=617

National Strategy for Neighbourhood Renewal

This is an action plan that sets out a National Strategy for Neighbourhood Renewal to narrow the gap between outcomes in deprived areas and other areas. It builds on the work of 18 policy action teams. The Strategy harnesses the hundreds of billions of pounds spent by the key government departments, rather than relying on one-off regeneration spending, and puts in place new ideas including Neighbourhood Management and Local Strategic Partnerships for empowering residents and getting public, private and voluntary organisations to work in partnership. Online. Available: http://www.neighbourhood.gov.uk/page.asp?id=908

Local Strategic Partnership (LSP)

This is a single, non-statutory, multi-agency body that matches local authority boundaries and aims to bring together at a local level the different parts of the public, private, community and voluntary sectors. It was developed to tackle deep-seated, multi-faceted problems, requiring a range of responses from different bodies. Local partners working through an LSP were expected to take many of the major decisions about priorities for their local area. Online. Available: http://www.neighbourhood.gov.uk/page.asp?id=531

Sure Start

A wide organisation encompassing the ideals of making life better for children and families in the community by improving childcare, early education and health and family support. Online. Available: http://www.surestart.gov.uk

Sure Start Scotland: http://www.scotland.gov.uk/Topics/People/Young-People/children-families/15939/3896

Sure Start Wales: http://www.surestart.gov.uk/aboutsurestart/help/contacts/wales/

Additional Sure Start resources

Sure Start (2003) Birth to three matters: a framework to support practitioners and carers. http://www.surestart.gov.uk/ensuringquality/birthtothreematters/

NESS: National Evaluation of Sure Start (2005) Implementing Sure Start local programmes: an in-depth study. Institute for the study of children families and social issues. Birkbeck College, University of London: http://www.surestart.gov.uk/_doc/1450-FE21F9.pdf

NESS: Towards Understanding Sure Start Local Programmes: summary of findings from the national evaluation. Online. Available: http://www.surestart.gov.uk/_doc/P0001077.pdf

A number of other Sure Start/NESS reports can be downloaded from this Sure Start publication website for example:

Lloyd N, O'Brian M, Lewis C (2003) Fathers in Sure Start local programmes. http://www.surestart.gov.uk/publications/?Document=370

Connexions

This was designed as a confidential support, information and advice structure for 13–19 year olds living in England. Online. Available: http://www.connexions.gov.uk/

The Children's Fund

This was launched in November 2000 as part of the government's commitment to tackle disadvantage among children and young people. The programme aimed to identify at an early stage children and young people at risk of social exclusion, and make sure they received the help and support needed to achieve their potential. Online. Available: http://www.everychildmatters.gov.uk/strategy/childrensfund/

Children's Centres

These were about developing integrated services for young children and their families to build on the foundation created by Sure Start. They would offer 'integrated early learning, care, family support, health services, outreach services to children and families not attending the centre, and access to training and employment advice'. Children's Centres will be models of multi-agency and partnership working. At the heart of a centre will be high-quality learning and full day care for children from birth. Online. Available: http://www.standards.dfes.gov.uk

National Service Framework for Children Young People and Maternity Services

The Children's NSF, published on 15 September 2004, sets standards for children's health and social services, and the interface of those services with education. Online. Available: http://www.dh.gov.uk/PolicyAndGuidance/HealthAndSocialCareTopics/ChildrenServices/ChildrenServicesInformation/fs/en

The Children Act (2004)

Online. Available: http://www.hmso.gov.uk/acts/acts2004/20040031.htm

Section 3

The influence on policies affecting health

It can seem quite daunting for practitioners to try and influence from their base work with clients and communities. However, their local knowledge is a key ingredient for successful policy development and implementation. Such information is generally welcomed by those planning public health strategies, as explained in Chapter 7. Policies may affect health for better or worse, and health programmes need planning carefully to ensure that services are beneficial, particularly in respect of reducing inequalities. This may involve plans that extend beyond the health service, so Chapter 9 draws on established health promotion theories to show how these approaches can also influence change. It is not always possible to measure a direct line of improvement from interventions directed at the social context in which community public health operates. However, as outlined in Chapter 8, evaluative research and systematic approaches to development can be used to improve health and wellbeing.

The influence on policies affecting health is associated with the following performance standards (Nursing and Midwifery Council 2004: p. 11):

1. Work with others to plan, implement and evaluate programmes and projects to improve health and wellbeing.
2. Identify and evaluate service provision and support networks for individuals, families and groups in the local area or setting.
3. Appraise policies and recommend changes to improve health and wellbeing.
4. Interpret and apply health and safety legislation and approved codes of practice with regard for the environment, wellbeing and protection of those who work and the wider community.
5. Contribute to policy development.
6. Influence policies affecting health.
7. Develop, implement, evaluate and improve practice on the basis of research, evidence and evaluation.

7 Planning public health strategies

Jean Rowe

Key issues

- Themes are discussed in terms of the health policy, public health strategies and the components that are necessary for health gain:
  - International, national and local policy requirements
  - Public health strategies
  - Public participation in health
  - Evidence-based strategies and outcomes
  - Public health roles in primary care.

Introduction

Until fairly recently, health policy in the UK was thought to be about how the health service is funded and the provision of medical care. Health is not just the realm of the health service, but engages all sectors of the society, government administration and the globalisation of the economy. The inter-relationships of all these factors play a part in both individual and population health. Changes in philosophy that have occurred within past few years acknowledge that it is not just the individual state of good or bad health that decides human survival, but also the social determinants of health (Wilkinson & Marmot 2003).

In recognition of these factors, which have been evidenced in large numbers of published documents, the United Nations has presented its Millennium Development Goals:

- eradicate extreme poverty and hunger
- achieve universal primary education
- promote gender equality and empower women
- reduce child poverty
- improve maternal health
- combat HIV/AIDS
- ensure environmental sustainability
- develop global partnerships for development.
  (UN 2005)

Health strategy

The broad-based NHS strategies are set by government and are based on party ideologies and what the electorate has mandated. The past few years have seen

162

a plethora of policy changes that have centred on the community, with the focus being on public health, partnerships and public participation.

Proposals for reconfiguration are underway for the possibility for primary care trusts (PCTs) to take on the responsibility for commissioning and securing services from a range of providers. Therefore, some of the traditional community services that were provided by PCTs can be provided by other organisations, including the independent and voluntary sector (Department of Health (DH) 2005a). Accordingly:

- commissioners will be actively seeking new and innovative ways to improve new services with a range of providers
- commissioners will assess what services should move away from direct PCT provision and at what pace
- where PCTs continue to manage services, decision making on commissioning and on provision will be separated in order to enhance contestability
- there is to be a reintroduction of practice-based commissioning similar to GP fundholding.

Practice-based commissioning

Under practice-based commissioning, GP practices will take on responsibility from their PCTs for commissioning services that meet the health needs of the local population. Commissioning practices or groups of practices will have the following main functions:

- designing improved patient pathways
- working in partnership with PCTs to create community-based services that are more convenient for patients
- responsibility for a budget delegated from the PCT, which covers acute, community and emergency care
- managing the budget effectively.
  (DH 2005a)

163

Evidence from the Wanless Report (2002) suggests that the NHS should take a whole-systems approach, including prevention, diagnosis and treatment, rehabilitation and long-term care. In order to direct resources efficiently and produce sensible incentives, appropriate structures need to be in place and seen from the user perspective.

Wanless (2002) looked at future funding models for the NHS and suggested that health needs should be focused on health promotion and disease prevention, and that generalising of National Service Frameworks for other diseases could cost less than anticipated. However, the report also says that development not considered to be cost effective should be abandoned.

Part of the challenge within the NHS is that services are reorganised in terms of the political ideologies and many decisions about resources need to be made for the long term; for example, the number of people to be trained, the skills they will require, the types of buildings likely to be needed and the information and communication technologies upon which the efficient operation of the system will depend (Wanless 2002).

Policy context

The Health Act 1999 mandated an emphasis on promoting health, reducing inequalities and social exclusion, working in partnership and involving communities. *saving lives: our healthier nation* (Secretary of State for Health 1999) and *reducing health inequalities* (DH 1999a) built on the previous requirements under

The Health of the Nation (DH 1992) targets. Providers are expected to take action on health targets at all levels, including the PCTs (DH 1997, 1998). Strategic Health Authorities are responsible for giving guidance and performance monitoring of the PCTs (England) on the national plan for the NHS (The NHS Plan) and National Service Frameworks. Explicit targets and objectives will be met by all PCTs and objectives carried out strategically. In the hierarchy of responsibilities, each unit of the organisation will adjust its focus to meet the national priorities. National priorities are based on people making healthier choices (DH 2005b). The six health priorities are:

1. Tackling inequalities.
2. Reducing the numbers of people who smoke.
3. Tackling obesity.
4. Improving sexual health.
5. Improving mental health and wellbeing.
6. Reducing harm and encouraging sensible drinking.
   (DH 2004a)

What has been recognised is that, in order to reduce the burden of ill health and narrow the health gap, all the major government departments must play a part. This has produced more cohesive arrangements for partnership working, with local authorities playing a major role with the primary care organisations in health promotion, prevention strategies and reducing inequalities in health through Local Strategic Partnerships in England and Wales, and Community Health Partnerships in Scotland. The Local Strategic Partnerships/Community Health Partnerships support work on the development of Health Improvement and Modernisation Plans.

The plans are based on the belief that, as well as modernising the NHS structurally, modernisation of the way in which services are planned is also necessary, which includes key partners like local authorities, local business, voluntary organisations, patients and the public.

Each health authority is obliged to produce a Health Improvement and Modernisation Plan to set the strategic framework for improving health, reducing inequalities and offering faster, more responsive services of a consistently high standard (DH 2002).

Cross-agency health targets

Health targets also need to be met and included in the floor targets for local government, e.g. Neighbourhood Renewal Schemes, Best Value in Local Government approaches, regeneration schemes, and for Children's Centres. The Children's Centres will have multi-professional and multi-agency systems to support children and their families. Partnerships with local government makes a lot of sense when working with communities, since the needs of older people and people with mental health problems, for example, may have to be met by many differing agencies, including the non-governmental organisations. It means that community nurses must take a more strategic and commissioning role, as well as delivering an appropriate safe service to the public.

Local Strategic Plans and Local Delivery Plans

The core objectives for health and wellbeing in relation to health improvement and modernisation programmes in England are:

- needs assessment
- resource mapping
- identification of priorities for action
- strategies for changes.
  (DH 2004c)

Inclusiveness will be sought through the widest possible involvement in planning from the outset, rather than consultation on a near final product.

The Scottish Executive strategy includes six priority areas:

- opportunities for Community Health Partnerships (CHPs; see Chapter 3) in terms of improving health
- linking clinical teams
- improving access
- developing leadership capacity
- developing skill and capacity for public involvement
- opportunities for Community Health Partnerships in terms of developing mental health services.
(Scottish Executive Health Department 2004)

All these priorities have to be translated into local action. Some of the issues will be of national concern, such as care of the people with enduring mental illness or how employers might put in place mechanisms, e.g. to reduce the level of absenteeism from the workplace. Some of the health improvement priorities will be locally sensitive to the ethnic mix and/or areas of high deprivation.

Both the *New NHS – modern dependable* (DH 1997) and *Saving lives: our healthier nation* (Secretary of State for Health 1999) stressed was user involvement in aspects in health. This area had been less well developed in the NHS but there were expectations that more work would be done to include what local people think about health and health services. The role of the users of health services became a priority in the NHS reforms in *The NHS Plan* (DH 2000).

Health care organisations have to work within a grand design, otherwise health planning and care delivery would be chaos. Each part of the organisation works within the overall strategy, but all levels have their own local strategy for delivery of a service. A public health strategy would be based on the local demography, births, infant mortality and childhood morbidity, deaths by age and cause, and incidence and prevalence of disease. The strategy would identify the potential to improve health and quality of life and, through co-ordinated health programmes, aim to reduce the impact of disease and disability for the population. It should identify gaps in the services so that either a new service can be developed or a plan made to organise services to deliver in a different way.

The NHS is a huge and complex organisation employing large numbers of people, many of whom are from professional groups and in particular nursing. Nurses are the largest professional workforce in the NHS and responsible for a majority of the care delivered within the NHS. Health care is also administered through the independent and voluntary sectors, both of which may have contracts with the NHS or work at the interface between their respect-ive organisations in order to care for people who have health needs. Community nurses therefore play a major role in delivering care and liaising with nurse colleagues, and many other organisations, for and on behalf of their clients and patients. Whichever organisation delivers care, it does so within a structural framework through an overall health care plan. The difference between the institutional care and community care is the mode or plan of delivery. For community nursing and health visiting, access to other parts of the health care system entails knowledge of the local systems, good communication, liaison, and negotiating care with other providers, as well as an intimate knowledge of the individual needs. But changes are affecting the workforce and more than 25% of community nurses, health visitors and district nurses are aged over 50 years. There are 13 000 health visitors and approximately 2500 school nurses, compared with 40 000 social workers for children and families and 440 000 teachers. Employers need to encourage this group to stay in work as this will impact on the care of people in the community (Health Development Agency 2004).

Setting the context – public health

Public health is about the health of the local population. Its origins lie in economic, social, environmental and ecological aspects of health and disease. Public health is both a collective and an individual issue. The health of the population is affected by health-sustaining policies of other government departments that are responsible for agriculture and food production, the fiscal system and transport. Inequalities and health outcomes have as much to do with community and individual resources as with an individual's genetic blueprint, and it is the reduction of health hazard that can help reduce the burden of disease. The wide range of these so-called 'determinants of health' is encapsulated in Dahlgren and Whitehead's diagram, shown in Figure 7.1.

Health draws on wider influences outside the control of the NHS: the local authority, community groups, business and commerce and the media. They are inter-related and affect health and wellbeing (Taylor et al 2002).

In order to decide that any health issue is a priority, information must be collected nationally and locally. The information then informs an agenda for action. However, data collection is complex. Huge amounts of information are collected by many differing sources, including the Public Health Common Data Set, the Office of National Statistics, the General Household Survey, local authorities, acute and community trusts, primary care and from studies carried out on the local population. Other sources of information and 'grey literature' used will be from university research. The collection mechanisms themselves are a problem, as data that meet the need of one organisation may not be presented in a useable way for another organisation. So health intelligence and information departments have the crucial task of analysing information and presenting it in such a way that health services can use it.

Public health reports

In England, public health departments within PCTs are required to produce an annual Public Health Report, focusing on health priorities and local epidemiology. It includes comparative national and local district data, and information on the health services' performance in relation to health targets set. Data from

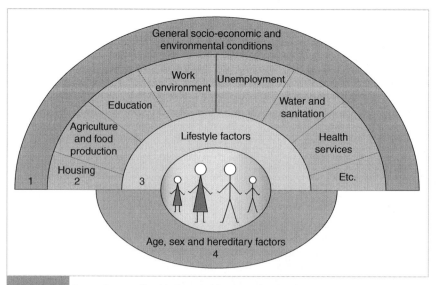

Figure 7.1 ● Determinants of health (from Dahlgren & Whitehead 1999)

the Health Protection Agency are included in the report. It is a public document and, therefore, is open for scrutiny by the public. Public health departments take a population approach and measure health at different levels by age group, condition-specific groups and disease prevalence. PCTs are responsible for assessing the health needs locally and, therefore, need support to take on this wider role. The assessment of need might include participative techniques, such as rapid appraisal through key informants, and may commission other *ad hoc* studies. Each information source gives a different standpoint, but what is higher on the public health agenda is the user perspective. It has the purpose of ensuring the longer-term health planning and identification of unmet health needs. Health intelligence, therefore, involves the bigger picture of health, which is about not only how resources are used for health services, but also how the total community impacts on health (Pearson 1998).

Public health and its responsibility for health improvement

Many new initiatives and financing streams can come either via the NHS or through local government for health improvement. The national priorities are heart disease and stroke, accidents, cancers and mental health. Some of these targets are now being met through funding via the National Service Frameworks. What is different now is that the environment in which health promotion is delivered is specified through identified settings – healthy schools, workplaces and neighbourhoods – with an emphasis a partnership approach.

Local authorities in some areas have merged functions with local PCTs. Programmes that have cross-funding may include:

- area-based initiatives
- neighbourhood renewal programmes
- healthy living centres
- local Sure Start programmes.

Concepts that underpin public health work

Public health approaches feature:

- identification of health needs and desired outcomes
- agreement on the most effective and acceptable action
- evaluation
- user perspectives
- knowledge of population health needs even when caring for individuals
- identified client groups
- whole communities
- geographical area
- emphasis on collective and collaborative action
- recognition of people as members of groups, not only as individuals
- a public health perspective that anchors clinical and non-clinical care in the social, organisational and policy aspects of health development
- a focus on health promotion enabling people to increase control over and improve their health combined with preventing disease.

(Standing Nursing and Midwifery Advisory Committee (SNMAC) 1995)

Health needs assessment

Health needs assessment is a methodology that reviews population health issues in order to produce a set of recommendations for action to improve health outcomes. The interventions have to be realistically acceptable to the population and the priorities are usually those that can reduce health inequalities.

Community-based needs assessment

Community-based needs assessment has three main approaches: sociology, epidemiology and health economics (Billings & Cowley 1995). Biomedical models of health have been the most prominent features of medical and nursing education but it was the inclusion of social aspects of health and disease in health visiting and school nurse education that gave them specialised knowledge and skills of public health in a wider context. Poverty and deprivation in childhood have a major impact in the health of adults.

Comment

Professor David Barker researched the evidence on the fetal origins of adult disease. In 1992 Barker's group originally examined cardiovascular mortality in men born in Hertfordshire, England, in the early decades of the century, on whom good records had been kept of size at birth and growth in infancy. Deaths from ischaemic heart disease were, indeed, more common in men who had been small at birth and at 1 year. At least seven such studies have shown that lower birth weight is associated with higher risks of later ischaemic heart disease and diabetes, or impaired glucose tolerance.

(British Medical Journal 2001 322; 375–376)

Needs assessment methods include the use of data and information to present a case for health improvement, service change or investment in a health programme. Much of the information gathered currently is used for the purpose of estimating total activity and total cost of services and really is an unsophisticated process for commissioning services. Careful consideration of community-based needs assessment is essential and should be carried out for an identified reason. According to research carried out by the London Health Economics Consortium (LHEC 1995), needs assessment has not had any major impact on purchasing decisions. The study found that purchasers and staff in primary and community services made a fairly accurate assessment of need in their local communities. But it did suggest that it may not be worthwhile going into detailed community enquiries, as needs may already have been identified by the local agencies. Local community nurses, in particular health visitors and school nurses, have long been required to produce community profiles, which have included a needs-based approach to their caseloads. What appear to be important in the process are: staff with good local knowledge of the area, good lines of communication and stable management structures within the organisation (LHEC 1995). Stable management structures do not appear to feature in the ever-changing policies.

Difference between need and want

To take a pragmatic view, need is about those things that are life sustaining, e.g. food, water, heat, shelter and health care. 'Want' may be a demand to have health and social care, which is felt to be a right in a modern society and which many older people may feel that they have invested in during their working lives. What may be more meaningful to ask is what people require. Requirements lie somewhere in between need and want, and may be about quality of the service (see also Chapter 13). It is a balance of competing demands and expectations. In the health services, users both need and want the good communications and staff to respond with respect to their human dignity, as often this is where users make value judgements of their care in terms of satisfaction or dissatisfaction. These are often related not so much to clinical interventions, but the way people are treated on a personal level (Stewart & Turner 1998, p. 142). Quality became a statutory duty for health service providers in the new NHS (DH 1998). Building on this, new standards for better health have now been set out, which must be met (DH 2004e). These are:

- safety
- clinical and cost effectiveness
- governance
- patient focus
- accessible and responsive care
- care environment and amenities
- public health.

Any strategy developed within the NHS should contribute to these standards overall. Proposed strategies are more likely to be acceptable if they help NHS organisations to meet their statutory duty in achieving these standards.

A strategy for health

What does a strategy involve? It is usually a corporate plan, which can be developed at a local or national level. Strategies can be developed to encompass a different size of area, or to focus on a specific topic or aspect of health. An example of a national level strategy focusing on one important aspect of health is the overall government strategy laid out in *Every child matters: change for children* (DfES 2004a), which is described in more detail in Chapter 4. This is a co-ordinated approach for the wellbeing of children and young people from birth to age 19 years. It includes the National Service Framework for Children, Young People and Maternity Services (NSF), which is a service specification that operates at a macro level, including all the elements required to meet the health needs for this part of the population.

The aim is for every child, whatever background or circumstances, to have the necessary support to:

- be healthy
- stay safe
- enjoy and achieve
- make a positive contribution
- achieve economic wellbeing.

Like all the NSFs, it was developed to tackle the fundamental issues of fragmentation, gaps and overlaps in the services that are delivered for children and young people. The contribution that community nursing and health visiting brings to this is vast, since they can offer so much to families in terms of identification of need, health promotion and prevention. However, a major concern for any strategy is the capacity of the workforce to meet the needs of children, young people and their families. By integration of the services and introducing core competencies for those working with the most vulnerable of children and young people, it is possible that practitioners can work across the boundaries of health and social care, allowing for more teaching and learning in a multidisciplinary setting. Shortages in the workforce have, in some cases, created opportunities for skill mix with the introduction of, for example, nursery nurses and child development workers into the local Sure Start programmes. There is a new statutory duty for local authorities that early years and child care will be part of an overall strategy as a result of the wider *Every Child Matters* agenda and the Children Act 2004 (HM Treasury 2004).

The Children Act 2004 also required Children's Trusts to be set up in all areas of England by 2008. Children's Trusts bring together all services for children and young people in an area, to focus on improving outcomes for all children and young people:

> 'People will work in effective multi-disciplinary teams, be trained jointly to tackle cultural and professional divides, use a lead professional model where many disciplines are involved, and be co-located, often in extended schools or children's centres' *Every Child Matters: Change for Children* (See http://www.everychildmatters/gov.uk/aims/childrenstrusts/).

Integrated processes will support Children's Trusts:

- joint needs assessment
- shared decisions on priorities
- identification of all available resources
- joint planning.

Alongside the development of shared decisions will be a process of joint commissioning, with pooled resources to ensure that those best able to provide the right packages of services can do so. There will be arrangements for governance and accountability for meeting statutory duties.

The whole system will have:

- leadership at every level, including front-line staff
- performance management driving an outcomes focus at every level, from area inspection to rewards and incentives for individual staff
- listening to the views of children and young people. (DfES/DH 2004a)

Community strategy for health improvement

The strategy could be a case for change, a new service, or a further development of an existing service and can involve major changes or relatively minor changes. But with any change, certain elements need to be in place. Even small changes can make a difference to the quality of care.

A useful model for thinking about a strategy is the Seven 'S' Model (Pascale 1990), the use of which is illustrated in Box 7.1. Included in the model are hard 'Ss' – structure, strategy, and systems – and soft 'Ss' – staff, skills, style and shared values. Marsh and Macalpine (1995) say that nurses tend to focus more on the soft 'Ss', but need to develop skills and include the hard 'Ss'.

Local level

Community nurses, health visitors and allied health practitioners collect and hold both quantitative and qualitative information that is very live. The caseload analysis presents a picture of local need and outcomes of services accessed by clients or patients. It can have the advantage of informing the local practice, but how does this fit with locality need? The aggregation of data and profiles of the practices in a locality or for the PCT has a local intelligence function so that community nursing and health visiting resources can be estimated. Equally, by gathering information, levels of unmet need can be obtained. The involvement of 'community matrons' in identifying need is a public health approach and a model for case management

---

Box 7.1

A community health strategy framework

Structure, strategy and systems

- The health issue/topic area – introduction
- The national policy requirements and regional guidance where appropriate
- Aims of the service/intended outcomes if known
- Service focus – primary/acute/tertiary care
- Service data/health need identified – justification for such a service based on epidemiology/national local needs analysis
- Evidence/research of effectiveness and health gain
- Evidence of intersectoral partnership support where appropriate and with whom
- Service evaluation and quality monitoring arrangements

Staff, skill, style and shared values

- Objectives for the service/scope for intervention
- Service group/professional group(s)
- Components of the service
- Underpinning principles
- Implementation plan – screening/prevention, care pathways, interprofessional issues/ service evaluation/patient/client charters
- Treatment and management of health care and voluntary sector support
- Staff support and management/clinical supervision arrangements
- Training and development
- Audit including service user perceptions

(DH 2005c). The approach involves assessing not only people on the caseload, but the wider population.

Community matrons must:

- identify people at risk in the population
- define the case management role
- involve users in the service design
- identify and involve the key stakeholders
- help skill-up the workforce
- identify and prepare supervisors and mentors
- establish a system of support the community matrons.
  (DH 2005c, p. 16)

The role of allied health professions is recognised as invaluable in the treatment and management for people with long-term medical conditions, particularly those living in the community. Patients can be taught: to become independent through rehabilitation, self-care and how they can prevent readmission to hospital (DH/Allied Health Professions 2005) (Figure 7.2).

Values in public health

The local authority and PCT/organisation must have a value system because it is accountable for the services that are commissioned and purchased on behalf of the local population. Central values are openness, fairness, equity, effectiveness, value for money and responsiveness (Ham et al 1993). Decisions have to be made on what the NHS will offer in terms of health care because resources are

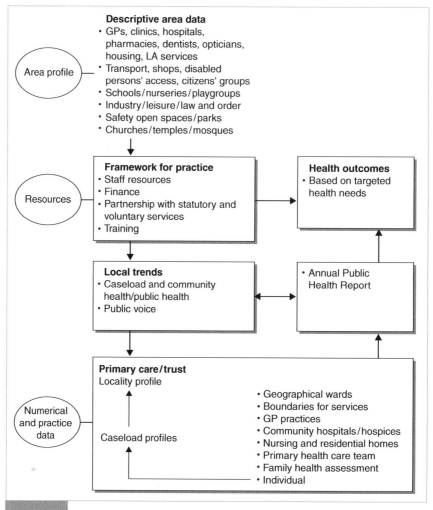

Figure 7.2 ● Community health aggregated data and community profile

limited. Likewise, local authorities must make decisions through the democratic processes. Decisions made may be on the basis of clinical efficacy and information provided through NICE will be able to provide information about new drugs and technologies that have increased opportunities for better health, but which also bring dilemmas in decision making. Patients are much better informed of the possibilities and will wish to have any life-saving treatments offered by the NHS. Decisions, therefore, must be considered on the balance of clinical possibilities, outcome probabilities and quality of life. Sometimes decisions made are reasonable, but may be unpalatable for patients.

Health impact assessment

More recently, health impact assessment or environmental impact assessments have been carried out within communities where major modifications to land, buildings and services are occurring within a community. These may challenge the health and wellbeing of the local community. Environmental impact assessments have been mandatory under the EC regulation since 2001 and include any plans or programmes for agriculture, forestry, fisheries, water and waste management and town and country planning (EC 2001). Some of the changes can be major, such as building a new housing development, or relatively minor, such as closing a local health or facility. More local authorities are now requiring an impact assessment, which can include a health component. Normally, health impact assessments are carried out to identify positive and negative impacts of changes so the communities have a voice in the decisions made about their local neighbourhoods.

The principles that underlie health impact assessment are:

- democracy
- openness
- equity
- sustainable development
- ethical use of evidence
- addressing inequalities.

Difference between health needs assessment and health impact assessment (Table 7.1)

The application of health impact assessments has been considered within several policy documents, including the Acheson Report (1998):
'All policies likely to have a direct or indirect effect on health should be evaluated in terms of their impact on health inequalities, and should be formulated in such a way that by favouring the less well off they will, wherever possible, reduce such inequalities' (Acheson 1998, p. 30).

Health impact assessment is defined as 'a combination of procedures, methods and tools by which a policy programme or project may be judged as to its

Table 7.1 ● Difference between health needs assessment and health impact assessment

	Health needs assessment	Health impact assessment
Starting point	Population	Proposal
Primary output	Informs decisions about strategies, service priorities, commissioning and local delivery plans and informs future HIAs and integrated impact assessments	Informs decision-making by advising how to maximise health benefits and reduce negative outcomes of a proposal or project, or change ways of working
Aims to take into account health inequalities and help health improvement	Informs health needs and health assets of different population groups within the community	Compares how proposals or projects may impact on the most vulnerable groups in population
Involvement of stakeholders	Always	Always
Involvement of community	Always	Ideally – depends on resources
Involvement of many sectors	Sometimes	Usually
Uses research methods	Always	Always
Based on determinants of health	Usually	Always

Adapted from (Quigley et al 2003)

potential effects on the health of the population and the distribution of those effects within the population' (WHO 1999).

Health impact assessments can be carried out prospectively, concurrently or retrospectively. In terms of assessing impact, it should preferably be carried out prior to any changes that are to occur. Importantly, if done early enough, the process should help influence and inform any key decisions that need to be recommended. Significantly, the process must include the members of the general public, as potentially they will be affected by any changes in policy, programmes or projects. It is an inclusive process that has at its core, enhancement of the positive impact of any decisions and reduction of any negative impacts on the health of the population (Taylor et al 2003).

Ethics approval

It is most important, even before going ahead with an impact assessment or any type of population enquiry, to think about whether ethics approval is needed. If there is any doubt, it is wiser to think that it may be needed. This always takes time and the committees only meet at certain times. Research protocols, consent form and explanatory letters have to be drafted to accompany the application forms. Even if the study is approved, the committee will expect feedback at certain points and notification of any changes made to the protocol.

Comment

Health visitors in Guernsey carried out a concurrent health impact assessment (HIA) aimed at reducing the health inequalities on the island. The States of Guernsey Board of Health and the Queens Nursing Institute funded the project. The question raised in the HIA was whether health visitors remaining attached to GP practices or returning to geographical working would be more effective in reducing health inequalities.

Findings for the population include:

- population wanted universal services, not targeted, for families and children
- enhanced continuity of services from antenatal period through school years
- valued home visiting highly
- less well off families would like the health visiting services to develop links with family centres further
- support introduction of family health plans
- health visitors needed to raise their profile and increase accessibility.

(Fant et al 2005)

Health promotion and public health

In 1985 the WHO identified international public health principles. These included peace and freedom from fear of war, equal opportunity for all, social justice, satisfaction with basic needs, public commitment and public support. In the Presidential address to the American Public Health Association, Levy outlined the public health values that are general: human dignity, health and wellbeing, quality of life, social justice and community responsibility. Public health needs a set of values and people who have leadership and vision. It is important that public health professionals develop skills to listen, educate and inform, advocate and develop partnerships (Levy 1998).

Health promotion departments may be stand-alone, but in some areas they have been merged with public health departments. They will be instrumental to the health strategy and planning of health programmes. Their role involves a broader influence, working with all other sectors that have a health remit and mutual interests. The strategic skills of health promotion specialists can help to forge closer links within and outside health organisations. Many inner-city areas have large populations from minority and ethnic groups, and there are health needs and health promotion concerns, especially uptake of services and cultural sensitivities. All areas have access to departments that offer resources and health information. Even if departments do not have all the specific information, they will be in touch with organisations that represent the public health concerns.

Public participation

Since publication of *The new NHS* (DH 1997) and *Saving lives: our healthier nation* (Secretary of State for Health 1999), the concepts of user involvement and, more recently, public participation have been increasingly important. Most people use the health services some of the time for both preventive and diagnostic services, or for a diagnosed medical condition. The NHS Plan (Secretary of State for Health 2000) requires Trusts to take more account of the views of the users and of the local population through representation on the Boards of Trusts, including the primary care trusts/organisations. The NHS Plan acknowledges the role of patient organisations and interest groups that do much to support people with medical and disabling conditions. Research commissioned by the Department of Health, to look at how people can be encouraged to participate in decisions about their own health care, recognised this as a complex concept. The conclusion of the research was that both health professionals and patients need support and training. Emerging themes suggest that patients would benefit from more information given in advance to prepare them for what may arise in the future course of their health care. Health professionals employ differing modes for discussion with patients, ranging from dictating the content of the consultation to facilitating a more negotiated decide the format of process by allowing patients to decide the format of the consultation and topics for discussion. However, there may be a wide range of types of decisions in routine practice situations and that patient's participation in decision making should not necessarily be equated with good decision making (Entwistle et al 2002).

Many user groups lobbied for more involvement in the health agenda, but often live a hand-to-mouth existence with constant worries about income and use of volunteers to get their needs met. Funding can often be short term, so that fund raising is a major preoccupation for these groups. The rise in the numbers of organisations that have mushroomed over the past 20 years or so might reflect the minimal power people had felt within the health care system; that decisions were made on their behalf without consultation. Much more consultation is carried out and the lay members of Trust Boards play an important role in ensuring that the community views are known.

The Expert Patients' Programme was set up in 2002 (DH 2004b) to allow people, particularly with long-term medical conditions, to understand and take more control over their lives. The programme helps people to communicate effectively with health and social care professionals, and to share decisions about how they wish to lead their lives.

Comment

Arthritis affects about 8.5 million people in the UK. This includes some 14 500 children.
Asthma is estimated to affect over 3.4 million people in the UK, including 1.5 million children (aged 2–15).
Back pain lasting more than a day was self-reported by 40% of adults in 1998. Fifteen per cent of back-pain sufferers said they were in pain throughout the year, and approximately 40% of back-pain sufferers consulted a GP for help.
Diabetes mellitus prevalence estimates vary, but there are thought to be in the region of 1.5 million doctor-diagnosed cases of diabetes in the UK.

> **Epilepsy** is the most common serious neurological disorder affecting more than 420 000 people or one in 130 of the UK population.
>
> **Heart failure** prevalence in the UK, based on morbidity studies in general practice, has been estimated to affect about half a million people.
>
> **Multiple sclerosis (MS)** is one of the most common diseases of the central nervous system. It is estimated to affect between 80 000 and 90 000 people in the UK. It usually strikes people when they are young adults.
>
> (DH 2004b)

National Patient Survey Programme

The patient experience Public Service Agreement (PSA) target for 2005–2008 is a key strategic driver. Each Trust and PCT is responsible for organising its own. The target is to 'Secure sustained national improvements in NHS patient experience by 2008, ensuring that individuals are fully involved in decisions about their health care, including choice of provider, as measured by independently validated surveys (HM Treasury 2004b, p. 14) '.

The PSA target requires sustained national improvements in patient experience by 2008, as measured by the national patient survey programme. Trusts are expected to use the results to identify how they can improve services for patients. Results of the survey must then be submitted to the NHS. The survey responses provide more detailed information on how patients feel about the service they receive, they form part of the assessment of trusts against the health care standards. The Health Care Commission will monitor the target, and the experience of black and minority ethnic groups will be monitored specifically as part of these surveys (DH Spending Review PSA).

Public safety

One of the public health issues that the NHS has to deal with is the issue of accidents and ill health due to environmental factors or failure to recognise danger in the home or workplace. Legislation exists to protect the workplace and human resources departments are responsible for ensuring training is available to staff. One of the major injuries within the health services is back injury, which can result in personal distress and huge costs to the services. Lifting and moving training, therefore, is an essential part of a clinical governance agenda.

176

Comment

Injuries

There were **220** fatal injuries to workers in 2004/05, a decrease of 7% on the 2003/04 figures. Around half occurred in two industries – construction and agriculture, forestry and fishing.

150 559 other injuries to employees were reported, a rate of 587 per 100 000 employees.

363 000 reportable injuries occurred, according to the Labour Force Survey, a rate of 1330 per 100 000 workers (2003/04).

Ill health

2.0 million people were suffering from an illness, which they believed was caused or made worse by their current or past work. **576 000** of these were new cases in the last 12 months.

Working days lost

35 million working days were lost over all (1.5 days per worker), 28 million due to work-related ill health and 7 million due to workplace injury.

(HSC Statistics 2004/05)

Any company with more than five employees is legally obliged to possess a comprehensive health and safety policy. Under the 1974 Health and Safety at Work Act, all employers and employees have a duty to protect themselves and the public, and report any risks in the work environment and places where the public would be entering the premises (Health and Safety at Work Act 1974). Equally, NHS employers are responsible for the safety of staff that work in the community where they are particularly vulnerable. Mechanisms are often set up to ensure that nurses working at night in people's homes do not work alone. The Health and Safety Executive will assess risk in the workplace; particularly if the there has been an accident or incident or if people are suffering the effects of poor workplace design.

Community nurses and health visitors also have a duty to protect their clients/patients and now that they have the powers to prescribe, they are clinically accountable for any action that they take as part of their role in prescribing. Whether community nurses are independent or supplementary nurse prescribers, the Medicinal Products: Prescriptions by Nurses Act 1992 and a set of principles for prescribing that should protect the public (National Prescribing Centre (NPC) 1999). For independent nurse prescribers, the list of medications and treatments must relate to their specific area of practice, but now, with supplementary prescribing, nurses are able to change dosages of medication where the patient already has been assessed and diagnosed for a specific condition, e.g. asthma and diabetes. Nurse prescribing is more appropriate in terms of patient and client safety in the community, e.g. district nurses are much more aware of the research evidence and treatment of leg ulcers. Community nurses, particularly in GP practices, quite often have the responsibility of the care of people with specific chronic illnesses and are able to monitor the patients on a regular basis. Nurses must ensure that they assess any risks with their patients when prescribing and develop plans with patients to confirm concordance (NPC 2003).

Duty of care

All health care staff have a duty of care towards their patients and clients, and care must be in the best interests of patients, their colleagues, themselves and the wider public.

Duty of care applies to registered and non-registered health services groups of staff.

Situations that may be in conflict with these principles might include:

- being able to undertake excessive or unsafe workloads
- being asked to implement questionable delegation of roles and tasks
- being able to follow potentially unsafe instructions
- being asked to work in unsafe environments for both staff and patients
- working in a situation where there is a climate of fear and where that prevents proper concerns being raised about patients for staff safety
- being asked to collude with inappropriate allocation of resources, which are not in the best interests of the patient.
  (UNISON 2003)

Patient advocacy

The establishment of the Patient Advice and Liaison Service (PALS) in each NHS Trust was designed to give the public more control over their lives, as it gives advice, information and access to other organisations that may support them with health issues. The PALS team can act as independent facilitator, handling personal and family concerns (NHS Plan 2000, p. 91). This service supports patient-centred care and complainants.

Participation models

Models of user involvement indicate that there is a continuum of involvement, which was developed by Arnstein, as described in Leonard et al (1997), which uses the concept of a ladder of participation. Each rung corresponds to a position of citizen power (see Figure 7.3).

Whilst citizen control might be difficult to manage in terms of accountability for delegated resources, the NHS Trusts have more user non-executive representation on their boards.

The International Association for Public Participation developed another model (2000) using five stages that increases the level of public impact. The stages each have specific objectives that involve the public:

- Informing – providing the public with balanced and objective information so they can understand the problem and possible solutions.
- Consulting – obtaining public feedback on analysis or decisions.
- Involving – work directly through the public and to ensure that the public understand issues and concerns.
- Collaborating – working in partnership with the public so that each action and decision including development of alternatives and preferred solutions.
- Empowering – final decisions made by the public.

Commissioning

Commissioning is an elaborate process that consumes many resources in terms of people and time. Information on existing levels of investment in services and the future funding allocation must be considered in the light of necessity.

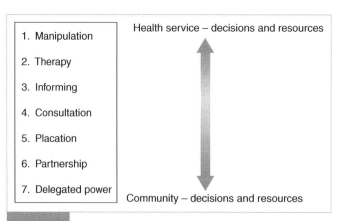

Figure 7.3 ● Public Participation Continuum

Box 7.2

Stages to public health action

1. Is there a health need and what is the question?
2. What is the social context of this health need?
3. What do the health data tell you about this need?
4. Are there any other sources of information, e.g. health or local authority?
5. Is the health need important enough to do something about?
6. What are people doing already?
7. What works and what does not work?
8. What do local people think and want to see happen?
9. Who else should be involved – from health, other agencies, and voluntary sector?
10. How will we know if we have made a difference?

(CPHVA 1997)

Commissioning can also result in disinvestment of some services, which, when reviewed, may prove to be ineffective.

Commissioning entails:

-   monitoring the performance of the assessment of health needs of the relevant population
-   developing strategies to meet that need
-   negotiating with providers to deliver services (NHS and other health care providers)
-   monitoring of that service, including the quality
-   reviewing services.

Strategic Health Authorities will have to support PCTs that serve larger populations to develop their public health infrastructure in partnership with local authorities. Working through a partnership approach with the local authority and community networks is where the community nursing and health visiting intelligence and perspectives are invaluable (see Box 7.2)

An estimate of costs needs to be developed to support any project or new service set up to ensure that any funders have a realistic idea of the potential for the services to be a pilot or, in the future, to be mainstreamed as part of a range of health care resources offered to a community (Figure 7.4).

Barriers

Many community nurses and health visitors find it difficult to think about measurement of outcomes, especially as they are very long term, e.g. prevention programmes in childhood that may have an impact in adult life.

Tracking long-term outcomes is made more difficult by constant restructuring, which can bring insecurity and changes in the configuration of the services and policies where practice is not embedded. Job insecurity and changes to job roles can inhibit new ideas. It is a rare event for good practice to be mainstreamed. Often, good practice is ignored and much time is spent on trying to find out why things have gone wrong. There is a need for good leaders in these situations.

Leadership in the community

With all the recent policy changes that have occurred in the NHS, local authorities and education, many more community nurses, health visitors and allied

---

PROPOSAL FOR A SERVICE DEVELOPMENT

☐ Name of provider ....

☐ Funding proposal to ....

☐ Total amount sought ....

☐ Period of project ....

☐ Health needs to be targeted ....

☐ Significance of health need ....

☐ Proposed service to meet health need ....

☐ New service ....

☐ Changes to present service ....

☐ Who else has been consulted/what other partners involved in the service

changes? ....

☐ What health benefits are anticipated from proposed service/changes? ....

....

☐ How will the service be evaluated? ....

☐ Explanation/justification for funding sought ....

☐ Key references ....

Financial profile

Staff costs

Posts	Grade	WTEs	Starting salary	Weighting	Overheads	On-costs	Total costs Year 1	Total costs Year 2

Total funds required

Non-recurring costs – equipment etc.	
Other recurring costs – specify	
Total for staff costs year 1	
Total staff costs year 2	
Grand total	

Figure 7.4 ● Proposal for a service development (from Leonard et al 1997)

health professionals have become involved with strategic changes and managing change. Many services have had to be re-designed in line with, for example, National Service Frameworks so that the services better meet the needs of the patient. This entails both innovation and risk within the NHS, factors that may be confounded by feelings of failure. As with any experiment or pilot, the outcome may be failure, in part, since this is how people learn, but often it appears that failure of one system tends to inspire yet another re-organisation. The present policies are laden with targets that have to be met by the services and, in particularly deprived communities, meeting certain targets can be very challenging. Nationally set targets may be less relevant to the local population, and resources and energy may get diverted from the need to deal with, for example, high levels of sexually transmitted infections or levels of drug taking in the local community (NHS Confederation 2001).

In 2003 the NHS set up the leadership programmes to help individuals and board members to take on lead responsibilities (Shaw 2003). This was to:

- build and strengthen leadership across the NHS
- ensure all top leaders have personal development plans and are supported in their career development
- provide information and support appointments and succession planning
- maintain links with former senior leaders who might wish to return to the service and to provide tailored development for newcomers
- improve the performance of the NHS.

The nurse leaders' programme has been set up for those people who are taking more responsibility and for those on the Trust Boards and Committees. It aims to enhance the confidence and skills to meet the challenges through work-based learning, mentoring or educational programmes. Leadership London developed a framework with building blocks for learning:

- articulating a vision
- embody values
- motivate
- take decisions
- encourage creativity
- value responsiveness
- release talent
- work across boundaries
- develop personal resources.

Teamwork

Some public health functions are devolved to locality level, and with this will be the need for good networking, partnership and teamwork. Critical to this will be accountability, equity, accessibility and effectiveness of the services for not only the registered population, but also the un-registered groups who live in communities. This is where community teamwork plays an important role in terms of being a safety net. Many of the homeless, asylum-seeker and refugee populations may be known to the services, but through differing access routes via the communities, accident and emergency departments, mental health, social housing sector, social services or through the voluntary sector.

Poverty and deprivation profiling need to be constituents of the overall process of profiling. In the case of people who are socially excluded, community nurses and health visitors will need to recognize that the effects of deprivation on health are considerable and inequalities can occur in any age group and for almost any disease group. Local authorities and public health departments have data on localities and communities that bear out much of what community practitioners see in practice. Many of the Sure Start areas were built around small geographical centres of population where there is deprivation and disadvantage in terms of childcare, family and community resources (see Chapter 6 for more information). The programmes applied not only to the inner-city areas but also to other areas in England with high unemployment and social deprivation. The aim is to ensure delivery of free early education for all 3- and 4-year-olds, and a feature of the Sure Start programmes is that they work in partnerships with other government departments, the voluntary sector and their communities. Responsibility for early education and childcare in Scotland, Wales and Northern Ireland rests with the devolved administrations. Sure Start local programmes and the Sure Start Children's Centres will deliver all the services for children and their families based on the outcomes of the early excellence centres and neighbourhood nurseries.

Skill mix

One of the challenges facing the community nursing and health visiting groups is the issue of recruitment and retention and maintenance of services. The numbers of qualified community nurses has been falling and many nurses are due to retire. Between 1999 and 2002, district nursing numbers dropped by 6% and health visitors dropped by 0.4% (DH 2003) In contrast, many of the new developments in health care and technology have meant shorter hospital stays with a rise in day surgery and day care for cancer patients. This has placed a burden of responsibility on community nurses, with rising workloads, and some of the work has had to be delegated to other grades of staff. Registered staff, therefore, face the issue of staff supervision and support, which is what their statutory body will expect them to take responsibility for in the interests of the patients. NHS managers have a Code of Conduct that states that the care of patients is their first concern and that they must act to protect patients from risk (UNISON 2003).

Public health teamwork

Where there is a health issue or problem for a specific condition or population group, then the public health expertise will be concentrated around the problem. It depends on the health issue and, therefore, brings together the most appropriate team skills. The members will come from very different agencies and will either advise or become the 'hands on' practitioners. This multi-disciplinary team works to a strategic plan that has a common aim and focus. The team must evaluate and review the outcomes, especially if an infection needs to be controlled or if it is a new service that might be commissioned if successful (see Figure 7.2).

The reality of teamwork is that it is not easy and involves complex relationships. Although it is thought to be a panacea for good practice, it involves commitment to make it work, and that takes time. The team members must share goals and vision, values and aspirations. Work is needed to plan procedures and protocols to ensure patients receive the most appropriate person to offer them care. Regular team meetings and effective communication will aid the support and recognition of each other contributions with a commitment by all members. Audit and reflection time must be built in to review the whole team performance (Vanclay 1998).

Role of the National Institute for Health and Clinical Excellence (NICE)

The function of NICE is to offer clinical guidelines based on the best available evidence. These guidelines help health care professionals in their work, but they do not replace their knowledge and skills. NICE is an invaluable source of information and research, and provides the NHS and the public with advice as to the best forms of treatment. The advice is not mandatory and can cause dilemmas for PCTs when resources for the more expensive drugs and technology are very limited. In terms of clinical effectiveness, evidence in some cases is difficult and there is always a possibility that because the evidence of effectiveness is not available or has not been researched, that services may be cut on that basis. There is also a

Table 7.2 ● Examples of public health teamwork

Community health problem	Public health team	Possible strategy for action
Outbreak of diarrhoea in a local nursing home	Director of public health PCT public health team Nursing team Communicable disease control team Registration and inspection team Environmental health infection control nurse	Notify PCT's Public Health Department Collect stool samples Isolate patients if possible Alert any visitors Advise on infection control Teach and advise care assistants Monitor any new cases
Large numbers of children in school with diagnosed asthma A decision made to look at best practice with possible outcome so that children can have their medication with them in school	Primary care group/ community health services Form teacher Head teacher Parent group School secretary School nurse Community paediatrician Director of education/ policy Special needs teacher Health promotion advisor	GPs, school nurses, community paediatrician, health promotion and Director of Education meet and discuss possible strategy Head teachers and staff meet to discuss their needs School governors, staff and parents meet to discuss how children can safely maintain their own care by having their medication with them in school Health staff and school staff develop an agreed protocol including what to do in an emergency situation Group to agree review date
District nurses wish to set up a leg ulcer clinic in the community Evidence from other areas suggests that community clinics have been very successful in improving healing rates	Lead nurse – professional development District nursing teams Research link with university Director of nursing Consultant in vascular surgery Community podiatrist Local patient transport service Locality manager Administrator Community pharmacists GP advisor PCT commissioning manager	Assess need through patient caseload profiles Identify the research evidence on venous leg ulcer management Discuss plan with Trust/ commissioning manager and draft proposal to include accommodation, equipment patient access. Draft patient protocols and patient information sheets – send out for comments as appropriate Identify budget for treatment and dressings Set up appointment systems and GP communications Service promotion leaflets Teaching programme for nurses Audit outcomes, and patient satisfaction and review service
The local hospital gynaecological ward sister has asked patients	Ward sister Liaison health visitor Consultant gynaecologist	Results of the patient survey shared with immediate team in ward Information gained from national

(Continued)

Table 7.2 ● (Continued)

Community health problem	Public Health Team	Possible strategy for action
if they would like some support following a miscarriage They agree that they do, but not in the hospital setting	National miscarriage support group Health centre manager Locality manager Health promotion manager	support groups Discussion with health centre manager *re*: evening accommodation and security Invitation flyer developed with health promotion support Plan for first evening meeting and facilitation Identify with parents what support they would like Discuss short pilot programme and review with group Identify materials and training needs for group to continue Review progress, budgets and future funding
The local GPs have many patients who come from the Punjab area in India There is a high level of diabetes and coronary heart disease Many of the older members of the community do not speak English Literature suggests that other similar programmes have been successful but not been tried with ethnic groups	PCT public health team GP practice Practice manager Practice nurses Health visitor (speaks Punjabi or accesses interpreter) Health promotion manager Diabetes sister Consultant cardiologist Coronary rehabilitation Sister Public health specialist PCG commissioning manager	Identify numbers of patients who have had a coronary event Arrange locality meeting with public health specialist Set up liaison with local cardiac rehabilitation nurses to refer patients for follow up at surgery Plan with practice managers to tag those patients who have had a coronary event in past year Set up appointments and protocols Plan lifestyle programme with health visitor/health advisor Pilot some clinics and record outcomes including patient satisfaction Write up results share with locality staff, and colleagues and commissioning manager Develop training for practice nurses

dearth of research in community nursing and health visiting, therefore, research on nursing questions is needed, and may break new ground.

Clinical governance

Clinical governance is a major feature of policy within the NHS and will include evidence-based practice, research, protocols and guidelines as a feature of service delivery. For practitioners there needs to be continual evaluation and reflection in practice through peer review. The Royal College of Paediatrics and Child Health

(RCPCH) have produced a useful document for the commissioners of services in child health and have ranked the evidence. These were graded as:

- statutory/legal requirements
- clear evidence for value
- of likely benefit in spite of lack of overwhelming evidence of effectiveness
- of common sense benefit only
- of doubtful value.

This is particularly useful as some areas of clinical practice have in the past been questioned as to their value and could, therefore, be deemed as unnecessary (RCPCH 1997). A strategy for clinical governance in practice, therefore, should include:

- management structures
- staffing
- access to clients
- applied research and development
- patient advice and information
- audit and outcomes measures
- training and support
- quality control systems, including IT
- resources
- facilities
- accommodation
- health and safety concerns and ethical practices.

Measuring health outcomes

Why measure outcomes? For practitioners it can demonstrate accountability and improvements in quality of services, and identify what is good or not about community practice; it can also aid risk management and justify more resources. But equally it can improve morale in cases where outcomes have never been demonstrated before. Measuring outcomes is a broad concept. Traditional ways of measuring outcomes has been through death rates associated with intervention or non-intervention. Health status can be measured via programmes of care. Examples could include immunisation levels for children and the elderly, smoking cessation in pregnant mothers or teenagers at school as a result of health promotion input, or healing rates of venous leg ulcers as a result of a clinically effective intervention.

Measuring outcomes for health has been a thorny issue for community nursing and health visiting and, in particular, for the groups of nurses, such as school nurses and health visitors, who have public health, prevention and health promotion as the major focus of practice. Their work will often have much longer-term outcomes for health gain, but staged outputs on objectives of health plans and proxy measures can still offer evidence of progress towards a stated goal. At the practice level, audit and review must be included and relevant to the area of work. It is naturalistic in that it will be from patients or clients themselves or from clinical notes. It need not involve complicated statistics. It is internally led but can be multi-agency. Audit and service reviews should feed into a cycle of change and practice development for staff. The quality model in Chapter 13 provides one way to achieve this. Audit can lead to an understanding of why people behave as they do, e.g. do not comply with medication or turn up for appointments. It can indicate whether it was about service administration or patient's perceptions of care received. Many people, and particularly patients, do not like to complain but may vote with their feet; therefore, it is important to find out the issues so that services can be improved and be more flexible.

Developing a proposal for a development project

Development funding may be available for community nursing and health visiting, health promotion and public health through, for example, Neighbourhood Renewal Funding, or through national nursing bodies. For proposals to be accepted, they must fit with the strategic aims for the NHS, local authority and local strategic partnerships with a modernisation theme.

Questions that may need to be asked are:

- Is it based on evidence of the need for change or improvement?
- What strategic direction or policy initiatives would be the focus (national and local health authority/LA)? Is it a commissioning priority?
- Has a literature search on the evidence been carried out?
- Is there anyone else developing a project or research around area?

One of the first things to do is to formulate an action plan and, if possible, discuss it with a research and development (R&D) officer, especially if there may be ethical issues to consider:

- Discuss ideas with other people.
- Is it a strategic priority locally and would it have employer support?.
- Draw up a skeleton of the idea.
- Identify support for the project by networking with possible stakeholders.
- Determine approximate resources required and planning framework for the project.
- Identify possible funding routes and submit project proposal to funding bodies.
- Form a steering group or project committee.
- Allocate responsibilities to members.
- Plan start date and pilot the project.
- Evaluate pilot and consider any changes as a result of pilot experience.
- Develop implementation and action plan with evaluation included in the process.
- Consider exit strategies where appropriate, i.e. future resourcing of project or service development.
- Develop strategy for dissemination including articles, workshops and conferences.

Fitting the brief in terms of funding

There are now multiple sources of information available through professional libraries, academic departments, and centres for clinical trials, but it does take time and energy to complete a search enquiry.

Steering groups

The steering group is a multi-professional team of people who will advise and monitor the progress of the project. They are extremely important, as they keep the motivation going within any project or programme, especially if it is a new development. The group needs to have representation with people who have appropriate clinical backgrounds and senior people in the organisation to get support. It is important that the steering group has the potential to influence and make decisions on behalf of the organisation.

Informing people

For the plan to be accepted and owned by all members, it is necessary to inform the organisation and the people who may be affected by your project or research. In some cases this may necessitate an impact assessment. If people are not well informed they are less likely to participate in its achievement. However, in some cases, information may need to be restricted if it may be part of some research.

Outline plan: critiqued by others

Once the outline plan is in place, ask someone, like the R&D officer (if there is one), other practitioners, and supervisors, to critique the plan. Often this is very helpful in preventing pitfalls in the early stages, especially if it is a first time. Other people can see things from different angles and practitioners may not have thought about some fundamental and pragmatic issues. Once it has been critiqued, more refining may need to occur in the protocol. Other people may need to be included as stakeholders.

Resources needed

Time is a great resource for people working in the health services and is often at a premium. When undertaking any developments or research, this is going to take more time than is envisaged. As a general rule, researchers need to spend one-third of the time on literature reviews, one-third of the time collecting and analysing data, and the final one-third writing the plan up. Funding bodies include European Funding through partnerships with other European countries, local government funds, the National Lottery and, locally, trustees schemes. For specific topic areas, grants may be available through professional organisations, charities and private companies.

Public health professionals

There is recognition that many other professionals work in the area of public health and not just the doctors working in public health medicine. The English nursing strategy, Making a Difference, identified health visitors, school nurses and midwives as having a major role in the public health function:

'Health visitors will lead public health practice and agree local health plans, school nursing teams will provide a range of health improvement activities, midwives are uniquely placed to improve health and tackle inequality through services to women and their babies.'

(DH 1999b, pp. 60–62)

Health visitors, school nurses, occupational health nurses and other professionals who work in community settings are only too aware of the health issues and the wider determinants of health. Principles identified and embodied in public health work in community nursing and health visiting include:

- Knowing what the health needs of the population are, not just those on your caseload, waiting in the surgery or on your list for visits.
- Making sure services are accessible to those with the greatest need.
- Working with others – not just those who work in the service – to do something about the wider determinants of health.
- Getting people involved in what you do.

- Being aware and ready to respond to infectious disease outbreaks and other threats to health.
- Using evidence – this is just as important in public health as in other care interventions.

(DH Nursing/Community Practitioners and Health Visitors Association 2003, p. 6)

Working as fieldworkers, many of the health issues these practitioners experience every day will be about low income, poor housing, lack of transport, poor access to affordable healthy foods, etc. Not only are these issues observed in the inner-city areas, but increasingly in rural farming areas. Social isolation and lack cohesive communities can reduce the possibilities of access to resources.

Recent proposals that PCTs might choose to concentrate on commissioning services, instead of continuing to employ the community practitioners who provide these grass-roots services (DH 2005a, DH 2006), have raised concerns about the potential for fragmentation. One organisation has claimed:

'If Primary Care Trusts divest themselves of the provider function, the huge numbers of unsung contributors to community health and wellbeing, the public health workforce will become further fragmented and disillusioned leading to a negative impact on public health.'

(United Kingdom Public Health Association 2005)

However the new proposals pan out in practice, the need to understand how public health strategies are developed and implemented will be increasingly important.

Conclusion

Change is inevitable within the health services, as can be seen by the rapidity and number of policy directives that are received by health professionals at regular intervals. Working with the public and in public health is exciting and challenging. It often means working with people who think that the government is concerned with being a 'nanny state' and that it is the people's right to choose, for example, whether they smoke or not. However, public health is about doing the right thing for the public good and that individual behaviour can affect the wider population. In a democracy, people have the right to express their opinion, and the role of public health is sometimes to acknowledge its political dimensions and health advocacy role. This may also make it very unpopular. By their nature, public health strategies ensure that the wider dimensions of health are explored. They stand a better chance for acceptance and sustainability if all stakeholders including community practitioners and the local population have their say.

 DISCUSSION QUESTIONS

- What are the dilemmas that community practitioners face when commissioning health care alongside GPs and social services?
- Primary care trusts have community practitioners on their Boards, but what and whom do they represent?

- How can community nurses and health visitors make sure that community profiling is part of the public health role and, if needs are identified, how can they change the strategic direction?
- What advantages or otherwise do community practitioners feel about the involvement of the user perspectives as described within The NHS Plan?
- To what extent does 'Facing the Future: a review of the role of health visitors' (Department of Health 2007) serve as a strategy for improving public health?

References

Acheson D 1998 (Chairman) Independent inquiry into inequalities in health report. The Stationery Office, London

Billings JR, Cowley S 1995 Approaches to community needs assessment: a literature review. Journal of Advanced Nursing 22: 721–730.

British Medical Journal 2001 The fetal origins of adult disease. Editorial. British Medical Journal 322: 375–376

Children Act 2004 HMSO, London

Community Practitioners and Health Visitors Association (CPHVA) 1997 Public health: the role of nurses and health visitors. CPHVA, London

Dahlgren G, Whitehead M 1999 Policies and strategies to promote equality in health. Health 21: Health for all policy framework for the European Union. WHO, Copenhagen.

Department for Education and Skills/ Department of Health 2004a Every child matters: change for children. TSO, London

Department for Education and Skills (DfES)/Department of Health (DH) 2004b National Service Framework for Children, Young People and Maternity Services. DfES/DH, London

Department of Health (DH) 1992 The Health of the Nation (CM 1986) HMSO, London

Department of Health (DH) 1995a Making it happen. Public health – the contribution, role and development of nurses, midwives and health visitor. Report of the Standing Nursing and Midwifery Advisory Committee. DH, London

Department of Health (DH) 1995b Primary care: delivering the future. HMSO, London

Department of Health (DH) 1997 The new NHS – modern, dependable (CM3807). DH, London

Department of Health (DH) 1998 Our healthier nation: a contract for health (CM3852). DH, London

Department of Health (DH) 1999a Reducing health inequalities: an action report. DH, London

Department of Health (DH) 1999b Making a difference: strengthening the nursing, midwifery and health visiting contribution to health and health care. DH, London

Department of Health (DH) 2000 The NHS plan. The Stationery Office, London

Department of Health (DH) 2001 Shifting the balance of power within the NHS: securing delivery. The Stationery Office, London

Department of Health (DH) 2002 Health improvement and prevention – National Service Frameworks: a practical aid to implementation in primary care. DH, London

Department of Health (DH) 2003 Statistical Bulletin 2003. DH, London

Department of Health (DH) 2004a Choosing health: making healthier choices better (CM6374). DH, London

Department of Health (DH) 2004b Choosing health: making healthier choices easier. DH, London

Department of Health (DH) 2004c National standards, local action health and social care standards and planning framework 2005/06–2007/08. DH, London

Department of Health (DH) 2004d Practice based commissioning: promoting clinical engagement. DH, London

Department of Health (DH) 2004e Standards for better health. DH, London

Department of Health (DH) 2004f The Chief Nursing Officer's review of the nursing, midwifery and health visiting contribution to vulnerable children and young people. DH, London

Department of Health (DH) 2004g The expert patient: a new approach to chronic disease management for the 21st Century. DH, London

Department of Health (DH) 2005a Commissioning a patient-led NHS. DH, London

Department of Health (DH) 2005b Delivering choosing health: making healthier choices easier. DH, London

Department of Health (DH) 2005c
Supporting people with long term conditions: liberating the talents of nurses who care for people with long term conditions. DH, Leeds

Department of Health (DH) 2006 The NHS in England: the operating framework. DH, Leeds

Department of Health & Allied Health Professions 2005 Working differently: the role of allied health professions in treatment and management of long term medical conditions. DH, London

Department of Health (DH) Nursing/Community Practitioners and Health Visitors Association (CPHVA) 2003 Liberating the talents of community nurses and health visitors. Best Practice Guidance. DH and CPHVA, London

Entwistle V, Watt I, Brugge C, Collins S, Drew P, Gilhooly K, Walker A 2002 Exploring patient participation in decision-making. Health Services Research Unit University of Aberdeen, Aberdeen

European Commission 2001 Directive 2001/42/EC on assessment of the effects of certain plans and programmes on the environment. EC, Luxemborg

Fant M, Roberts-Davis M 2005 Concurrent health impact assessment of recent and proposed future changes in the health visiting services on Guernsey QNI/Health and Social Services. A States of Guernsey Government Department, Guernsey

Ham C, Appleby J 1993 The future of the NHS. NAHAT, Birmingham

Health Act 1999 HMSO, London

Health and Safety at Work Act 1974. HMSO, London, ch 37

Health and Safety Commission (HSC) 2005 Health and safety statistics 2004/05; National statistics, HSC Publications, Sudbury

Health Development Agency (HDA) 2004 Strategic Health Authorities/workforce directorates and the mid-life age group: using the evidence to take action, NHS/HDA, London

HM Treasury 2004a Choice for parents, the best start for children: a ten year strategy for childcare. HMSO, London

HM Treasury 2004b Spending review: public service agreement 2005–2008. Chapter 3 Department of Health Objective IV; 7 p. 14. HMSO, London

International Association for Public Participation 2000 The IAP2 Public Participation Spectrum. International Association for Public Participation, Denver, USA

Leonard O, Allsop J, Taket A Wiles R 1997 User involvement in two primary health care projects in London. Social Science Research Papers No. 5. South Bank University/College of Health, London

Levy BS 1998 Creating the future of public health: values, vision and leadership: 1997 presidential address. American Journal of Public Health 88: 188–192

London Health Economics Consortium 1995 Community based needs assessment. test bed sites study: overview paper and summary of findings. Report to the steering group. School of Tropical Hygiene and Medicine, London

Marsh S, Macalpine M 1995 Our own capabilities: clinical nurse man-agers making a strategic approach to service improvement. Kings Fund/Nursing Development Units, London

National Prescribing Centre (NPC) 1999 Sign post for prescribing nurses – general principles of good prescribing. Prescribing Nurse Bulletin 1. NPC, Liverpool

National Prescribing Centre (NPC) 2003 Supplementary prescribing: a resource to help health professionals to understand the framework and opportunities. NPC/NHS, Liverpool

NHS Confederation 2001 Leading edge: 2. Aligning what we say and how we behave. Rethinking performance management. October 2001. NHS Confederation, London

Pearson V 1998 Who needs needs assessment? Assessing health needs and integrating public health into locality commissioning. In: Dixon M et al (eds) The locality commissioning handbook. Radcliffe Oxford pp. 60–68

Quigley R, Cavanagh S, Harrison D, Taylor L 2004 Clarifying health impact assessment, integrated impact assessment and health needs assessment. NHS/ Health Development Agency, London

Royal College of Nursing 2004 Vision of the future nurse supplement: the future nurse: trends and predictions for the nurse workforce. RCN, London

Royal College of Paediatrics and Child Health (RCPCH) 1997 The essentials of effective community health services for children and young people: report of a working party. November 1997. RCPCH, London

Scottish Executive Health Department 2004 Community health partnership development guidance. Scottish Executive, Edinburgh, 13 January 2004

Secretary of State for Health 1999 Saving lives: our healthier nation (CM4386). HMSO, London

Secretary of State for Health 2000 The NHS plan: a plan for investment, a plan for reform (CM4818–I). HMSO, London

Shaw T 2003 NHS leaders: a career development and succession planning scheme. NHS, London

Standing Nursing and Midwifery Advisory Committee (SNMAC) 1995 Making it happen. Public health: the contribution, role and development of nurses, midwives and health visitors. HMSO, London

Stewart R, Turner I 1998 Achieving quality in residential care and nursing homes. In Mason C (ed.) Achieving quality in community health care nursing. Macmillan, London

Taylor L, Gowman N, Quigley R 2003 Influencing the decision making process through health impact assessment. Health Development Agency, London

Taylor L, Blair-Stevens C 2002 Introducing health impact assessment (HIA): informing the decision-making process. HDA/NHS, London

The Medicinal Products: Prescriptions by Nurses Act 1992 (c.28). HMSO, London

UK Public Health Association 2005 Sins of commission? Response from the UKPHA

to 'Commissioning a Patient Led NHS' Document. UKPHA, London

UNISON 2003 The duty of care: a handbook to assist health care staff carrying out their duty of care to patients, colleagues and themselves. UNISON, London

United Nations 2005 Millennium development goals: blue print for the worlds' countries. UN Web Services Section, Department of Public Information United Nations

Vanclay L 1998 Teamworking in primary care. Nursing Standard 12(20): 37–38

Wanless D 2002 Securing our future health: taking a long-term view final report. Her Majesty's Treasury. HMSO, London

Wilkinson R, Marmot M (eds) 2003 Social determinants of health: the solid facts, 2nd edn. WHO Regional Office for Europe, Copenhagen

World Health Organization (WHO) 1985 Targets for health for all. WHO, Geneva

WHO European Centre for Health Policy 1999 Health impact assessment. Main concepts and suggested approach. Gothenburg Consensus Paper. WHO Regional Office for Europe, Copenhagen

Further reading

Marmot M, Wilkinson RG (eds) 2006 Social determinants of health, 2nd edn. Oxford University Press, Oxford

This book discusses the power of the socio-economic determinants of health and its relationship with health inequalities. It also has chapters that link the evidence of physiological stress to factors in early life and social and cultural influences on health.

Naidoo J, Wills J 2004 Health promotion: foundations for practice. Baillière Tindall, London

Since the publication of the first edition there has been a significant policy shift within the UK that makes this book even more important for an increasing number of health care professionals. In addition, the rise of evidence-based health care makes this book's focus on the dilemmas and challenges that underpin health promotion (i.e. where is the evidence and how is health promotion practice informed by it?) even timelier.

Resources
National Institute of Clinical Excellence/Health Development Agency

This is the independent organisation responsible for providing national guidance on the promotion of good health and the prevention and treatment of ill health. On 1 April 2005 NICE joined with the Health Development Agency to become the new National Institute for Health and Clinical Excellence (also known as NICE).

It has taken on the functions of the Health Development Agency to create a single excellence-in-practice organisation responsible for providing national guidance on the promotion of good health and the prevention and treatment of ill health. Its guidance is for those working in the NHS, local authorities and the wider public, private and voluntary sector.

Kings Fund Successful Nurse Leader: Developing skills for career success

This is a 5-day programme for nurses run by the Kings Fund, which help nurses take on new levels of responsibility and respond to changes within their work environment.
Website: http://www.kingsfund.org.uk/leadership

NHS Expert Patient Programme (EPP)

The EPP provides training opportunities for people with chronic conditions, such as arthritis, asthma, hæmophilia, heart disease, stroke, manic depression, diabetes mellitus, endometriosis and others, to develop skills to 'self-manage' their condition more effectively.

UKPHA

The UK Public Health Association is a charity launched in 1999 whose membership includes practitioners and specialists who promote the public's health and wellbeing. It works with other organisations, both nationally and internationally, to the develop public health policy. It is open to all individuals who share the UKPHA values and aims.
E-mail: info@ukpha.org.uk

Understanding effectiveness for service planning

8

Peter Griffiths

Key issues

- The effectiveness of a service is its ability to achieve desired outcomes
- Evidence for effectiveness should not be confused with efficacy: the impact of an intervention in ideal circumstances, as opposed to in everyday practice
- Direct evidence of effectiveness for public health interventions is often lacking, and decisions must often be made on the basis of a range of available evidence
- Evidence that is available is often ignored
- The evidence-based health care paradigm identifies the randomised controlled trial (RCT) as the strongest form of evidence for service effectiveness
- The reality of many complex health care interventions means that RCTs may only provide evidence of *efficacy* in all but the simplest cases
- RCTs may sometimes be impossible for public health interventions
- The decision about the ideal type of evidence for many public health interventions is more complicated than it is for simple drug treatments
- The idea of a clear hierarchy of evidence must be disputed
- *No* form of evidence (qualitative or quantitative) can be rejected out of hand when determining the effectiveness of public health interventions
- *Any* form of evidence must be critically appraised rather than taken at face value

Introduction

Surely effective public health care is good health care? It does what is intended to do, which is to restore or promote health or to prevent illness. The difficulty arrives when it comes to deciding the appropriate outcomes, the appropriate ways of defining them and the appropriate way of determining whether the desired outcome has been achieved. This is the problem of determining effectiveness. It is often at its most problematic when dealing with complex, multi-faceted interventions, which have multiple outcomes and operate through complex mechanisms. Many public health interventions undertaken by public health practitioners are of this type. Public health practitioners are increasingly expected to contribute to service planning too, perhaps as members of a Primary Care Trust (PCT), or in a working group for one or more aspects of a Local Strategic Partnership (LSP) or Local Delivery Plan (LDP) (see Chapters 3 and 7). How can they choose which services will best meet the health needs? Those seeking evidence to use in planning public health services need to consider the type of evidence needed and the value of that evidence very carefully, prior to putting any intervention into effect.

Much of the debate about effectiveness is fuelled by competing approaches to scientific enquiry and arguments about the nature of human knowledge and experience. Those who are tempted to paddle in these turbulent philosophical waters are advised to bear in mind that at the heart of the effectiveness debate lies a simple purpose. To put it most plainly, we wish to determine whether our actions had an effect and whether that effect was that which we intended. For public health interventions, the desired effect is 'health', construed in its broadest sense to encompass a range of human experiences from the relief of physical illness through to positive aspects of wellbeing in individuals or groups.

We begin with a definition of effectiveness drawn from the paradigm of evidence-based health care (EBHC), going on to examine this paradigm and the approaches to determining effectiveness. The chapter then moves on to an examination of approaches to evaluation, beginning with a consideration of the role of experimental/quasi-experimental approaches. After examining the limitations of the experimental approach, alternative and complementary approaches to evaluation will be examined, which in turn emphasise the need to consider the full complexity of public health interventions when seeking evidence for their effectiveness. Finally, we will consider the role of guidelines in the delivery of effective public health.

Defining effectiveness

Muir Gray (2001) offers a simple definition of effectiveness. The effectiveness of a health care service or professional is the extent to which desired outcomes are achieved *in practice* (p. 185). Effectiveness is distinguished from quality, which is seen as the adherence to (best) standards of care delivery. Although you might generally expect that standards of care be set in order to deliver the most effective care possible, this is frequently not the case. One reason for this is that the effectiveness of many health care interventions is simply not known. In many cases (perhaps all) the goal is not necessarily the most effective care possible for a specific problem, but that which yields the best effect within parameters that are dictated by financial resources and decisions about allocating resources across a range of interventions for a variety of problems. Further, since the effects of health care interventions are generally multi-faceted, the most effective approach to care depends upon the value ascribed to different outcomes, which varies across individuals and groups. Effectiveness must also be distinguished from efficacy, the impact of an intervention in ideal circumstances, as opposed to everyday practice.

Should the distinction between quality and effectiveness seem unconvincing, it may help to consider an alternative framework for defining quality in health care. According to Donabedian, a health outcome is, '. . . the effect of care on the health and welfare of individuals or populations' (Donabedian 1988, p. 177). Donabedian's work distinguishes outcome from process ('. . . care itself') and structure ('. . . the characteristics of the settings in which care is delivered') (1988, p. 177). Although the validity of any quality indicator is predicated upon a relationship between that indicator and some dimension of patient health or wellbeing, it is frequently the case that this relationship is hypothetical (Donabedian 1966). Quality in the structures and processes of care is not necessarily based on a proven link to outcomes, i.e. effectiveness (see Chapter 13 for more information about quality).

A hypothetical example might illustrate these differences. Suppose that we designed a fall-prevention programme for elderly people. We choose to implement it through individualised visits to people identified as at-risk by a specially trained public health practitioner. The programme consisted of an assessment of risk in the home, advice on exercise and feedback to the GP about any risks to the individual from their medication regime and the need for any further medical assessment.

A research study demonstrates that the programme dramatically reduces the number of falls experienced by the target group when compared to an appropriate comparison group who do not receive it, and it is deemed a success. Such a research study would almost certainly have at its core a randomised controlled trial in which clients are randomly allocated to receive the fall-prevention programme or a control intervention, which would probably be simply GP follow-up. At this point the programme has been identified as having efficacy, since it has worked, albeit in these special circumstances. A range of such studies have, in fact, been done, which provide some evidence for a health/environmental risk factor screening assessment and individually tailored interventions in preventing falls (Gillespie et al 2003), although research has not generally examined the specific contribution of public health practitioners.

Let us further imagine that the National Service Framework for older people or a similar policy framework identifies this service as representing quality care for at-risk elderly people. The quality of a preventative health service for elderly people might now be judged, in part, by whether practitioners offered this programme.

Unsurprisingly, when an intervention like this is implemented in everyday practice, its effectiveness may be not nearly so dramatic as identified in the original research. Imagine this (hypothetical) intervention when implemented routinely. The intervention would be but one of many activities undertaken by the public health practitioner. As relatively few specialise in working with elderly people, other professionals might become involved in delivering the intervention. It might be that few of those involved received specific training or the nature of the training may vary in extent and quality and the clients they see are not so carefully assessed prior to referral as were those who took part in the research. Under these circumstances, although defined quality standards may be met, this 'quality' provision may not deliver the same outcomes. We will return to these distinctions between aspects of quality later, but for the moment the important points are that neither quality services nor evidence of efficacy necessarily guarantee effectiveness.

Evidence-based health care

Evidence-based medicine has been defined as '. . . the conscientious, explicit and judicious use of current best evidence in making decisions about the care of individual patients' (Sackett et al 1996, p. 71). The approach is not, however, restricted to decisions about medical care nor to the care of individual patients. EBHC is more broadly defined in terms of decision making about the health care of individual patients, groups of patients and populations (Muir Gray 2001) and it is this broader term that is used here. Although the particular set of practices and principles that represent the current EBHC movement emerged into the mainstream of practice only during the mid 1990s, its advocates claim illustrious ancestors.

Origins in public health practice

The link between public health practice and EBHC is firmly established. Authors in the area often seek to establish its lineage by tracing its roots to the pioneering studies including the epidemiological work of Semmelweiss and Oliver Wendel Holmes, both of whom identified the role of health care practitioners in causing puerperal fever through lack of basic hygiene (Rangachari 1997). Systematic observation allowed Holmes to discern that incidence of puerperal fever seemed to be in clusters that were associated with particular physicians and concluded that these physicians were transmitting the disease-causing agent from one woman to another. Semmelweiss' comparison of infection rates in women cared for by doctors (who did not wash their hands when attending to women after post-mortem examinations) and midwives (who were not contaminated in this way) is held up as an early prototype for today's randomised controlled trials (RCTs).

If Holmes and Semmelweiss are claimed as its grandfathers, Archie Cochrane, an epidemiologist who worked on the earliest RCTs conducted by the Medical Research Council in the UK, could be said to be the father of today's EBHC movement. After a lifetime spent working on studies of effectiveness he complained, 'It is surely a great criticism of our profession that we have not organised a critical summary, by specialty or subspecialty, adapted periodically, of all relevant randomised controlled trials' (Chalmers 1997). For Cochrane, an unbiased synthesis of evidence from good-quality studies is the true endpoint of health research. He campaigned for effective health care to be free in the National Health Service (NHS), but equally argued that interventions with no evidence of effectiveness should not be offered unless as part of a well-designed research programme.

Use of evidence

At the heart of the EBHC movement lie two simple premises. Many interventions lack evidence of effectiveness and much existing evidence of effectiveness is not put into practice. For practitioners and policy makers alike, the most significant aspect of this problem will be the identification and utilisation of existing evidence, since action can rarely be delayed until new research is commissioned to answer a question. Even where the main action is to undertake or commission research or implement pilot projects to be evaluated, it is to be hoped that such action would be based on an appraisal of the existing evidence-base (or lack thereof).

Muir Gray (2001) reduces the problem of identification and utilisation of evidence of effectiveness to a simple algebraic formulation (which I suspect he would not wish us to take too literally). In his formulation the decision-maker's performance as an 'evidence-based decision-maker' is proportional to motivation (to utilise evidence) and competence (in identifying, appraising and interpreting evidence). It is inversely related to barriers which, in Muir Gray's account, are lack of resources for accessing evidence (Figure 8.1).

Muir Gray's term 'motivation' covers a complex set of cognitive processes, which are often touched on in studies of research utilisation. In the extreme case it has been frequently argued that practitioners will simply disbelieve or disregard evidence if it does not accord with pre-existing beliefs (Hunt 1996, Jones 1997, Rodgers 1994). Within the paradigm of EBHC, these complex factors are essentially irrational, in that they will tend to lead the individual toward making an incorrect decision (or to be sufficiently unmotivated as to make no decision at all).

$$\text{Performance} = \frac{\text{Motivation} \times \text{Competence}}{\text{Barriers}}$$

Figure 8.1 ● Algebraic account of research utilisation (after Muir Gray 2001)

The experiences of the early pioneers Semmelweiss and Wendel Holmes illustrate that the power of rational argument alone is not enough to ensure that evidence is implemented. Semmelweiss was eventually dismissed from his job in Vienna and forced to return to his native Hungary, after failing to find further work. Wendel Homes was the subject of considerable scorn from eminent practitioners for many years, before his findings were finally accepted. One detects a whiff of anti-semitism in the treatment of Semelweiss and it is clear that the perceptions of the messenger have considerable impact upon people's willingness to listen to the message. This is a complex topic, and one that is well outside the remit of this chapter, although readers might like to consult two excellent reviews of implementing evidence that have been commissioned by the NHS in recent years (Greenhalgh et al 2004, NHS CRD 1999).

There is, however, one issue of substantive import that must be addressed prior to moving on. I would not wish to ally myself to an extreme relativist pos-ition on knowledge. Absolute relativism has little place in a practice discipline where all parties must accept (if only on pragmatic grounds) that individuals do not completely construct their own realities. Events such as survival and death are of fundamental significance and subject to external verification. However, this does not necessarily mean that the evidence available for rational scrutiny is not subject to interpretation. What one party may perceive as useful evidence may not necessarily be seen as such by another. The questions asked about health care practice are selective and the answers that are published are also filtered and selected according to particular world views. It is not that practitioners are free to construct any version of reality that they choose, but equally the available evidence cannot be said to simply purvey objective 'truth' in any absolute sense either (Griffiths 2005).

Much of the research on research utilisation implies that disbelieving the evidence of research is always an essentially irrational phenomenon. Certainly, experience suggests that a blanket refusal to believe research evidence based on a sophisticated rational appraisal of its limited utility is rare. However, the distinction between effectiveness and efficacy identified earlier should serve as a warning that the implications of a particular piece of evidence for practice in a particular setting are often far from clear. Thus, lack of motivation might, in part, be a product of the lack of utility practitioners find in evidence offered to them for making decisions about effectiveness. We will return to this later when considering the formulation of evaluations. For now, we will consider the model decision maker who is motivated to find evidence for effectiveness and is willing (at least in principle) to implement it. What follows is based squarely within the EBHC paradigm. The reasons for this are twofold.

First, the literature on evidence-based practice clearly describes the basis on which many health care policy and practice decisions can be, and are, made. Indeed, although by no means ubiquitous (see Sheldon et al 1996), the EBHC model is probably now the dominant one in current health services research and research policy. Certainly, the majority of initiatives that resulted from the UK's NHS research and development and information strategies in the early 1990s (e.g. the Centre for Reviews and Dissemination; the National Institute for Health and Clinical Excellence, which now incorporates the former Health Development Agency; the Health Technology Assessment programme; Health Scotland, which combines the former Health Education Board for Scotland and Public Health Institute for Scotland and the National Library for Health; see Box 8.1) seem to adhere broadly to the tenets of the model. The second reason is that the model's critique of many aspects of current ('evidence less') practice is compelling, as are some of the solutions offered. The following sections will describe the nature of the evidence that the evidence-based decision-maker is urged to use in order to ensure patients and clients receive the most effective health care.

Box 8.1

The UK's NHS strategy for identifying effective intervention

In the UK, a number of initiatives were developed to provide evidence for practice and health care management. Key to these initiatives was making information readily available to 'consumers' of research. The worldwide web has been used as a mechanism for disseminating information on effectiveness and the initiatives themselves. The web addresses for four of the key initiatives are:

- Centre for Reviews and Dissemination – http://www.york.ac.uk/inst/crd/
- National Library for Health – http://www.nlh.nhs.uk/
- National Institute for Health and Clinical Excellence – http://www.nice.org.uk/
- Health Technology Assessment programme – http://www.hta.nhsweb.nhs.uk/
- Health Scotland – http://www.healthscotland.com/

Hierarchy of evidence

Imagine we wish to implement a programme to control head-lice in children. In the first instance the question appears to be a simple one. What is the most effective treatment of head-lice? Clearly, in order to determine the relative merits of any one treatment we would wish to compare it with the alternatives (including non-pharmacological approaches). The treatment that led to the highest number of children being free of head-lice would be the most effective. So a carefully controlled comparison is what we require.

In evidence-based practice, the ideal single study design for answering this form of question is the (well-conducted) RCT. There is a clear and explicit hierarchy of evidence. There is some discussion of the relative merits at the lower end of the hierarchy, but for a single study there is no serious debate as to the superiority of the RCT. Best of all is a systematic review of good-quality RCTs encompassing all of the valid evidence (see below).

A physicist is able to create a vacuum in order to control extraneous factors, such as air resistance, to determine whether the acceleration of a pebble subjected to gravity is the same as that of a feather (it is!); no such parallel vacuum exists in health care interventions. Since in health care we cannot remove extraneous variables (differences in the characteristics of people), the RCT allows variation arising from these factors to be dealt with by distributing groups of people randomly, to different treatment groups. The probability of any differences between groups prior to the intervention is precisely modelled by probability theory, as are individual variations in response to treatments. Statistical-significance testing allows chance variation to be quantified and potentially discounted (certainly over repeated replications). Thus we can account for the play of chance and attribute any differences between groups at the end of the study that are in excess of what might be seen purely by chance to differences in the effects of the treatments people received.

The problem of using non-random groups to compare the effectiveness of interventions is clear when considering a hypothetical comparison of two head-lice treatments. Imagine treatment X is the most expensive pediculocide on the market. If we simply compared those children whose parent bought and used treatment X with those who received the extremely cheap treatment Y it is difficult to determine what caused any observed differences in louse infestation. Treatment X may appear more effective because it is more diligently applied by parents who have invested heavily in treatments. Alternatively, treatment Y might appear more effective because it tended to be bought by parents who thought they ought to treat 'just in case', but had in fact seen no lice. The permutations are endless, but just about any pattern of outcomes could be accounted for by explanations other than differential effectiveness in treatments.

Only when treatment X is compared to treatment Y in a well-conducted RCT can differences between the two groups be confidently attributed to the treatment itself. In the paradigm of EBHC, the ideal form of research evidence for answering a question such as this is thus the RCT. This, then, is the type of evidence that decision-makers should seek in order to answer their effectiveness questions.

However, evidence from RCTs is not always available. In some cases randomisation to groups may be practically or technically impossible. In these cases, other comparative designs, such as cohort studies (where outcomes of comparable groups with and without exposure to the intervention are compared), case control studies (where known cases, e.g. those exposed to an intervention or experience, are compared to matched controls) or 'n of 1' trials in which an individual (or group) is exposed to one or more interventions intermittently (in random order), may be considered. The natural experiment on head-lice treatment comparing those who simply chose to use different treatments would constitute a (rather poor) cohort study. Studies of disease causation must generally be cohort studies, since randomisation to the causal agents of disease is frequently impossible and almost never ethical. The individual case report, or series of case reports, where the effectiveness of the intervention is illustrated by a change in status before and after exposure to an intervention or agent, with no comparison whatsoever, is seen as evidence, which is so weak as to be negligible in most cases.

Many public health interventions are delivered at a level of service organisation where randomisation of individuals to receive 'treatments' would not be possible. For example, if one wished to investigate the impact of an initiative aimed at promoting self-care within a community using multiple sources of dissemination, including distribution of a self-help/self-assessment guide, it would be highly problematic to randomise individuals. The aim of the intervention is to disseminate information within a community. An 'ideal' design here would probably be one in which the unit of randomisation was at the level of the community itself (for example, a whole town) and effectiveness was measured in terms of population outcomes rather than at the individual level. However, widespread policy initiatives are often implemented without extensive piloting. In such cases, and in the UK NHS Direct is an example of a national initiative that has many of these features, it may be that the only available comparison is with a historical cohort prior to the implementation of change.

In cases where non-randomised studies are conducted, a judgement on the quality of the evidence produced is generally made upon the extent to which the study has managed to control bias. A study on the effectiveness of primary care trusts (PCTs) might attempt to adjust (in statistical terms, 'control') for differences in the age and socio-economic status of individuals in the lists of practices involved in the study.

Complex techniques of design and analysis are deployed to improve the validity of results from such non-randomised (quasi-) experiments (Cook & Campbell 1979). All are essentially designed to control for the effect of extraneous causes that might lead to differences between groups, and thus to increase the confidence with which cause can be attributed to the intervention under investigation. In essence, the endeavour is to make the quasi-experiment as much like the RCT as possible. Thus, alternative study designs represent no shift in the paradigm. Rather they represent best fixes for technical problems that mitigate against the use of an RCT.

Nonetheless, two of the leading authors in the field offer the following observations: 'With the data usually available for such studies, there is simply no logical or statistical procedure that can be counted on to make proper allowances for uncontrolled pre-existing differences between groups' (Lord 1967, p. 305 cited in Cook & Campbell 1979). In other words, nothing really beats a good RCT, a point emphasised by Muir Gray (2001): 'The main abuse of a cohort study is to assess the effectiveness of a particular intervention when a more appropriate method would be an RCT' (p. 150).

Yet, as we have seen, in some cases the only available design to measure effectiveness is in fact a quasi-experiment. The criticism of the quasi-experiment and associated analysis techniques is offered here largely to establish their inherent imperfection and associated uncertainty. Unlike the true RCT, such uncertainty cannot be precisely quantified and thus the influence of other factors cannot be discounted simply by replication, and reduction of the probability of 'random' error accounting for the findings.

Critical appraisal

The first step in seeking evidence of effectiveness is thus to seek reports of appropriate primary research (or, ideally, systematic reviews of all such research – see below). In general, this will be from an RCT or, for complex interventions such as many public health initiatives, a quasi-experiment, cohort study or, occasionally, a case-control study.

Clearly, having identified studies that can provide answers to questions of effectiveness, it is important to assess the validity of the studies themselves. Not all RCTs are properly conducted and reported. Most texts on evidence-based practice provide critical appraisal guidelines for varying types of study designs. Those given by Greenhalgh (2001) and Muir Gray (2001) are both typical and usable, with details of how they should be applied. Box 8.2 gives an outline of key points to be considered.

Accumulation of evidence increasing precision

At the pinnacle of the hierarchy of evidence is the systematic review, which should represent an unbiased synthesis of all the (valid) evidence available for the effectiveness of an intervention. In a classic paper, Antman and colleagues (1992) criticised the traditional 'review' article for providing biased accounts that fail to properly represent the current state of evidence. Thus, the emphasis of the EBHC movement on the use of systematic reviews might at first seem perplexing.

The word 'systematic' is key. The systematic review should contain an explicit statement of its objectives and methods. This should include the techniques used for searching the literature and identifying all relevant studies, the criteria for selecting studies for the review, a description of how the criteria were applied and an explicit method for synthesising the findings of the studies. The systematic review is conducted with the rigour expected of primary research and the validity of a review is judged by similar criteria (Egger & Smith 2001, Shea et al 2001).

The logic of the systematic review is to eliminate the effect of 'random' variation between different settings and participants, in order to determine a precise, numerical, estimate of 'true' effect. However, while the RCT allows precise quantification of uncertainty, the lack of control over extraneous variables intrinsic in other study designs means that quantitative estimates of effect from systematic reviews of these studies imply a rather spurious confidence in the success of statistical control (Egger et al 2001). Nonetheless, the systematic search and appraisal of all relevant research studies, which is at the heart of the systematic review, clearly represents a major advance from selective reviews, which can present a significantly misleading picture of the weight of evidence in a particular area (Egger & Smith 2001).

Box 8.2

Critical appraisal for studies of effectiveness

Appropriateness of design

In identifying evidence for effectiveness, the first stage is to determine whether or not a particular study design is appropriate to answer a question about effectiveness. Clearly there must be some form of comparison.

In general, the study design should be the strongest possible. Cohort studies are viewed as weaker evidence than randomised controlled trials (RCTs) and case-control studies as weaker still. Although we question the absoluteness of this hierarchy later in this chapter, it is still important to consider. If the design is not appropriate there is no point in reading the study.

The paper should then be scrutinised to identify the description of the intervention under study and what it is to be compared with. Adequate description is essential in order to determine if the evidence is useful.

Finally, it is crucial to identify the actual outcomes studied and how they were measured. If a paper claims an intervention is 'effective', it is important that it is clear that a reader knows precisely *what* it is effective for.

Applicability

A study report should be scrutinised in order to identify the particular population studied. An intervention that was tested on one group or in one setting may not work in another. Evidence that cervical screening programmes are effective in university students says little directly about the effectiveness of a similar programme in a council estate. It is also important to consider the 'control' condition to which an intervention is compared. Crudely, an intervention that improves health, compared to no services at all, cannot be assumed to be effective compared to some other services.

Bias

In appraising any comparative design it is vital to establish that comparison groups were similar in every way but their exposure to the treatment. In an RCT this is achieved through properly concealed randomisation, complete follow-up and analysis of outcomes on the basis of the groups to which people were randomised to (irrespective of treatment received) – so-called intention to treat analysis. In non-randomised studies possible bias must be discussed and the authors must demonstrate that groups did not differ in terms of all important prognostic factors.

Outcomes assessment

Outcomes should ideally be assessed by someone with no knowledge of the intervention received by an individual or group (although this is not always possible). For retrospective studies, there are additional problems associated with identification of both the outcome and the exposure or otherwise to the intervention. In these cases it is vital that both outcome and intervention are assessed using a standardised approach that uses clearly-defined criteria.

However, in areas where the available body of research is disparate and weak, or the questions to be addressed intrinsically multi-faceted, a systematic review in this form does little to advance knowledge, except insofar as it clearly delineates the weakness of the evidence base. Increasingly, efforts are being made to apply systematic approaches to complex questions using various types of evidence in attempt to organise knowledge from diverse sources, particularly in the face of complex questions (Forbes & Griffiths 2002). A particular issue in the face of scant evidence is the extent to which there is a poor correspondence between what has been researched and what occurs in practice. Reviews that incorporate a survey of practice in addition to a review of research, such as the UK's Social Care Institute of Excellence 'Knowledge Reviews', enable the reader to identify not only the evidence base, but also, crucially, the practices about which questions can be asked.

Studies of efficacy vs. effectiveness

The emphasis of the evidence-based practice approach to critiquing evidence of effect is on determining that observed differences between groups are caused by the intervention rather than by chance. This is an important component of any answer regarding a question of effectiveness. Indeed, it may ultimately be the most important answer. However, confidence in the answer comes at a price, which may considerably reduce its utility. A quick review of our hypothetical RCT for head-lice treatments can illustrate one way in which such utility is limited. Even in the case of such a simple question, which can be reduced to one of treatment effect, it is far easier to answer the question of 'efficacy' than truly answer the question of 'effectiveness'.

In an experimental study, the factors that lead people to participate in the study may make them more or less likely to utilise the treatment in a particular way. In the earlier example of an RCT of head-lice treatments, I hypothesised that the expensive treatment might induce a particular diligence among parents using it. In a trial they would be given the medication and so this difference between different medications would not become apparent. Conversely, because they are in a trial, parents may be more likely to continue using a medication when in the 'real world' aspects of the application might deter 'proper' use. The circumstances of an RCT may often mean that the application of an intervention is in many ways atypical. The factors which determine the success (or lack of it) of the interventions may be masked by the very act of experimental control, which deals with 'extraneous' factors by attempting to balance the probabilities of them occurring in each group to be compared. Even where such balance is successfully achieved, there is no guarantee that the extraneous factors do not interact differently with different treatments to produce different effects.

In an RCT application, regimes will be strictly standardised to ensure proper control and a fair comparison. But our expensive treatment X may have a less noxious odour than treatment Y. Under the controlled conditions of the study this may have little effect, as people adhere to the application-regime specified, but may well lead to ineffective use of Y in other circumstances. Thus, application of Y will be improved by inclusion in an RCT while the use of X would be much the same in or out of it. The very fact that efficacy and effectiveness are not the same thing should point to a need for a wider consideration of the mechanisms through which interventions operate.

The EBHC paradigm is thus subject to a bias wherein questions of effectiveness are, in fact, often answered by information about efficacy. Quasi-experiments may often be more suited to addressing real-life situations through the use of pre-existing groups and patterns of behaviour or intervention, but are associated with an unquantifiable imprecision and susceptibility to bias. There seems to be an inevitable conflict between the internal validity associated with an RCT and the higher external validity but lower internal validity of the quasi-experiment.

Most public health interventions are not at all like simple medical treatments. Evidence about efficacy should only be accepted in the absence of direct evidence of effectiveness. In some cases, this may mean accepting weaker evidence of effectiveness over and above more robust evidence of efficacy. Nonetheless, a well-designed study can strive to minimise bias and grapple squarely with the question of effectiveness. However, it is unlikely that RCTs (or quasi-experiments) alone can fully answer these questions even in the simplest medical treatments.

We will now move on to consider the determination of effectiveness from the perspective of a body of applied research that examines programmes in action – evaluation. Evaluation as a discipline holds a promise to both broaden our focus on outcomes, as we attempt to assess the value of those outcomes, and to directly address effectiveness, since evaluation research is generally associated with programmes of care targeted at individuals or populations, rather than the efficacy of specific treatments.

Evaluation and public health interventions

Øvretveit (1998) outlines four different evaluation perspectives. The experimental perspective focuses on establishing cause–effect relationships and predictable patterns of outcome. Its model research design is the RCT, although, as we have seen above, alternative quasi-experimental approaches exist, wherein pre-existing groups are used for comparison and to determine the effect of the intervention.

The economic perspective focuses on the use of resources. Although Øvretveit differentiates between the experimental and economic perspectives, in reality the essential difference between the two lies in the chosen outcome measures. Evaluations range from simple costing exercises and cost minimisation (where the cost of two interventions is compared to see which is cheaper) through to more complex approaches aimed at combining costs and some measure of effectiveness (Box 8.3).

Øvretveit's (1998) remaining evaluation perspectives are the 'developmental' and the 'managerial'. The developmental perspective sees the purpose of evaluation as guiding change and developing or improving the interventions that are the subject of evaluation. The role of the evaluator is as much to feed back information to guide the development of the intervention process, as it is to accumulate generalisable evidence. The managerial perspective focuses on the implementation of policies and processes defined by those with a supervisory or regulatory function.

These distinctions are, in my opinion, somewhat arbitrary. However, they do serve to introduce the idea that there may not be one single answer to the question of effectiveness. Rather, it may depend on precisely what question is being asked, which may, in turn, depend upon who is asking it. Øvretveit also identifies a range of possible 'stakeholders', such as patients (or recipients of interventions), practitioners, managers, politicians and health researchers.

The priority, indeed value, ascribed to a given outcome (effect) may differ according to the position of a given stakeholder and thus the views of the effectiveness

---

Box 8.3

Types of economic evaluation

- Cost minimisation – the cost of two interventions is compared to see which is cheaper
- Cost effectiveness – a cost is put upon improvements in an outcome associated with the intervention, for example, cost per life saved for a cancer screening programme
- Cost utility – the outcome is given a value, so rather than simply measuring lives saved a measure of quality of life is introduced and costs are set against a measure, such as a 'quality adjusted life year' or 'health day equivalent'
- Cost benefit – a monetary value is attached to both the intervention (cost) and the outcome (benefit). Since both benefits and costs are measured in the same terms, it is theoretically easy to see if the benefit is greater than the cost. The reality of putting a monetary value on (for example) a year of life is somewhat more complex

of a programme may differ. It is in the nature of public health interventions that there is a potentially large number of stakeholders, including (but not limited to) all those mentioned above. A naive 'scientific' approach does not, at first, seem compatible with accommodating these perspectives. Science seeks truth, not opinion; facts, not values. A sweeping critique of experimental perspectives made by Guba and Lincoln (1989) not only reiterates the limitations in determining effectiveness outlined above, but also adds an inability to accommodate multiple perspectives to the charge.

Guba and Lincoln (1989) reject experimental evaluation as a tool for exploring the perspectives and values of stakeholders. They argue for the need to accommodate qualitative, descriptive and interpretative methods to answer such questions. Clearly there is considerably more to evaluation than the simple determination of an 'effect'. The context of any action in the social world (including public health interventions) is usually a complex one and the effect of the intervention will be valued differently by different parties. More significantly, interventions themselves will be mediated by individual values and perceptions, as well as the social (and economic) context the individual finds themselves in.

For example, campaigns aimed at promoting breastfeeding that are based solely on the beneficial effects for the baby may be successful in some contexts but fail in others, due to a failure to address the competing motivations that lead some women to choose not to breastfeed and others to give up in the face of adversity. The results of the experimental evaluation of head-lice treatments described might be very different if conducted in an area that introduced a campaign to involve the whole community in 'bug-busting' techniques (Fee et al 2000), which involve encouraging everyone to routinely wet-comb their children's hair at each wash to reduce the spread of infestation. It would be extremely difficult to unravel whether the relative infestation rates were simply due to application of one treatment or another, or were in part dependent on reduced exposure to head-lice because of changes in prevalence in the surrounding area. The choice of treatments to be considered is also not value free. There is evidence about the effectiveness of pediculocides and some about 'bug busting', but no evidence from trials about any other approach (Dodd 2001). The choice of treatments to consider is mediated by many factors, but must at least in part be because there is a company marketing the product. This is not to say the research itself is necessarily biased, but a simple alternative treatment (which may or may not be effective), such as shaving, has not been researched at all and is virtually not mentioned (Lwegaba 2005) possibly in part because it was long regarded as socially unacceptable (although this may now have changed with changing fashions in some parts of the world) and in part because there is no product to sell.

However, this critique does not in itself negate the value of experimental approaches for determining differences between groups in terms of achieving (particular) goals. Qualitative research approaches can ask participants direct questions concerning effectiveness, but if the aim is to determine the effectiveness of one intervention relative to another, any evidence obtained this way must be weak in terms of our certainty that any perceived differences in effect are, indeed, caused by the intervention.

Nonetheless, Guba and Lincoln's critique raises a vital counterpoint to the experimental approach. Questions of effectiveness are essentially questions of how to achieve change. A broader range of approaches is needed in order to explore the context and mechanisms that lead people to make particular decisions or choose particular behaviours in the face of public health interventions. The possible acceptability of shaving for head-lice would not best be explored in a RCT, but this knowledge might be a powerful explanation of why a programme involving it did or did not work. There is an apparent contradiction here. Approaches to evaluation that can shed light on how something works appear to be weak in determining whether something works. However, determining effectiveness using the experimental perspective will generate little knowledge of the mechanism through which change occurred (or why it failed to).

A resolution to this apparent contradiction is proposed by the advocates of 'realistic evaluation' (Pawson & Tilley 1997). Essentially, they argue that a range of research techniques is valid and necessary in order to evaluate fully the context, mechanism and outcome of social interventions. Although their work is primarily based upon research in the area of penal reform, the arguments can easily be transferred to a public health context. An ideal realistic evaluation would explore all aspects of context, mechanism and outcome. It is necessary to understand how programmes affect people ('mechanisms') and under what circumstances ('context'), in order to fully understand how to achieve a particular effect ('outcome'). This daunting endeavour may, perhaps, be moderated by an analysis of what is already known in relation to each of the three components, in order to determine the priorities for any given evaluation.

Where little is known about effectiveness (outcome), however, it is difficult to avoid the need for some kind of comparative (quasi-experimental or experimental) study. Nonetheless, lack of knowledge about outcomes does not remove the need to evaluate other aspects of a programme. In some cases the priority may reasonably be on examining mechanisms (or to return to Donabedian's framework, process) because the link between process and outcome is well established.

The true value of a realistic evaluation is in allowing an accumulation of knowledge on effectiveness that has sufficient context and mechanism information to allow the selection of appropriate interventions for particular circumstances. Where generalisation is not a prime concern, outcome information may be all that is required and the experimental approach alone may be appropriate. However, given the limitations associated with experiments and quasi-experiments identified earlier, it becomes harder to promote these as the sole means for assessing effectiveness in the absence of detail on the setting in which the study is carried out.

More fundamental limitations can arise from taking a purely experimental perspective. Of even more concern to the limits of knowledge generated from RCTs is the danger of limiting interventions to those that can only be evaluated by this 'gold standard' measure of effectiveness. In order to develop an RCT, the outcomes of interest must be measurable. The measurable effect of the intervention must occur over a timescale within which it is realistic to run an experiment. Finally, it must be possible to deliver the intervention to individuals or discrete clusters of individuals, so that randomisation to comparison groups can be achieved. While this may be technically possible for any intervention that is targeted at individuals, it is simply not achievable in the case of many public health interventions where the programme may be diffuse (such as an advertising campaign) or be anticipated to have effects over a long period, which may not be discernible at an early stage (for example, Sure Start – see Box 8.4). While it may seem farcical to neglect potentially beneficial interventions simply because they cannot be evaluated by an RCT, this phenomenon has been observed in a number of settings, for example AIDS education programmes in Australia (Kippax & Van De Ven 1998).

Perhaps the most important limitation of evidence-based practice is not that its seeming objectivity provides incorrect answers but that the processes and outputs of evidence-based practice can obscure the range of possible questions to be asked (Forbes & Griffiths 2002). The selection of questions is not value free and while some of the selection process may equate to our own value systems (e.g. scientifically plausible, socially acceptable from our own perspective) other aspects of it may not (e.g. research backed by the possibility of finding an effective product that can be marketed, socially acceptable from other perspectives). In this sense the critique of evidence-based practice by post-modernists is clearly true: there are no absolute answers to questions of effectiveness and many different readings of the evidence base for practice are possible (Freshwater & Rolfe 2004).

Box 8.4

Sure Start

In the UK in the late 1990s the government launched the 'Sure Start Programme', which aimed to support families with young children and reduce social exclusion. The key to the programme was to provide early interventions aimed at preventing later difficulties and thus to provide the children with a 'sure start'. Rather than identifying a single intervention or set of interventions, the programme invited 'trailblazers' to develop packages and approaches to care that adhered to a number of key principles. These included delivery of a service that involved all families within a locality, provision of long-term support (rather than 'one-off' interventions), parental involvement, co-ordination and streamlining of services and improved access to services (Department of Education and Employment 1999).

Some of the research on which the programme was based has been the source of considerable controversy within the world of education. In the USA a number of 'Headstart' programmes were set up, to prepare children for school through various activities, such as preschool groups, sometimes combined with family support through home-visiting and other activities (Cowley 1999). Early studies using rudimentary quasi-experimental designs led to ambiguous results, which could be analysed in a number of ways to show a positive effect, a negative effect or no effect (Cook & Campbell 1979). Later RCTs seemed to show a positive early effect on school performance, which then tailed off over time (Barnes McGuire et al 1997). Thus the programme was scaled back, as long-term benefits were not demonstrated. However, later reassessments showed that by the time the children came to leave school it appeared that fewer of those who had received the Headstart package had dropped out or were identified as 'delinquent' and more went into jobs (Lazar & Darlington 1982). The programme may have had the ultimately intended effect, but the presumption that this could be measured by sustained performance in school tests was erroneous.

This of course presents a significant problem for evaluating 'Sure Start', as it may be that the benefits are not easily measured in the short term. Furthermore, the insistence on universal involvement in a defined area rules out randomisation of individuals, while the absence of a prescribed single intervention makes randomisation of 'clusters' impossible, as a particular programme will exist in only one site. The variation in programmes over localities provides ample opportunity to explore 'context–mechanism–outcome' configurations, as advocated by Pawson and Tilley, but necessitates the acceptance that ultimately the evidence on outcome cannot be as strong as would be provided by an RCT. Of course, the alternative would be no evidence on outcome, because such a programme ultimately cannot be evaluated by an RCT.

Early results of impact and implementation studies from the National Evaluation of Sure Start are available on http://www.ness.bbk.ac.uk/ and more information is given in Chapter 6.

However, in abandoning the endeavour of pure objective science it is important to recognize that this does not simply mean that any belief is equally valid or that individual beliefs can be used to simply discount evidence like some metaphysical trump card. The basic issues of reliability, internal and external validity still stand and the rules for determining them are largely unchallenged by even the most strident post-modern critique (Griffiths 2005). Nonetheless, in seeking to accumulate evidence for effectiveness, it is important to start from the interventions that are to be tested rather than shaping interventions to research designs. It is important to consider the range of questions that could be asked and not simply consider the evidence about those questions to which answers are offered. The nature of the intervention and existing knowledge about it should define the information that is most important to determine in evaluations and the range of possible methods to be deployed in gaining it.

Role of guidelines

Guidelines, or rather (clinical) practice guidelines, are defined as systematically developed statements to assist in making decisions about appropriate health care for specific circumstances or problems (Field & Lohr 1992, Sackett et al 1997). Sackett goes further in his definition by insisting that a guideline should bring together the best external evidence to guide decisions (Sackett et al 2001). As we would not wish to advocate anything less than the best evidence, clearly Sackett's definition should be taken. However, the evidence that is to be admitted into clinical guidelines by the adherents of evidence-based practice is, of course, limited to that which is recognised as valid by that paradigm. Sackett is perhaps rightly sceptical of guidelines that are based simply upon expert opinion, insisting instead that they be developed and reported with the same rigour that is demanded of systematic reviews. Many producers of guidelines and recommendations follow a more or less explicit approach to reviewing the evidence and generally make the evidence base upon which recommendations are made explicit. However, in many cases, the complex interplay of value judgements and evidence means that the evidence base behind guideline-based recommendations or policies (such as those emanating from the National Institute for Health and Clinical Excellence and the National Service Frameworks) is far from clear. Further, evidence of effectiveness can identify what will happen if a certain strategy is employed, but it cannot determine whether it should actually be done. It is important in assessing a guideline to consider not just the evidence, but also the value judgements that have been made. Ultimately, to judge the relevance of a guideline, it is essential to determine how values have been considered and whose perspectives the values may represent.

The previous discussion in this chapter suggests that the nature of the evidence that should be admitted into guidelines for public health may differ markedly from that which might be regarded as legitimate for medical-treatment guidelines. Where there is good evidence from RCTs or quasi-experiments then these should form the core of any guideline. However, the utility of any such evidence for public health interventions can only be assured if it is be accompanied by information of the context and associated mechanisms.

Public health interventions are generally multi-faceted and complex. It will rarely be possible to prescribe the precise way an intervention should be delivered to ensure success, and thus it is important to include information from a range of research perspectives in a guideline, in order to guide practitioners and policy-makers to the nuances and detail that may be vital in ensuring success, or that may suggest that one strategy rather than another would be most appropriate in their particular circumstances.

Guidelines may represent the best available accumulation of evidence of effectiveness, but a lack of evidence on mechanism and context may limit their utility in determining the best approach in a particular situation. Thus, although systematic reviews of effectiveness and synthesis of evidence into single estimates of effect may seem appealing, it is also vital to explore the reasons for and nature of variation across studies, in order to understand the necessary conditions of success. Such evidence must come from a range of appropriate research designs.

If such contextual information seems to be a nicety, which in truth could be dispensed with, consider the following example drawn from the history of public health. In 1854 there was a major outbreak of cholera in London that was centred on an area close to Covent Garden. The area was supplied with water by means of a pump at Broad Street. Suspecting this to be the source of the infection, a local doctor, John Snow, removed the handle from the pump and miraculously ended the outbreak. If we disregard for a moment everything learned since 1854 about the mechanism of transmission of cholera, consider the evidence for control of cholera, which John Snow's act provided. To end an outbreak of cholera, one must remove the handle from a water pump.

This evidence (not provided from an RCT) was quite compelling. However, although there have been few outbreaks of cholera in London in recent years, I would speculate that this strategy would no longer work and so John Snow's remarkable achievement is confined to history. However, let us add the context: the pump was people's prime water supply. A mechanism: cholera is transmitted by water. More context: nearby water sources were not infected. While neither the mechanism nor the context is in itself evidence for effectiveness, it is this information and only this that allows John Snow's evidence of effectiveness to have a broader utility. The context and mechanism information tells us precisely the circumstances where exactly the same intervention would still work (where water is supplied from a contaminated pump but nearby sources are clean). Perhaps even more importantly, it gives us a very good idea of how one might go about planning effective interventions in quite different contexts. We should not assume their effectiveness (human capacity for ingenious self-harm being what it is) but we may be confident in using the knowledge to guide us.

Perhaps there is a danger in utilising such an extreme example. However, I believe it is not absurd, in particular since the contexts and mechanisms for social change are, if anything, even more changeable and context-bound than Victorian water supply. With a continuing improvement in the overall health of the population and the increasing implication of complex social structures (as opposed to simple material deprivation) in determining relative health disadvantage, it is likely that public health interventions will resemble Sure Start more often than John Snow's elegant solution to the cholera epidemic.

A short note on the philosophy of science

For the 'positivist', true scientific knowledge enables the scientist to exercise precise control over future events by the knowledge of predictive laws. These laws:

> '. . .enable one to know what will happen under specified conditions, so that what is wanted may be brought on . . . by making sure the necessary circumstances do come about.'
>
> (Pratt 1978, p. 76)

Such theories are evaluated not by their ability to describe a reality, but by the accuracy of their predictions. Since 'cause' cannot be observed, the pure positivist equates it with a constant conjunction of the 'cause' and the 'effect'. There is no distinction to be made and it is the accuracy of the predictions, not the assumptions, which lead to scientific credibility under this model (Pratt 1978). The key to positivist science is control and manipulation, prediction and measurement.

Precise prediction and control leading to universal 'laws' have long been seen as redundant by many social scientists (Gergen 1982). Since public health services (and researchers) are unlikely to achieve such precise control over antecedent variables to allow the consummate control implied by positivism to come about, it may be time to abandon the pure endeavour of positive science in this arena too. Even in the case of such concrete and controllable interventions as removing handles from water pumps, the nature of the intervention is changed as the world changes around it. The causal link between the two has been broken, but this simply serves to illustrate that the mechanism of cause had a substantial importance in and of itself. In this regard it is worth remembering that all health services are essentially transient historical constructs.

However, this is no reason to abandon the attempt to differentiate chance associations from real ones and hence the rejection of the RCT specifically, and empirical research generally, in no way follows from this shift. Acknowledging the complex and changing nature of the social world makes a preoccupation with cause more, not less important (Cook & Campbell 1979). Following Gergen's proposals for social science, research should serve to point out influences on behaviour, expose assumptions that have not proved useful and enlighten us as to possibilities and probabilities. Much of the evidence for effectiveness in public health practice will be in this form, rather than universal scientific laws. Although experimental and quasi-experimental studies are still crucial, with this changed perspective they provide but one part of the necessary evidence, not all of it.

Conclusion

The effectiveness of a service is its ability to achieve desired outcomes. Evidence for quality of a service does not necessarily establish that it is effective unless there is an established link between a particular care process and a particular outcome. This is frequently not the case. Evidence for effectiveness should also be distinguished from efficacy: the impact of an intervention in ideal circumstances as opposed to everyday practice. This distinction is particularly relevant to many public health interventions, which are complex and multi-faceted.

The EBHC movement has developed in response to an increasing recognition that many health care interventions lack evidence for their effectiveness, and that many decisions about health care are made without recourse to evidence, even when it is available. A clear hierarchy of evidence suggests that the best evidence for effectiveness stems from a RCT. However, many public health interventions are not readily subjected to an RCT and so other types of research evidence must be sought. In this chapter we also suggested that, in fact, the RCT may be better suited to providing evidence for *efficacy* rather than *effectiveness*. Decisions about the ideal type of evidence for many public health interventions are more complicated than for simple drug treatments. Evidence for the relative effect of one intervention compared to another will come from a suitable comparative design, but the ideal design will be different for different types of intervention. In some cases the superior external validity of a non-randomised study may give it precedence over a randomised study. In other cases randomised studies may be impossible. In all cases the research must be critically appraised rather than simply taken at face value.

In order to be truly useful in making decisions for public health interventions, any evidence for effectiveness will need to be accompanied by descriptions of the context and mechanisms that are thought to be relevant to the programme's success (or lack of it). Any decisions need to be made in the context of information about social values, but, specifically, when looking at evidence of effectiveness it is important to remember that the production of evidence is selective. This is not a simple matter of deliberate bias or even research fraud (although such things occur), but a complex issue of the social processes that leads to the selection of questions to be researched and the publication of answers. It may be just as important to consider what has not been addressed by available research as what has.

It is only with consideration of this wider set of information that informed decisions about generalisation of evidence can be made in a complex and changing social world. Thus, while comparative empirical research must form a crucial part of the evidence for effectiveness, it is but a part of the necessary evidence. I would ultimately question the idea of a rigid hierarchy of evidence. However, the EBHC paradigm does provide much useful guidance for those seeking to determine what services are effective. Perhaps most importantly it urges us to do so!

DISCUSSION QUESTIONS

- Are health policies made on the basis of evidence? Discuss with reference to a recent policy development that affects your area of practice.
- How could evidence for the effectiveness of a universal health visiting service be obtained?
- Can evidence of effectiveness be obtained without a comparison group?

References

Antman EM, Lau J, Kupelnick B, Mosteller F, Chalmers TC 1992 A comparison of results of meta-analyses of randomized control trials and recommendations of clinical experts. Treatments for myocardial infarction. Journal of the American Medical Association 268(2): 240–248

Barnes McGuire J, Stein A, Rosenberg W 1997 Evidence based medicine and child mental health services. A broad approach to evaluation is needed. Children and Society 11(2): 89–96

Chalmers I 1997 Assembling comparison groups to assess the effects of health care. Journal of the Royal Society of Medicine 90: 379–386

Cook DC, Campbell DT 1979 Quasi-experimentation: design and analysis issues for field settings. Houghton Mifflin Co, Boston

Cowley S 1999 Early interventions: evidence for implementing Sure Start. Community Practitioner 72(6): 162–165

Department of Education and Employment 1999 Sure Start: making a difference for children and families. Department of Education and Employment Publications, Sudbury, UK

Dodd CS 2001 Interventions for treating headlice. The Cochrane Database of Systematic Reviews 2001, Issue 2. Art. No.: CD001165.

Donabedian A 1966 Evaluating the quality of medical care. Millbank Memorial Fund Quarterly: Health and Society 44(2): 166–203

Donabedian A 1988 Quality assessment and assurance: unity of purpose, diversity of means. Inquiry 25: 173–192

Egger M, Smith G 2001 Rationale, potentials and promise of sytematic reviews. In: Egger M, Smith G, Altman D (eds). Systematic reviews in health care. British Medical Journal Books, London, pp. 3–22

Egger M, Smith G, Scneider M 2001 Systematic reviews of observational studies. In: Egger M, Smith G, Altman D (eds.) Systematic reviews in health care. British Medical Journal Books, London, pp. 211–227

Fee J, Briault V, Long J 2000 A community approach to reducing head lice infection. Community Practitioner 73(2): 477–480

Field M, Lohr K 1992 Guidelines for clinical practice: from development to use. National Academy Press, Washington DC

Forbes A, Griffiths P 2002 Methodological strategies for the identification and synthesis of 'evidence' to support decision-making in relation to complex health care systems and practices. Nursing Inquiry 9(3): 141–155

Freshwater D, Rolfe G 2004 Deconstructing evidence-based practice. Routledge, Abingdon

Gergen JK 1982 Towards transformation in social knowledge. Springer Verlag, New York

Gillespie LD, Gillespie WJ, Robertson MC, Lamb SE, Cumming RG, Rowe BH 2003 Interventions for preventing falls in elderly people. The Cochrane Database of Systematic Reviews 2003, Issue 4. Art. No.: CD000340

Greenhalgh T 2001 How to read a paper. The basics of evidence based medicine, 2nd edn. British Medical Journal Publishing Group, London

Greenhalgh T, Robert G, Macfarlane F, Bate P, Kyriakidou O 2004 Diffusion of innovations in service organizations: systematic review and recommendations. Millbank Quarterly 82(4): 581–629

Griffiths P 2005 Evidence-based practice: a deconstruction and postmodern critique: book review article. International Journal of Nursing Studies 42(3): 355–361

Guba E, Lincoln Y 1989 Fourth generation evaluation. Sage, Newbury Park, CA

Hunt JM 1996 Barriers to research utilization. Journal of Advanced Nursing 23(3): 423–425

Jones JE 1997 Research-based or idiosyncratic practice in the management of leg ulcers in the community. Journal of Wound Care 6(9): 447–450

Kippax S, Van De Ven P 1998 An epidemic of orthodoxy? Design and methodology in the evaluation of the effectiveness of HIV health promotion. Critical Public Health 8(4): 371–386

Lazar I, Darlington R 1982 Lasting effects of early education: a report from the consortium of for longtitudinal studies. Monographs of the Society for Research in Child Development 47: 2–3, serial number 195

Lwegaba A 2005 Shaving can be safer head lice treatment than insecticides. British Medical Journal 330(7506): 1510

Lord F 1967 A paradox in the interpretation of group comparisons. Psychological Bulletin 68: 304–305

Muir Gray J 2001 Evidence based healthcare: how to make health policy and management decisions. Churchill Livingstone, London

NHS CRD 1999 Getting evidence into practice. Effective Health Care Bulletin 5(1). (whole issue) Online. Available at http://www.york.ac.uk/inst/crd/ehc51.pdf

Øvretveit J 1998 Evaluating health interventions. Open University Press, Buckingham, UK

Pawson R, Tilley N 1997 Realistic evaluation. Sage, London

Pratt V 1978 Philosophy of social science. Methuen, London

Rangachari P 1997 Evidence-based medicine: old French wine with a new Canadian label? Journal of the Royal Society of Medicine 90: 280–281

Rodgers S 1994 An exploratory study of research utilization by nurses in general medical and surgical wards. Journal of Advanced Nursing 20: 904–911

Sackett DL, Rosenberg WMC, Gray JAM, Haynes RB, Richardson WS 1996 Evidence based medicine: what it is and what it isn't. It's about integrating individual clinical expertise and the best external evidence. British Medical Journal 312(7023): 71–72

Shea B, Dube C, Moher D 2001 Assessing the quality of reports of sytematic review: the QUROM statement compared to other tools. In: Egger M, Smith G, Altman D (eds) Systematic reviews in health care. British Medical Journal Books, London, pp. 122–142

Sheldon TA, Raffle A, Watt I 1996 Department of Health shoots itself in the hip. Why the report of the Advisory Group on Osteoporosis undermines evidence based purchasing. British Medical Journal 312(7026): 296–297

211

Further reading

Elkan R, Kendrick D, Hewitt M et al 2000 The effectiveness of domiciliary health visiting: a systematic review of international studies and a selective review of the British literature. Health Technology Assessment 4(13): 1–339

A systematic review of evidence for health visiting that illustrates the merits of using diverse sources of evidence while maintaining the rigour of a systematic review. The report discusses the difficulties of generalising evidence across widely differing health care settings. This is interesting and important reading, both as a direct source of evidence and as an example of how to bring together evidence for complex interventions.

Gomm R, Davies C (eds) 2000 Using evidence in health and social care. Sage, London

A good general introduction to the use of evidence in practice and for planning services. The text deals with a wider range of issues than most introductory texts. Its focus on health and social care makes it more relevant to public health practitioners than many evidence-based medicine texts.

Greenhalgh T 2001 How to read a paper. The basics of evidence based medicine, 2nd edn. British Medical Journal Publishing Group, London

An extremely readable, user-friendly guide to finding, appraising and using evidence. This book covers all the basic issues of evidence-based health care in a practical manner.

Greenhalgh T, Robert G, Macfarlane F, Bate P, Kyriakidou O 2004 Diffusion of innovations in service organizations: systematic review and recommendations. Millbank Quarterly 82(4): 581–629

Although not a public health topic, this review is both an exemplar of an adaptation of the method of systematic review to complex topics and directly useful reading to practioners seeking to implement change.

Pawson R, Tilley N 1997 Realistic evaluation. Sage, London

A review of the history of evaluation research and a description of a new approach, 'realistic evaluation', which offers a solution to the problems of accumulating evidence for complex interventions. The critique of previous approaches is scathing and irreverent and the case for realistic evaluation perhaps overstated. However, anyone wishing to acquaint themselves with the state of the art in service evaluation should start (and perhaps finish) with Pawson and Tilley.

Public health and health promotion

9

Pauline Pearson

Key issues

- This chapter addresses notions of health, public health, health promotion and primary health care, and some of the important overlaps and distinctions between them
- Distinctions between the 'medical' model of health – that health is the absence of disease – 'social health' – the ability to fulfil social roles – and lay definitions of health, are outlined
- The ways in which public health nurses, health visitors and other workers in the field negotiate between the various views of health in practice are discussed
- The main theoretical perspectives underpinning health promotion work in practice are described, for example, DiClemente and Prochaska's (1982) Behaviour Change cycle, Becker's (1974) Health Belief Model, organisation theories of transformational change, and Economic Theory, locating these in relation to work with individuals, with groups and organisations and at a policy level
- Brief examples from practice are given. These include a pilot scheme to provide warfarin-monitoring sessions through a GP practice, lunch-time health fairs to identify the health needs of young adolescents and work with a housing department

Introduction

Since the beginning of movements to promote and maintain the public health, it has been necessary for those engaged in practical, hands-on activity to think about explanations for the situations they encounter, and to ground their responses in appropriate frameworks. There has grown up a substantial body of theory in relation to the promotion of health, which supports and can enhance public health practice. This chapter first of all looks at the notions of health, public health, health promotion and primary health care, and teases out some of the important overlaps and distinctions between them. Some of the distinctions that have been made between medical, social and lay definitions of health, and the way in which public health nurses, health visitors and other workers in the field have negotiated between the various views are investigated. Consideration is given to some of the main theoretical perspectives underpinning health promotion work in practice, locating these in relation to work with individuals, with groups and organisations and at policy level. Finally, some brief examples of partnership working from practice are given, which are related to relevant performance standards.

What is health?

Before considering 'public health' or 'health promotion' it is important to briefly consider definitions of health. Ask three people the meaning of 'health', and each may give a different answer. One may say, 'It's when you're not ill'. Another may say, 'It's when you can get around and do what you have to do'. A third may suggest that it is when you feel good about yourself. Each of these views has been described in numerous research studies (Blaxter 1982, Cornwell 1984, Mayall 1986, Pearson 1991).

The first is often described as the 'medical' model of health – that health is the absence of disease. It is described in this way because health is seen as the absence of pathogens and disease processes. Medical interventions are frequently geared to avoiding or destroying pathogens or arresting disease processes.

The second view can be described as the 'functional' model of health – often used in relation to people with disabilities or older people. Difficulties arise with this model in a society where the boundaries of everyday function and the technological supports available are changing rapidly, and where activists have strongly put the case for a 'social' model of disability, which makes clear that it is the product of society's inability to adapt and respond to impairments, demonstrated in function (French 1993). An extension of this idea is the notion of 'social health' – an ability to fulfil social roles. This is in many ways the obverse of Parsons' (1951) idea of the sick role, in which being 'ill' confers exemption, for a period, from social roles.

The third view suggests that how people feel about themselves is more important than impairment or a disease process. The World Health Organization (1946) in its constitution brought together these ideas when they stated that health was, 'a state of complete physical, mental and social well-being and not merely the absence of disease or infirmity'. While this has been criticised as Utopian, it has the merit of integrating the three most common conceptualisations.

Health is thus not one but a number of ideas, which operate in different people's minds at different times in considering how the health of the public may be promoted and maintained.

What is public health?

Asked where 'public health' began as a concept, many health professionals will date its birth to the days of the Broad Street pump, and John Snow's single-handed determination to find and deal with the cause of a raging cholera outbreak in 1854. Alternatively, they may point to the work of Florence Nightingale, pulling together and laboriously presenting data on the incidence of infection and death among soldiers in the Crimean War, and later in the poorer areas of her day, and suggesting strategies to bring about change, the results of which are well-known. There is no doubt that in those early days of Queen Victoria's reign, the burgeoning of the Industrial Revolution, the shift of populations into cities and the movement of patterns of work from those linked to natural cycles to those tied to supply and demand, among many other factors, all generated patterns of health experience that began to concern many people, and led them to begin to think about the way in which a society creates health.

My personal vote for the key person behind the original public health movement is Edwin Chadwick. Chadwick's *Report on the sanitary condition of the labouring population of Great Britain* (Chadwick 1965) was seminal. He was a civil servant who drew together the reports of a range of local informants to produce a hard-hitting analysis of the morbidity created by overcrowding, lack of sanitation, long working hours and lack of leisure space or opportunity. Presented to the House of Lords in 1842, this led to demands for change. From these emerged the first Public Health Act in 1848.

At the beginning, public health was driven by concerns about visible suffering and high death rates. In the modern context these are the concerns of the 'Third' world (two-thirds of the world). In India, for example, only around 40% of households have toilet facilities even today, despite extensive government investment programmes. Provision of access to clean water has been more successful, though work now needs to be done to prevent build-up of waste water, which attracts mosquitoes and undermines progress on malaria. Polio is still relatively common, though intensive community education programmes and national immunisation drives are beginning to pay off, with 70% of 1-year-olds fully immunised against polio (UNICEF 2003).

In Victorian Britain, much less was known about the mechanisms of disease than is the case today, but careful analysis of large bodies of data enabled those who wanted to begin to identify possible relationships. If urban death rates for all socio-economic groups exceeded those for rural populations, then something about cities was bad for people! If a particular community was experiencing excessive morbidity from cholera, then something must make that area more susceptible, or it must be exposed to risk more often. From there it was a combination of trial and error and painstaking detective work on the ground. Theories about infection were in their infancy, but were to grow and become one of the central planks of public health workers' thinking up to the beginning of the NHS and to some extent beyond.

Towards the end of the 19th century, lady sanitary inspectors (the forerunners of health visitors), supported by a cadre of locally recruited women, were employed in Salford to take action on the ground to improve hygiene and take all appropriate action to prevent or curtail outbreaks of disease. Despite Chadwick's recognition of the importance of leisure, which bore fruit in some major cities in the form of great public parks, public health at this time was primarily about the prevention and control of infection, to ensure that the workforce in the new factories, male and female, and the soldiers fighting in a variety of wars, would be fit enough to maintain acceptable levels of productivity. It was in essence about preventing disease (a medical model) and maintaining a level of health within society, which enabled it to meet its economic obligations.

The next stage in the development of public health as a concept emerged at the beginning of the 20th century, when difficulties were encountered in obtaining enough fit recruits to fight in the Boer War. The technology of warfare was changing, and larger numbers of men were required. Too many of those volunteering had poor eyesight, were undersized, or had deformities produced by rickets and other nutritional deficiencies. The government responded by refocusing some of its efforts into the welfare of children. In particular, if children could be adequately nourished, and mothers guided to make a point of this, then the young men of the future would be equipped to go to war. Infant welfare clinics were opened across the country during and after the First World War; some, indeed, served as memorials within their communities. Babies were weighed and measured regularly, and advice on nutrition and budget-management became part of the package offered by the health visitors; much as Florence Nightingale had suggested many years earlier. Screening of vision, height and weight was undertaken with school-age children, though until the advent of the NHS, visual defects were responded to according to income (could glasses be afforded?), rather than need. Sanitary inspection branched out into issues about housing quality. Public health work had now expanded to include screening and the promotion of a healthy diet and housing. Its purpose now included establishing, as well as maintaining, health within society. There was some recognition of environmental and social contributions to health, though the predominant model was medical.

The NHS was born in 1948, with an underlying philosophy of equity in provision and entitlement to care, together with notions about providing cure/care for all, largely associated with a medical model of health. To some extent, *public* health lay outside this agenda, since many of those involved in its delivery – health visitors, school nurses, directors of public health – did not join the NHS, but remained within the local authority setting. At the same time, developments were occurring in ideas about behaviour and psychological theory. Skinner (1953) and other behaviourists were working on ideas about animals which would lead to new conceptualisations about human behaviour. Over the next few decades, Becker and colleagues (1974) were pulling together theories about people's health beliefs and examining the reasons why people take up or stop behaving in ways that damage health. Social theory was also developing rapidly, with sociologists looking at the development of professions, the functioning of communities and at marginal groups (Whyte 1993), while social policy was being driven forward by people such as Richard Titmuss (1970).

However, changes in patterns of service delivery were slow. In 1974, the NHS took in community health services, and at the same time set in place structures in which professionals began to be consciously 'managed'. Emphasis began to be placed on policies and protocols. Record systems were revised. The 'nursing process', a model originating in hospital settings and relating to the management of one or more problems, was widely promoted and taken up by many community practitioners; for example, in the form discussed by Clark (1986). In 1979, the political context changed. Margaret Thatcher came to power and over almost the next two decades proclaimed that there was 'no such thing as society'. Clearly, public health work had to reinvent itself to respond to the mood of the day.

In fact, two paths emerged. One, most clearly seen in the 1992 *Health of the nation* document, took up the medical model and proceeded to look, in the main, at individuals' behaviour, focusing on the responsibility of each individual to contribute to improving health targets, and the need to provide individuals with the 'information to help make the right choices' (Department of Health (DH) 1992, p. 22). Though there was a suggestion that other agencies might play a part in promoting the health of the public through the notion of 'healthy alliances', this idea was poorly developed, and little was done to follow it up, except to some extent in local authorities who picked up the idea of health-promoting schools. The other main deficit of policy at this time, again clearly seen in the *Health of the nation* document, was the failure to acknowledge poverty and socio-economic factors as significant in shaping people's health experience. The second pathway followed the community development ideas, which had flourished a decade or more earlier, and built on a salutogenic model of health (Antonovsky 1996), in which the key to a healthy population is that it has the resources for health. While the first approach was dominant, becoming increasingly so in government thinking, many community development projects were also set up during this time. Though many were short-lived, for example, Strelley in Nottingham (Boyd et al 1993), some (such as Castlemilk near Glasgow and Meadowell on Tyneside) survived into the 21st century.

Public health in general remained locked into these models, though there were some pioneers who began to look at what was known as the 'new' public health (Ashton & Seymour 1988). This rests on a model that draws on the World Health Organization's definition of health, acknowledging that health is a product of many factors, and that work to promote and maintain health requires a balance between individually focused work and work at the level of society. Like John Ashton, who was involved in the development of the Healthy Cities Initiative (Ashton et al 1986), Steve Watkins, Director of Public Health in Stockport, was a pioneer of this new way of looking at public health. Against the grain of policy at the time, he facilitated the establishment of an integrated public health service in Stockport, which offered community-based health development work, as well as large-scale intervention programmes (Watkins 1994, 1996).

By 1997, when a landslide victory unseated the Conservative government of 18 years, politicians had begun to acknowledge that the individualistic model alone was not sufficient, and that 'health variations' (inequalities in health) required attention at a more structural level. The new government set in place a range of initiatives, which demonstrated that promoting and maintaining the health of the public was now a central plank of the government's policies. *The new NHS: modern dependable* (DH 1997) shifted commissioning towards a health-oriented model and more firmly into primary health care. Late in 1998, the Acheson Report on 'inequalities in health' (Acheson 1998) and the publication by the Home Office of a Green Paper called *Supporting families* (Home Office 1998) gave further momentum to the shift to a psychosocial model of health. In the closing year of the millennium, the White Paper *Saving lives: our healthier nation* (DH 1999) highlighted the importance of community development approaches and of looking at environments (school, work and community), as well as the management of disease processes. It made clear the potential contribution of midwives, health visitors and school nurses, among others, to achieving this, building on their work with families and communities. In 2004, Derek Wanless, a financier, completed a review of the issues involved in maximising the health of the population, highlighting the need to tackle old problems in new and more imaginative ways, and to act appropriately on emerging problems (Wanless 2004). Most recently, the government has published *Choosing health: making healthy choices easier* (DH 2004). This is concerned with ensuring informed choice for all and supporting individuals and communities in making healthy choices. It also emphasises the need for partnership working across the complex network which influences the health of individuals and communities: statutory and voluntary agencies, advertisers, manufacturing industry, retailers and the media.

Future directions for public health?

Where will public health work move in the future? In Western societies one of the most significant health issues of today is mental ill health. Stress-related conditions are one of the commonest reported causes of work-related sickness absence. Unemployment too is associated with reduced psychological wellbeing, and a greater incidence of self-harm, depression and anxiety. Around one in six people in England of working age experience mental ill health at any given time (DH 1999). In the wider world, there is a need to promote the human rights of people with mental health problems, particularly those who are subject to involuntary detention (Council of Europe 2000).

The future health of our population is grounded in the health of today's children and young people. There has been increasing recognition, for example, in the National Service Framework for Children (DH and DfES 2004), that the social, economic and environmental contexts in which children grow up make a significant difference to their health experience. Policy has moved away from a focus on health screening and developmental reviews to programmes of support to children and their families, such as Sure Start, which are intended both to help to address the wider determinants of health and to reduce health inequalities. However, recent work (see for example Belsky et al 2006) suggests that programmes of this sort may be more effective for children and families with some economic and social resources than for those with few.

In the UK and Europe, public health work is likely to be influenced by the development of education about risk assessment and communication: a two-way process in which 'expert' and 'lay' perspectives interact and inform each other. 'Whole systems' interagency collaboration is increasingly recognised as a way to enable local people and others with a broad spectrum of expertise and resources for meeting health needs. As technology continues to develop, it seems likely too that work to promote the health of communities and populations will be enhanced by the integrated and interactive use of developing technologies in identifying and targeting health needs.

A major challenge for the delivery of a healthy population in the 21st century will be shortages and changes in the health care workforce. In the UK, demographic change is rapidly altering the workforce available to promote and maintain health. The traditional roles of health professionals in many areas of both primary and secondary care will need to change significantly over the next few years. Movement is already being seen in the development of accessible primary care facilities based in stores and supermarkets, the establishment of 'health trainers' to give local support and focused information on health, and the move to generic 'children's workers' at the interface between health, education and social care. Such changes are likely to accelerate. As around one-fifth of health visitors and school health advisers retire in the next few years, there will be a significant increase in the workload of those who remain. This will require professionals who are educated to embrace new roles and work with health care assistants, children's workers and health trainers who will be educated to take over more routine activity. In the wider world, there is a global shortage of around 4.3 million health workers (WHO 2006). Significant under-provision in the poorest areas of the world, for example, critically low provision of doctors, nurses and midwives in sub-Saharan Africa, will have a major impact on population health. Recent work by the Joint Learning Initiative has shown that countries where these professions represent fewer than 2.5 per 1000 population achieve less than 80% coverage of measles immunisation or of deliveries by skilled birth attendants, with consequent poor health outcomes. Action to improve health will require recruitment and training of many more health workers.

Promoting health

While the promotion of the health of the public is an intrinsic element of 'public health', it is often confused with other closely related concepts. The World Health Organization (1984) suggests that it may be defined as 'the process of enabling people to increase control over, and to improve, their health'. The process of promoting health may be undertaken in a variety of ways. Most often people think of health promotion in terms of, firstly, health education and, secondly, prevention. Tannahill (1985) highlights a third, overlapping, component, which he calls health protection. Each of these elements is discussed below.

Health education

Health education can be defined as giving people information about living healthy lifestyles and the skills to understand and use this information. In the early part of the 20th century, before the development of social and psychological theory, manuals gave detailed instruction on healthy living, with little concern about how real people might put the instructions into practice in real contexts (Board of Education 1928). In the later part of the 20th century, through to the present day, educational theory has developed further. Health educators have become aware, for example, that different styles of presentation of information may be effective for different audiences. Ewles and Simnett (1985) describe five different approaches to health education, which are listed in Box 9.1.

Those engaged in health education can look more closely at ways of engaging their target audiences and assess the impact their activity has, not only on knowledge and attitudes, but also on behaviour. Health education programmes have also drawn increasingly on the developing theory of marketing. For example,

> ## Box 9.1
>
> ## The five approaches to health education
>
> 1. Medical – the promotion of medical interventions to prevent or ameliorate ill health
> 2. Behaviour change – to encourage the adoption of a 'healthier' lifestyle
> 3. Educational – provision of information to underpin decision making, exploration of values and attitudes and skill-development
> 4. Client-directed – working with clients' own identified health priorities
> 5. The social-change approach – involving political or social change to alter the physical or social environment.
>
> Adapted from Ewles & Simnett 1985

Kaner et al (1999) describe the use of a marketing approach in introducing a brief intervention programme for problem drinkers into general practice. The purpose of health education may range from purely educational through empowerment and personal growth to a more 'radical–political' approach.

Prevention

The relationship between prevention and health promotion is more complex than it seems. The idea of prevention has been clearly linked to a pathogenic concept of health. Leavell (1953) sets out the inter-relationship clearly, identifying three levels of prevention and linking them to different levels of disease process. His model assumes that where there are no symptoms of disease, but exposure is possible, then primary preventive action is required, for example, immunisation programmes. Where early symptoms exist, but disease may remain at a subclinical level (in other words may not have reached a point where the individual has presented it to a health professional), then secondary preventive action is required – for example, through screening for cervical cancer or for glaucoma – to enable action to be taken to arrest the progress of the disease. Where disease processes are established, tertiary prevention aims to minimise further damage; for example, through the provision of cardiac rehabilitation programmes for post-MI patients. However, though this model is widely used in discussions of health-promoting activity, its base in a pathogenic framework limits its usefulness. Wass (2000, after Brown 1985) has suggested a development of Leavell's model, which superimposes three further components on the original. Figure 9.1 shows that she suggests that the primary prevention level is also the primary health promotion level; geared to eradicating health risks at the individual level. She then suggests that there are two further levels of health promotion: secondary health promotion, which is concerned with raising individual quality of life, and tertiary health promotion, which is concerned with effecting enduring social change.

The introduction of a level beyond the individual reflects the experience of most community nurses. An alternative model of health promotion put forward by Kelly and colleagues (1993) suggests that there are in fact four levels at which health-promoting activity takes place: individual, organisational, social and environmental. While these are useful ways of conceptualising what is going on, they do not fully reflect the complexity of practice, where interventions may be made consecutively with the individual and his or her context at the same time as advocating social change. Individual practitioners may be carrying out activities that fit into several levels at once.

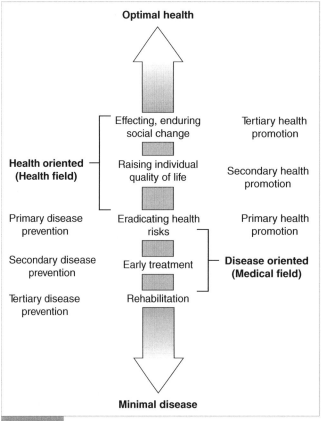

Figure 9.1 ● Beyond disease prevention (Reproduced with permission from Wass A 2000 developed from Brown 1985, pp. 332–333)

Health protection

Health protection is understood, within Tannahill's (1985) model, as comprising decisions by 'local, national or international government or other influential bodies', for example, industrial or commercial organisations, which 'will positively promote health'. Examples might be the passage of seat-belt legislation, taxation on cigarettes or the voluntary installation by car manufacturers of additional safety features.

The building of healthy public policy formed an important element of the Ottawa Charter for Health Promotion (World Health Organization 1986). This suggested that health promotion through policy might involve legislation, fiscal measures, taxation and organisational change, to produce policies that would foster greater equity. The Charter linked health protection, the use of politics to create an environment that is safer and in which healthier choices are easier to make, to strengthening community action and developing personal skills. This fitted with the balance inherent in the 'new public health' agenda. Health protection alone might be seen as paternalistic, or at least imposed. Nevertheless, it is worth comparing this approach with the work of early public health pioneers, such as Chadwick, who sought to make a difference to the lives of the poor through policy development.

Where does primary health care fit?

Primary health care is 'essential health care made accessible at a cost a country and community can afford, with methods that are practical, scientifically sound and socially acceptable' (World Health Organization 1978). The Alma-Ata Declaration goes on to state that primary health care is based on principles of equity, participation by the community, an intersectoral approach, appropriate technology and affordable costs. Despite the inter-relationships between the notions of primary care espoused by the World Health Organization and the ideas about public health and health promotion set out above, little has been done to explore how these operate on the ground. The context in which they relate is changing rapidly. Around 890 000 people consult their GP or practice nurse each day, and there are over 300 000 other community contacts with NHS staff each day. Although they are undergoing almost continual change, there is a duty on primary care organisations to work through Local Strategic Partnerships to improve the health of the people they serve. From 2004, Primary Care Trusts (PCTs) were allocated increased funding to give greater priority to areas of high health need, and encouragement to focus their work on tackling key lifestyle issues; in particular smoking, obesity, alcohol consumption and sexual health. Further policy moves appear to be shifting the balance of planning health improvement further from those who provide services. Nevertheless, in practice it is often general practitioners and community nurses, especially health visitors, who must find ways of identifying and meeting health needs for the populations with which they work.

Bhopal (1995) advocated a much stronger public health role for general practitioners, but also identified some of the barriers to this in existing patterns of work, not least their tendency to focus on disease management. As far back as 1977 it was recognised that health visiting revolved around four key principles: the search for health needs, stimulation of awareness of health needs, facilitation of health-enhancing activities, and influence on policies affecting health (CETHV 1977). More recent reviews suggest that these principles remain valid, and could underpin the implementation of recent reforms. However, an increasingly contract-led environment has led to many health visitors being unable to do more than routine surveillance visits, with some thus losing their ability to respond flexibly to a perceived health need. Recent work (Pearson et al 2000) has examined how far programmes of education successfully prepare community nursing practitioners to carry out a public health role, and some of the factors that help or hinder this once they have qualified. Some of the key difficulties appear to be in the articulation of what public health work means at the grass-roots level, and in the production of an effective model to bridge the practice-to-commissioning divide.

Primary health care is also about equitable provision and the promotion of health for *all*. Yet there is ample evidence that most inequalities in health have either remained the same or widened over recent decades. The Acheson (1998) report sets out 39 recommendations, backed by 529 references, which the committee suggests should be priority areas for action to reduce inequalities in health in England. Most do not relate directly to NHS services. However, they do highlight the importance of ensuring that communities most at risk of ill health have good access to effective primary care, and that effective partnerships between health and social care providers are nurtured. In the White Paper *The new NHS modern, dependable*: (DH 1997) the importance of including 'a strong public voice' was emphasised. User choice is a fundamental principle of *Choosing health* (DH 2004). It is, therefore, important to consider in more detail some of the ways in which medical, social and lay definitions of health differ.

Distinctions between medical, social and lay definitions of health

Some of the different views of health that exist have been set out above. While initially the medical perspective was dominant, an alternative set of perspectives on health, which has rather different implications for health promotion, derived from the rapidly developing social sciences over the 20th century. The development of psychology as an academic discipline led to the conceptualisation of 'normal' and 'abnormal' behaviour. Alongside this, developmental psychology took shape, indicating 'normal' patterns of development. The notion of health as related to functional or developmental 'adequacy' was highlighted. This idea has been used in many health-related intervention studies as the basis of an outcome measurement for health promotion at some level. What proportion of the population can achieve an adequate Barthel score (Collin et al 1988) following intervention from a multidisciplinary early-discharge team (Rodgers et al 1997)? What proportion of children achieves 'normal' language development following an intensive programme of health visiting (Cox & Hill 1993)? One of the key issues here is the question of value judgements. What is adequate, or normal, and for whom? Community practitioners who have transferred from the inner city to the outer suburbs, or vice versa, have anecdotally highlighted the different framing methods that they had to develop in relation to these judgements. In one area it may be seen as developmentally normal for a child to be beginning to construct sentences by 24 months, whereas in a neighbouring area the perceived norm may be later. In dealing with subgroups of a larger population, judgements of this sort will be common. In addition, a behaviour that is broadly harmful to health, such as smoking, may be defined, by a subgroup of society, as functional: to produce smaller babies, or to reduce stress, or both. The measures of health that emerge from this grouping of perspectives tend to relate at an individual level either to the level of independence (of function) or to the level of capacity (in terms of development towards an optimal state). Functional and behavioural problems or developmental delay can also be looked at in relation to population measures, such as incidence, to determine whether particular interventions lead to significant reductions.

Promoting health in this context may link to wider debates, such as the role of parenting as an antecedent in positive or negative patterns of behaviour, and to the development of initiatives and interventions that build on this approach. The Sure Start initiative seeks to intervene directly with young families to help them achieve effective parenting and to prevent poor literacy, child abuse and crime (DfEE 1999). Work to manage sleep problems (Kerr et al 1996) and other behaviour problems can be located within a psychological framework, though it is important to remember that low self-esteem may impact on the ability of any individual to successfully alter their behaviour, or to sustain altered behaviour.

The development of sociological theories about health and health care has been considerable, and is addressed in many other texts. Sociologists have sought to make sense of the ways in which health is understood by individuals and society as a whole. Of particular relevance to an exploration of promoting health is how the literature highlights ways in which health is socially constructed. Classically, Zola (1973) describes the way in which mental health problems are differentially presented in different ethnic groups, based on different perceptions of everyday behaviour, rather than any objective standard. This highlights both the need to review existing diagnostic and treatment standards for equity, but also more widely the need to test understandings with patients and carers as well as professionals. Cornwell (1984) interviewed a sample of people living in part of the East End of London about their health and health care. She looks at individuals' definitions of health and says that her (lay) respondents see health as 'functioning in a socially accepted way'. They perceive a moral imperative to conform, and in particular to seek relevant help or seek to avoid known risk factors. Where individuals are seen as not conforming, they are seen as blameworthy in relation to their illness. Parsons (1951) described the notion of the 'sick role,' which required an individual to take appropriate action to get better when ill. Cornwell's work appears to somewhat extend this to place an obligation to avoid risk, if possible. Using this framework, health promotion might be construed as social control, seeking to facilitate conformity. For example, Look After Your Heart classes (Rowland et al 1994) provided information about patterns of behaviour in relation to food and exercise that were appropriate to reduce the risk of heart disease, but could be seen, at least implicitly, as disapproving of other behaviours. Following the Coronary Heart Disease NSF (DH 2000) they were superseded by a range of other initiatives with a philosophy of choice and empowerment, so that the current initiatives encouraged through Local Strategic Partnerships and Healthy Living Centres include walking groups, provision of local (sometimes mobile) fruit and vegetable supplies and jogging buddies.

Cornwell goes on to identify three lay conceptualisations of illness: 'serious illness' (for example myocardial infarction or a cerebrovascular accident), 'normal illness' (which might include measles or mumps) and 'health problems that are not illness' (a category into which many problematic aspects of child and family health might fall). Alongside this, several studies (Blaxter 1982, Mayall 1986, Pearson 1991) have highlighted three lay conceptualisations of health, touched on earlier.

Health can be seen as 'not being ill', bearing in mind the ways in which illness may be viewed. Health may also be seen as functional by lay people, being able to achieve day-to-day tasks effectively, or in relation to children achieving appropriate developmental function. Finally, health may be seen as related to emotional wellbeing. Socio-emotional wellbeing incorporates ideas of 'happiness' and contentment, and the avoidance of the fear of crime, drugs and violence. In one survey of a local community to ascertain health needs, most lay people suggested reductions in crime and increases in shops and facilities long before exercise classes or information provision.

Because these different understandings of 'health' exist between different agencies and professional groups, and between professionals and lay people, health promotion in practice requires public health nurses (and others) to negotiate these in their work and come to a shared view, before intervention can occur. In the next section, ways in which the negotiation process works are discussed, before the theories that may underpin interventions are described, and examples given.

Negotiating perspectives

Negotiation between these ideas can arise at an individual or family level. For example, a patient who smokes and has high blood pressure may be depressed. She may be a single parent, living in vulnerable, poor-quality accommodation, harassed by violent neighbours. She may have several children, some of whom are experiencing developmental problems. Different agencies and professionals are likely to utilise different models. The GP is likely to focus on medical and behavioural ideas of health, looking at screening for and reduction of cardiovascular risk through medication or behavioural intervention. The health visitor may prioritise exploring issues to do with parenting, self-esteem and community safety, using social and psychological concepts of health, an approach that sees the family, the community and the wider environment as key players in the health of this person. Provided these models are viewed as complementary rather than in conflict or overriding each other, the GP and the health visitor can operate effectively as a health-promoting 'team'. Within the wider context, different models may also be seen to operate. The local school or nursery would probably build on a behavioural approach and prioritise intensive work with the children to facilitate their development. The housing department might take a risk-based approach to this family's housing needs, possibly looking at this in relation to severe psychological or physical risk only. If these different perspectives are recognised, they can be used to build up an action plan addressing health holistically.

At a community level, agencies and professionals may also negotiate health promotion activity from different perspectives on health. In looking at the health needs of a community, local GPs may work from the traditional medically focused base of identifying specific morbidity and mortality figures for that area. Health visitors may use social and behavioural approaches to prioritise access to healthy food choices, parenting problems and community safety concerns. School nurses may build on behavioural ideas to highlight high-school exclusion rates and incidence of bullying. All of these ideas may be negotiated in the primary care organisation or local health group, prioritised, and appropriate action planned, within the construction of the Health Improvement Programme or the Local Strategic Partnership.

One important issue in the debates around health promotion is the question of targeting. What is the evidence on the relative effectiveness and feasibility of targeting individuals or population groups? In practice, a judicious combination may be best. Where an intervention is specific and has a clear value, whole population groups can appropriately be targeted. For example, it is now commonplace to offer all babies immunisations against diphtheria, tetanus and polio, among others, at an early age (see Chapter 14). The protective effect of this is well described, and side-effects are few. However, there has been more debate about other interventions. One example of targeting populations for health promotion is the routine 'over 75 check', which became mandatory for practice teams to offer during the Thatcher government. This was offered to everyone in the relevant age group, but was rapidly found to be of questionable value. There was an initial positive effect, particularly in relation to services such as chiropody, and in increased morale (echoing Luker, 1982, who demonstrated a positive psychological impact of health visitor visits to older people). However, longer-term morbidity and mortality effects reduced the impact of the check, and further resources were required to provide an effective longer-term service, essentially with regular follow-up (McEwan et al 1990).

Attempts to develop effective postal screening tools also had mixed success. Targeting individuals for health promotion interventions requires not only an effective intervention, but also an initial screening exercise to highlight people as appropriate recipients of an intervention. One study that has looked at health promotion in relation to alcohol use (Kaner et al 1999) relies on the use of a validated screening tool to pick out those patients whose alcohol consumption level is at risky levels or worse. The doctor or nurse then targets these people for a 'brief intervention'. However, in this instance, there is no intervention with people who are not yet drinking to excess, so the health promotion is focused on secondary rather than primary prevention.

Theoretical perspectives underpinning health promotion work in practice

Work with individuals

One of the theoretical frameworks most commonly used in looking at effective health promotion is that of DiClemente and Prochaska (1982). This was originally

> **Box 9.2**
>
> ## Stages of change
>
> - Precontemplative: not even thinking about making a change in this area
> - Contemplative: the idea of change has been triggered – perhaps by an event, a coincidence, a conversation or an advert – but the individual has no plan for its achievement
> - Motivated/planning change: at this stage the individual has begun to plan how he can make a specific change, setting goals for doing more exercise, giving up smoking or eating more healthily. At this stage he will also be considering the factors that will either help or hinder in this, for example peer pressure, breaking routine
> - Putting change into action: change goes into action – the plan begins
> - Keeping change going (or) relapsing: the individual has to operate strategies to maintain the new behaviour, working to overcome adverse effects of change, such as stiffness after exercise, or exacerbation of cough on giving up smoking. In many cases, the individual relapses back to previous patterns of behaviour. He requires reassurance that this is normal. Many people will need to go around the cycle perhaps three or four times before achieving successful change.
>
> Adapted from DiClemente & Prochaska 1982

developed in work with alcohol-dependent people. It rests on the idea that an individual will only change his behaviour when he is ready, having weighed up the pros and cons for him, and will only sustain change when he has reviewed the implications of change and found ways of managing them and making them acceptable. The behaviour–change cycle, as it is commonly known, identifies a series of stages (Box 9.2) through which the individual will pass on the way to a new way of behaving.

The theories that underpin the behaviour–change cycle include Becker's (1974) Health Belief Model, which indicates some of the ways in which individuals may be moved from a precontemplative to a contemplative state, or from a contemplative to a planning stage, as well as indicating the factors that may help to sustain behaviour. Another important linked theory is Skinner's (1951) Stimulus–Response Theory, which developed ideas about ways of reinforcing and extinguishing certain sorts of behaviour by offering rewards or punishments. In the context of the behaviour–change cycle this indicates the importance of looking for the rewards and 'punishments' delivered by different behaviours: the comfort of a familiar chair by the fire versus the run in the cold and rain.

Work with groups and organisations

Increasingly, policy development is moving towards the promotion of health within communities or across organisations and institutions. Theoretical development in this area has taken place in the study of urban regeneration and in organisational and community development. Much of the thinking has been located in other countries and cultures. The elements of theoretical development have predominantly been in two areas.

First, attention has been paid to the involvement of people within communities and organisations in decisions about change. The importance of public participation in the process of seeking to achieve and maintain health is a central tenet of the 1978 Alma-Ata Declaration on Health for All by the year 2000 (World Health Organization 1978). In the UK it was the Griffiths Report on NHS management in 1983 that first set out the policy shift towards consumerism. While this was seen as empowering people by increasing the choices open to them in a market model of health care, more recent policy shifts have also been motivated by notions of transparency, autonomy, equity and justice. It is now believed by those guiding policy that:

> 'Successful action to reduce inequalities and to promote health can only be taken with the active participation of the communities and individuals that have been excluded from the benefits available to more affluent members of society'.

> (NHS Executive 1998)

The World Health Organization (1991) set out the overall benefits of community involvement and participation in health care as fivefold: increased coverage of the population; increased efficiency through better coordination of resources; increased effectiveness through more relevant goals; increased equity through greater recognition of need; and increased self-reliance as a result of increased opportunities for people to control their lives. As noted earlier, in the White Paper *The new NHS modern, dependable*, the importance of including 'a strong public voice' has been emphasised (DH 1997).

Second, the way in which organisations and systems operate to bring about change has been explored, and theories constructed about how and why to achieve successful change. For example, Nelson and Wright (1995) suggest that 'stakeholders' and 'transformation' are key concepts within this process. They indicate that these concepts are related to the introduction of ideas from North American organisational management, which view organisations as made up of free-floating actors (stakeholders) with interests that they pursue by a process of bargaining. Transformation is seen as the structural change that results from this.

Work at policy level

Health promotion work at the level of policy appears to be driven by theories on a different scale. Economic theory is perhaps influential in the slow pace of change in relation to advertisement of cigarettes, while it was used effectively in the move to seat-belt legislation. Ideas about potential economic benefit remain among the strongest drivers for health promotion policy: European health policy, in particular, seems to demonstrate concern for the economic benefits of health promoting activity. In the UK, the Treasury led the move to pump-prime Sure Start initiatives to the tune of £540 million, when faced with massively rising costs of juvenile crime, mental illness and drug use in young people, a trend that the evidence suggested could be reduced or even reversed by early interventions focused upon the most disadvantaged 5% of the preschool population (see Chapter 6).

Examples from practice

To conclude this section, a few examples of health promotion work in practice are described. First, at the individual level, a practice nurse working in a large primary care team in Gateshead noticed that many patients of the practice were experiencing difficulties with warfarin treatment. She highlighted two main problems. The first related to the outpatient clinic at which levels were monitored, which had long waiting times and very brief consultations. The second was that people remained uncertain, despite attendance at the clinic, about how they should adjust their dosage according to their day-to-day needs. The practice nurse read up on warfarin. She talked to the GPs and to the consultant haematologist running the outpatient clinic. Then she set up a pilot scheme to provide warfarin-monitoring sessions through the practice, within very strict protocols.

The patients were keen to attend, and appreciated having a local service with clear appointments. They continued to ask questions about their dosages, many of which she could not initially answer. However, she found out the answers, and after a while produced a number of leaflets that addressed particular issues that recurred. Evaluation of the service showed that not only was this seen as more accessible and helpful in addressing individual questions – partly through longer consultations – but it was also cheaper than the standard option.

An example that takes place at the level of a local school involved issues of both participation and of successful work to change an organisation's culture. Two school nurses in Newcastle worked together to identify the health needs of young adolescents through lunch-time health fairs, at which students were encouraged to put their questions into an anonymised box. Considerable concerns about sexual health and development, as well as mental health, were highlighted. However, offers of discussion with the nurses failed to generate many takers: consultation with young people suggested that sessions would be more effectively located off the school premises, after school hours. When sessions were set up at a local clinic after school hours, these proved to be well-used. Feedback from students enabled the school to reduce bullying and other threats to mental health.

Health promoting policy has not always been recognised. The examples that exist are often those where an individual city or county has been influenced by relatively small-scale initiatives that challenge traditional ways of thinking. One such example arose out of the secondment of a health visitor and later a district nurse to the Housing Department in Newcastle City Council. She was exploring housing patterns across the city and decided to visit all the sheltered housing units. As a result, she discovered a number of issues, ranging from training deficits for sheltered housing wardens to decision making by housing officers. Wardens complained of the 'TWIT' syndrome: The Warden Is There. They were often cast in the role of semi-formal carer for an increasingly frail group of people, while in reality having a very limited knowledge base. This was addressed by collaborative sessions with local district nurses and social workers, and contributed to the development of a new organisational structure for wardens, including a 24-hour centralised control room, and greater use of a mobile service as back-up. Housing officers often made their decisions about housing in the virtual absence of health information. They were encouraged to make links with local health professionals to facilitate appropriate sharing of knowledge, and more timely and suitable placements.

Conclusion

This chapter began by setting out some definitions. In particular, it was asserted that health is not one, but a number of ideas, which operate differently in different people's minds at different times, as they consider how the health of the public can be promoted and maintained. The historical development of ideas about health and its promotion and maintenance have been outlined, and set in the context of political change. At various points along the way, public health work has reinvented itself to respond to the mood of the day. The related notions of health promotion, health education and of primary health care have been explored, and different perspectives on these described.

Negotiation of perspectives within primary care groups or local health groups, in the construction of a Health Improvement Programme, have been outlined. Evidence on the relative effectiveness and feasibility of targeting individuals or population groups has been described. Theoretical frameworks have been set out in relation to individuals, groups and at policy level, linking ideas about participation and organisational change. These theories are illustrated in practice using some examples.

DISCUSSION QUESTIONS

- In considering how the health of the public may be promoted and maintained, what theories and models are most important to you?
- Wass (2000) and Kelly and colleagues (1993) have sought to describe health promotion activity as a range of levels. How far do their suggestions fit in with practice in your area?
- What is your view on the appropriateness of targeting health promotion interventions with individuals or population groups? Why?
- In your own context, can you identify examples of health-promoting activity at the individual, community and policy levels?

References

Acheson D 1998 Independent inquiry into inequalities in health. HMSO, London

Antonovsky A 1996 The salutogenic model as a theory to guide health promotion. Health Promotion International 11(1): 11–18

Ashton J, Seymour H 1988 The new public health. Open University Press, Buckingham, UK

Ashton J, Grey P, Barnard K 1986 Healthy cities: WHO's new public health initiative. Health Promotion 1(3): 319–323

Becker MH (ed.) 1974 The health belief model and personal health behavior. Thorofare, New Jersey

Belsky J, Melhuish E, Barnes J, Leyland A, Romaniuk H and National Evaluation of Sure Start Research Team 2006 Effects of Sure Start local programmes on children and families: early findings from a quasi-experimental, cross sectional study. British Medical Journal 332: 1476–1481

Board of Education 1928 Handbook of suggestions on health education. HMSO, London

Bhopal R 1995 Public health medicine and primary health care: convergent, divergent, or parallel paths? Journal of Epidemiology & Community Health 49(2): 113–116

Blaxter M 1982 Mothers and daughters: a three generational study of health attitudes and behaviour. Heinemann Educational Books, London

Brown V 1985 Towards an epidemiology of health: a basis for planning community health programs. Health Policy 4: 331–340

Boyd M, Brummell K, Billingham K, Perkins E R 1993 The public health post at Strelley: Nursing Development Unit,

Nottingham. Community Health NHS Trust, Nottingham

Chadwick E 1965 Report on the sanitary condition of the labouring population of Great Britain (reprint of Chadwick 1842). Edinburgh University Press, Edinburgh

Clark J 1986 A model for health visiting. In: Kershaw B, Salvage J (eds) Models for nursing. John Wiley & Sons, Chichester

Collin C, Wade D, Davies S, Horn V 1988 The Barthel ADL Index: a reliability study. International Disability Studies 10: 61–63

Cornwell J 1984 Hard-earned lives: accounts of health and illness from East London. Tavistock Publications, London

Council for the Education and Training of Health Visitors (CETHV) 1977 An investigation into the principles of health visiting. CETHV, London

Council of Europe 2000 White paper on the protection of the human rights and dignity of people suffering from mental disorder, especially those placed as involuntary patients in a psychiatric establishment. Council of Europe, Strasbourg

Cox J, Hill S 1993 Tackling language delay: a groupwork approach. Health Visitor 66(8): 291–292

Department for Education and Employment 1999 Sure Start. DfEE, London

Department of Health (DH) 1992 The health of the nation: a strategy for health in England (CM1986). HMSO, London

Department of Health (DH) 1997 The new NHS: modern, dependable (CM3809). HMSO, London

Department of Health (DH) 1999 Saving lives: our healthier nation (CM4386). HMSO, London

Department of Health (DH) 2000 National Service Framework for Coronary Heart Disease. HMSO, London

Department of Health (DH) 2004 Choosing health: making healthy choices easier (CM6374). HMSO, London

Department of Health and Department for Education and Science 2004 National service framework for children, young people and maternity services: Core standards. Department of Health, London

DiClemente CC, Prochaska JO 1982 Self-change and therapy: change of smoking behavior: a comparison of processes of change in cessation and maintenance. Addictive Behaviors 7(2): 133–142

Ewles L, Simnett I 1985 Promoting health: a practical guide to health education. John Wiley, Chichester

French S 1993 Disability, impairment or something in between? In: Swain J, Finkelstein V, French S, Oliver M (eds) Disabling barriers – enabling environments. Sage, London

Home Office 1998 Supporting families. Home Office, London

Kaner E, Heather N, McAvoy B, Lock C, Gilvarry E 1999 Intervention for excessive alcohol consumption in primary health care: attitudes and practices of English general practitioners. Alcohol and Alcoholism 34(4): 559–566

Kelly MP, Charlton B, Hanlon P 1993 The four levels of health promotion: an integrated approach. Public Health 107: 319–326

Kerr SM, Jowett SA, Smith LN 1996 Preventing sleep problems in infants: a randomized controlled trial. Journal of Advanced Nursing 24(5): 938–942

Leavell HR 1953 In: Leavell HR, Clark EG (eds) Textbook of preventive medicine. McGraw-Hill, New York

Luker K 1982 Evaluating health visiting practice. Royal College of Nursing, London

Mayall B 1986 Keeping children healthy: the role of mothers and professionals. Allen & Unwin, London

McEwan RT, Davison N, Forster DP, Pearson P, Stirling E 1990 Screening elderly people in primary care: a randomised controlled trial. British Journal of General Practice 40: 94–97

Nelson N, Wright S 1995 Participation and Power. In: Nelson N & Wright S (eds) Power and participatory development: theory and practice. Intermediate Technology Publications, London

NHS Executive 1998 In the public interest: developing a strategy for public participation in the NHS. Department of Health, Wetherby, UK

Parsons T 1951 The social system. Free Press, New York

Pearson P 1991 Clients' perceptions: the use of case studies in developing theory. Journal of Advanced Nursing 16: 521–528

Pearson P, Mead P, Graney A, McRae G 2000 Evaluation of the developing specialist practitioner role in the context of public health. University of Newcastle, Newcastle upon Tyne

Rodgers H, Soutter J, Kaiser W, Pearson P, Dobson R, Skilbeck C, Bond J 1997 Early supported hospital discharge following acute stroke: length of stay and three month outcomes. Clinical Rehabilitation 11: 280–287

Rowland, L. Dickinson E, Newman P, Ford D, Ebrahim S 1994 Look after your heart programme: impact on health status, exercise, knowledge, attitudes, and behaviour of retired women in England. Journal of Epidemiology and Community Health 48(2): 123–128

Skinner BF 1953 Science and human behavior. Macmillan, New York

Tannahill A 1985 What is health promotion? Health Education Journal 49: 10–12

Titmuss R 1970 The gift relationship: from human blood to social policy. Allen & Unwin, London

UNICEF 2003 http://www.unicef.org/infobycountry/india_india_statistics.html [accessed 15/08/05].

Wanless D 2004 Securing good health for the whole population. HMSO, London

Wass A 2000 Promoting health: the primary health care approach, 2nd edn. Elsevier Australia, Marrickville

Watkins SJ 1994 Stockport health promise. Stockport Health Authority, Stockport Metropolitan Borough Council

Watkins SJ 1996 Health 2000: four years to go. 8th Annual Public Health Report for Stockport. Stockport Health Authority, Stockport

Whyte WF 1993 Street corner society, 4th edn. University of Chicago Press, Chicago

World Health Organization 1946 Constitution. World Health Organization, Geneva

World Health Organization 1978 The declaration of Alma-Ata. International conference on primary health care, Alma-Ata, Kazakhstan. World Health Organization, Geneva

World Health Organization 1984 Health promotion: a discussion document on the concept and principles. World Health Organization, Copenhagen

World Health Organization 1986 Ottawa charter for health promotion. World Health Organization, Ottawa

World Health Organization 1991 Community involvement in health development: challenging health services. World Health Organization, Geneva

World Health Organization 2006. The world health report 2006 – working together for health World Health Organization, Geneva

Zola IK 1973 Pathways to the doctor – from person to patient. Social Science and Medicine 7: 677–689

Further reading

Allott M, Robb M (eds) 1998 Understanding health and social care: an introductory reader. Sage Publications, London

Although this book is a very broad reader, it is an excellent resource in thinking through the context of public health and health promotion, primarily from a sociological perspective. It is a collection of papers gathered from a range of sources. The two particularly relevant sections are Section 2 (Where Care Takes Place) and Section 5 (Contexts of Care: Policies and Politics), but there are also pieces exploring empowerment, professionalism, and social control among others.

Naidoo J, Wills J 1998 Practising health promotion. Baillière Tindall, London

This book addresses health promotion practice. It is well presented with good use of case studies, activities and discussion points. It considers the policy context in which health promotion takes place, although is slightly dated due to the fast pace of change. One of its particular strengths is the 'challenges in practice' section. In this, the research base provided is helpful – for example, in looking at the prevention of coronary heart disease and stroke – reference is made to reports of the OXCHECK study amongst others, though again, this material dates quickly.

Popay J, Williams G (eds) 1999 Researching the people's health. Routledge, London

This book is particularly helpful in exploring ways in which researchers can help practitioners to identify the health needs of the people they work with. It includes sections on the theory and methods of health needs assessment and on ways of involving the public in this. It is well referenced and includes a number of practical examples.

Section 4

The facilitation of health-enhancing activities

The principle of facilitation draws attention to the fact that this form of public health work is rarely concerned with doing things 'to' or 'for' individuals. Instead, the focus remains on setting up systems and activities that enable people to act in ways that enhance health (for example, breastfeeding, as in Chapter 10). Community public health operates primarily through partnership and by promoting the population's health and wellbeing, but some elements of health protection are still required. These may involve service policies and procedures, including the safeguarding of children (Chapter 11) or protecting employees within a work environment.

Leadership for health and wellbeing is a pre-requisite of all public health work, but it is not the exclusive domain of senior management. In community public health practice, the concept is more subtle and egalitarian, as explained in Chapter 12, although no less skilled for all that. Also, it is notoriously difficult to assure service quality in situations where the outcomes are long term and preventive, but the model outlined in Chapter 13 provides a mechanism for achieving this. Working with individuals in the interest of the health of a wider population inevitably raises ethical concerns at times, and can create personal dilemmas. Chapter 14 provides a clear direction for practitioners faced with queries about immunisation, which has been one such 'hot topic' in recent years, as on occasions in the past.

The facilitation of health-enhancing activities is associated with the following performance standards (Nursing and Midwifery Council 2004, p. 12):

1. Work in partnership with others to prevent the occurrence of needs and risks related to health and wellbeing.
2. Work in partnership with others to protect the public's health and wellbeing from specific risks.
3. Prevent, identify and minimise risk of interpersonal abuse or violence, safeguarding children and other vulnerable people, initiating the management of cases involving actual or potential abuse or violence where needed.
4. Apply leadership skills and manage projects to improve health and wellbeing.
5. Plan, deliver and evaluate programmes to improve the health and wellbeing of individuals and groups.
6. Manage teams, individuals and resources effectively.

10 Breastfeeding and public health

Sally Kendall and Francesca Entwistle

Key issues

- Breastfeeding makes a significant contribution to public health
- Public health policy focuses on the prevention of disease and does not recognise the contribution to positive health that breastfeeding can provide, particularly in relation to women's own perceptions of the benefits to health
- The incidence and prevalence of breastfeeding in the UK continues to be low relative to other countries and there are marked variations according to age, socio-economic group and region
- There are many factors, including cultural barriers and breastfeeding in the workplace, that make it difficult for women to breastfeed beyond the first few weeks of life
- There is great scope for health professionals (especially health visitors and midwives) to promote and support breastfeeding

'If a new vaccine became available that could prevent one million or more child deaths per year, and that was moreover cheap, safe, administered orally, and required no cold chain, it would become an immediate public health imperative. Breastfeeding can do all of this and more, but it requires its own 'warm chain' of support – that is, skilled care for mothers to build their confidence and show them what to do, and protection from harmful practices. If this warm chain has been lost from the culture or it is faulty, then it must be made good by health services.'

(Lancet 1994)

Introduction

Historically, there was only one way to nourish infants: by putting them to the breast, be it the natural mother or a wet nurse. Prior to the Industrial Revolution, most babies received human milk. Although we know from early literature that babies were often fed additional weaning foods that may not be approved of today, nonetheless pre-19th-century infants could expect to benefit from milk that was designed for them. This provided protection against diseases and the emotional closeness that is provided through breastfeeding that, in the 20th century, became known as bonding or attachment. After the Industrial Revolution, social and economic change directly impacted on family life and influenced infant feeding practices significantly, so that by the post-war years of the 1960s and 1970s, breastfeeding rates among UK mothers fell significantly. Today, breastfeeding rates in the UK have improved markedly, but vary enormously across social and geographical areas. This fall and gradual rise of breastfeeding has, it is argued, been a significant factor in both infant and maternal health and, therefore, played an important role in the public health debate.

This chapter will explore how and why the natural act of breastfeeding has become a public health issue. We will explore the history and politics of breastfeeding, the policies that have evolved to encourage and support women to breastfeed their infants, the evidence to support the public health benefits of breastfeeding and the research that supports the promotion of breastfeeding. We also include some discussion around women and the factors influencing the choice to breastfeed.

Historical background

Prior to the 19th century, breastfeeding or wet nursing were the most accessible and natural ways to feed a baby. Whilst it is known that substitutes were used and provided, via a sheep's horn for example (such as goats milk and flour with water), the majority of infants would have received human milk. Breastfeeding became a public health issue during the 19th century. As the Industrial Revolution began to have a major effect on the economy in Western Europe, infant mortality was at an all time high. As agriculture declined, urban living became a necessity for many in the search for work, and poor housing, overcrowding, squalor and the attendant scourges of infestation and infection, such as cholera, typhoid and syphilis, took their toll on as many as 250 infants per 1000. As Gabrielle Palmer (1993) reliably informs us in her book *The politics of breastfeeding*, the movement of industry away from cottages and family-based units in the rural areas and into the urban settings had a serious economic and social outcome for women and their children. Whereas child rearing and infant feeding had been a natural part of the daily life of the cottage industrialist, the move to a capitalist economy, where the means of production was centrally based in a factory, meant that women who had to work to live did not have the flexibility during the working day to breastfeed their infants. Protection from infection, as well as the provision of essential nutrients and the ability to manage their own fertility were thus limited for women working in industrialised societies. Breastfeeding as the natural method of feeding, therefore, became increasingly redundant as entrepreneurs, such as Henri Nestle, realised the niche market for artificial feeding and started to produce dried milk powder to replace breastfeeding. Prior to this time, the only alternative to breastfeeding had been wet-nursing – the practice of hiring another breastfeeding woman to feed the infant. This in itself had been a source of respectable income for many women who gained both stability and status by breastfeeding the babies of noble women. The vast majority of women, however, fed their own babies and not only was infant mortality *lower* in most areas before the Industrial Revolution (about 150 per 1000), women were able to take advantage of the contraceptive effects of lactation to space their families. Indeed, Palmer (1993) remarks on the fact that noblewomen often had much larger families, miscarriages and stillbirths than working women, as they did not tend to breastfeed their own babies. The daughters of the cottage industrialists would have been brought up not only as skilled helpers in the cottage industry, but as able mothers who would have no difficulty in breastfeeding her own children alongside the hard and often long working day.

Combining work outside the home with child rearing, within an economy that was driven by capitalism and controlled by patriarchy, deprived women of the power they had had to determine the health and future of their offspring. The only way to maintain some independent means of sustaining themselves and their children was to work in the factories and mills. Whilst breastfeeding continued in rural areas to be successfully sustained, it declined in the urban populations as artificial milks and their contaminants flooded the market, this was seen by many women as the only viable alternative. Public health officials such as Dr Reid (cited by Palmer, 1993), who exhorted women to return to the natural feeding of their infants, over-looked the fact that most women were powerless to do so and, thus, the moral debate over breastfeeding versus artificial feeding was inaugurated. Women who breastfed were seen as harlots, fallen women who wet-nursed to make a living or impoverished women of little moral worth. Working women, for whom breastfeeding was increasingly impossible, were selfish beings who worked to make their own lives better and had little care for their children. Women in the 19th century were in a Catch-22 situation and the legacy of this continues for women today, where arrangements to breastfeed or express milk in the workplace remain unusual and breastfeeding in public can still cause a moral outcry. Indeed, the influence of Westernised economic thought can now be seen to be infiltrating traditional agricultural economies in the developing world. Maher (1992) describes how in one North African tribe women have been almost forced into artificial feeding by the change from a self-sufficient agriculture to a cash-crop economy. The men command the power in the community through the sale of cash-crops in the urban markets, and they retain the profits. The women can only maintain a degree of power by using some of the wealth to purchase formula milk for their infants, a practice that is undoubtedly reinforced by Westernised marketing methods. To breastfeed means to surrender access to the means (and ends) of production, which the women themselves have played a major part in producing.

In today's Western civilisation it would be inaccurate and false to directly attribute infant mortality rates to the decline and rise again of breastfeeding – there have been so many other major public health and social reforms. However, there are many public health benefits associated with breastfeeding, which will be discussed later in this chapter, and breastfeeding continues to be a political issue demanding considerable structural and economic changes if the cost benefits to the public are to be truly realised and those babies who are most in need are to receive the benefits of breast milk.

The Innocenti Declaration

The Innocenti Declaration was signed by 30 governments (including the UK) in 1990, and states that 'all women should be enabled to practise exclusive breastfeeding and all infants should be fed exclusively on breast milk from birth to four to six months of age.'

The Declaration calls on all governments by 1995 to 'enact imaginative legislation protecting the breastfeeding rights of working women'.

The importance of this international declaration cannot be over-emphasised in terms of how pubic health policy and practice within the states that signed the declaration have been, or could have been, developed. It has been the guiding principle of the work of UNICEF in working across countries to develop the Baby Friendly Initiative and thus to enable organisations and practitioners to promote and sustain good breastfeeding practice and policy. This is enshrined in the Ten Steps to Successful Breastfeeding (UNICEF 1996).

The purpose of introducing such declarations and plans internationally is to promote and support breastfeeding to enable both mothers and babies to realise the full health benefits of breast milk, both physical and psychological. As suggested in the introduction, breastfeeding rates have declined since the industrial revolution, and particularly since the Second World War and the economic boom of the 1960s. Against this, the evidence for the public health benefits of breastfeeding has become increasingly more convincing and sophisticated. It has also become possible through better data-collection systems to identify more precisely what the prevalence of breastfeeding is across the UK and where there might be a need for more targeted support.

Incidence and prevalence of breastfeeding in the UK

How popular is breastfeeding in the 21st century in the UK? Without a doubt there has been a significant shift from the 1960s and 1970s when, not only was bottle feeding seen to be the most efficient and proper way to feed a baby, but also the feminist movement (ironically) probably contributed to women liberating themselves from their bodily functions and the perception that breastfeeding was domination by men, which tied them to the home. Surveys of infant feeding are conducted every 5 years by the Office of National Statistics (ONS) and these provide a rich data-base of information on infant feeding practices, which reveal differences around the country that may be linked to public health issues.

The most recent survey was conducted in 2005 and early results were published in 2006, with reference to the previous 2000 survey. The Health and Social Care Information Centre (IC) randomly selected a sample of over 19 848 women from registrations of births compiled by the General Register Offices of England and Wales, Scotland and Northern Ireland. Of these, a total of 62% responded to an initial questionnaire when their babies were between 6 and 10 weeks old. These were followed up by further questionnaires when the babies were 4–5 months and 8–9 months old. The IC defines the incidence of breastfeeding as the proportion of babies who were breastfed initially, even if they were put to the breast only once. Prevalence of breastfeeding is defined as the proportion of babies who were wholly or partially breastfed at specific ages. These definitions have been used since the 1975 survey and are, therefore, helpful for comparative purposes. However, they do disguise the fact that some babies may only be breastfed for a very short time and, in relation to incidence in particular, these babies are counted in the same way as babies who were exclusively breastfed from the moment of birth. The health benefits of exclusive breastfeeding for 6 months as recommended by WHO (2002) are, therefore, difficult to extract from the ONS/ IC data. However, as Table 10.1 shows, there has been an overall increase in the incidence of breastfeeding since 1995. The obvious issue that these data draw our attention to is one of difference in the incidence of breastfeeding between the UK constituent countries, breastfeeding being highest in England and lowest in Northern Ireland; however, breastfeeding rates in Northern Ireland between 2000 and 2005 rose more significantly than any other country (9% vs 6 and 7% in Scotland and England and Wales). There are regional variations within these figures; for example, the incidence of breastfeeding in London and the South East in 2000 was 81%, compared with 61% in the North of England (Hamlyn et al 2002). There have been significant overall increases in breastfeeding initiation since 1990: in England and Wales this increase represents 13% of new births, in Scotland 20% and in Northern Ireland 27%. Clearly, the changes have been proportionally greater in Scotland and Northern Ireland, but these countries started from a lower baseline.

Breastfeeding rates for Wales were available for the first time in 2005 and showed an initiation breastfeeding rate of 67%.

The prevalence of breastfeeding also indicates positive changes since 1995 (see Table 10.2). However, it is important to note that breastfeeding drops dramatically after 6 weeks and that these figures include babies who are receiving other forms of nourishment as well as breast milk. Again, health benefits over time are

Table 10.1 ● Incidence of breastfeeding by country

	Percentage breastfed initially			
	England and Wales	Scotland	Northern Ireland	United Kingdom
1990	64	50	36	62
1995	68	55	45	66
2000	71	63	54	69
2005	77	70	63	76

(Source: Bolling K 2006)

Table 10.2 ● Duration of breastfeeding for those who breastfed initially by country

Age of baby	Percentage breastfed initially							
	England and Wales		Scotland		Northern Ireland		United Kingdom	
	1995	2000	1995	2000	1995	2000	1995	2000
	Percentage still breastfeeding							
Birth	100	100	100	100	100	100	100	100
1 week	86	85	84	83	79	72	85	84
2 weeks	81	80	79	78	73	66	80	79
6 weeks	65	65	66	67	56	51	65	64
4 months	42	45	45	50	27	30	42	44
6 months	32	34	35	40	19	21	32	34
9 months	21	19	24	23	11	11	21	19

(Source: Hamlyn et al 2002)

236

difficult to extract unless exclusive breastfeeding is counted and identified as the independent variable. Finally, the ONS measures duration of breastfeeding, which is defined as the length of time a baby is breastfed from initiation to weaning, but again includes other forms of nutrition. The figures suggest that there has been a small decrease from 21% to 19% of babies across the UK who continue to receive breast milk at 9 months of age. However, the differences between UK countries is not so marked between 6 and 9 months, except that Northern Ireland babies appear to stop feeding dramatically after 6 months compared with the rest of the UK. Unfortunately, data are not systematically collected beyond this period so there is little national evidence of the effects of long-term breastfeeding. (These data will be available for 2005 with the full report due for publication in Spring 2007.)

The ONS/IC survey also provides an interpretation of the data that demonstrates significant positive correlations between incidence, prevalence and duration of breastfeeding and social class, age and education of the mother. Overall, younger mothers from lower social economic groups who completed their education by 16 are less likely to initiate breastfeeding than older, longer-educated women from better-off backgrounds. This is true across all UK countries, particularly Scotland and Northern Ireland. The Acheson report (DH 1999b) on inequalities in health identified the differences in prevalence in breastfeeding among different social groups and called for policies to address these differences. This was subsequently re-emphasised by HM Treasury and the Department of Health in the cross-cutting review of inequalities in health (DH/Treasury 2002), which recognised that promoting breastfeeding was one way in which infant morbidity and mortality rates among the most disadvantaged in our society could be improved. Interestingly, evidence from a study undertaken by the Institute of Education (Dex & Joshi 2005) has found that mothers from black and ethnic minority groups are more likely to breastfeed their babies for longer than white women, even when low income is taken into account. Their longitudinal study of 19 000 children born in 2000 and 2001 found that 49.4 of white mothers breastfed their infants for at least a month, compared to 68.6 of Indian mothers, 67.1% of Bangladeshi mothers and 82% of black mothers.

In order to address pubic health targets adequately, these breastfeeding data are critical to the interpretation and understanding of local health needs within primary care trusts and strategic health authorities, alongside other correlates of health improvement, such as smoking behaviour and teenage pregnancy. To realise the necessary health improvements, account has to be taken by public health analysts and practitioners of the co-variates affecting health behaviour and, ultimately, public health outcomes. The positive changes in breastfeeding rates should be correlated with other health data and some epidemiologists – notably Howie and colleagues (1990) – have conducted some rigorous analyses of these possible relationships.

Public health benefits of breastfeeding

Across the world, it has been estimated that over a million babies per year die from diarrhoea as a result of unsafe formula-feeding techniques, and that babies who are bottle-fed in poor conditions are 25 times more likely to die than breastfed babies (Baby Milk Action 2006, citing WHO). In relation to gastroenteritis, Bauchner (1986) found from a review of over 40 studies since 1970, that breastfeeding had a protective effect. Howie (1990), in a study of 618 children in Dundee, found that babies who breastfed for 13 weeks were not only protected from gastroenteritis but also that the benefits lasted for up to 1 year.

Breastfeeding has also been identified as a protective factor in sudden infant death syndrome (Savage 1992) and shown to be important in protection in the longer term from diseases such as Crohn's disease (Kolezko et al 1989) coeliac disease (Akobeng et al, 2006) and insulin-dependent diabetes (Metcalf et al 1992). Clearly, the initiation and continuation of breastfeeding should lead to significant health gains and cost savings within the health services. These studies have been ground breaking in setting a pubic health agenda around breastfeeding and in recent years have been supplemented by a series of systematic reviews that have found unequivocal evidence for the pubic health benefits of breastfeeding and for exclusive breastfeeding up to 6 months of age.

Most of the evidence on the public health benefits of breastfeeding is predicated on its relationship with the reduction of risk for certain diseases for either baby or mother. However, an alternative approach to public health is to consider the health promoting effects rather than the disease prevention effects of an intervention on its own. The White Paper *Choosing health* (DH 2004a) referred to areas for health improvement and outlined proposals for a 'third way' of both managing and preventing ill health. The paper acknowledged the social and economic causes of ill health, recognising that there are real inequalities in health, confirmed in *Tackling inequalities in health* (DH/Treasury 2002). The White Paper sets out to achieve public health improvements through reductions in smoking, improving diet and nutrition and preventing obesity, promoting mental health and promoting sexual health. Such initiatives are linked to serious diseases such as cancer and heart disease, but *Choosing health* sets out a series of salutagenic proposals that, if fully implemented, would promote and improve the conditions within which people make health choices, not just warn of the risks of disease associated with that choice. For example, nutritional improvements were located within a whole series of initiatives within schools and nursery schools, including free fruit for 4 to 6-year-olds and the development of the Healthy Schools Standard (DfES 2004), and Healthy Start (DH/NHS 2005) that replaces the Welfare Food Scheme by introducing vouchers that can be exchanged for healthy foods (full roll-out of this initiative expected by the end of 2006.) Improvements in mental health were considered in the light of many determinants, such as age of young men dying from suicide and postnatal depression, alongside social disadvantage and deprivation. Social support and advice for young parents, such as Sure Start and the development of Children's Centres and Children's Trusts, were also recognised in *Choosing health* as being crucial to the improvement of public health.

Choosing health was an advance on previous government consultations on public health because the focus was away from the immediate risks of disease towards a more integrated approach to tackling the issues that determine health and illness. It is within such a framework that the promotion of breastfeeding has an important position because of the many known health-promoting effects of breastfeeding. The next section of the chapter provides an overview of recent evidence that supports the public health benefits of breastfeeding, with a particular emphasis on evidence that supports the UK government's aim to reduce obesity in childhood and, thus, in the longer term prevent the diseases associated with obesity, such type 2 diabetes and coronary heart disease.

In the public spending review of 2005, the government introduced Public Service Agreements (PSAs) across all departments on which they are to deliver. For example, the Department of Health (DH) introduced a PSA target to halt the year on year increase in obesity among children under 11 by 2010. Recent indications suggest that this target will not be met. One in four children is obese, the Health and Social Care Information Centre (Health and Social Care Information Centre 2005) survey of 2000 children found: from 1995 to 2004, obesity among boys aged 11–15 rose from 14% to 24% and girls from 15% to 26%. The rate rose slightly in the 2–10 age group. Interestingly, the DH also introduced a PSA target that breastfeeding would increase by 2% per year:

'Deliver an increase of 2 percentage points per year in breastfeeding initiation rate, focusing especially on women from disadvantaged groups.'

(DH 2002)

These two targets are inextricably linked, as demonstrated in the Healthy Start initiative. *Choosing health* potentially provides an integrating policy framework within which to build healthy public policy that enables and empowers individ-uals and families to benefit from health-promoting activities. However, there are challenges and barriers in the implementation of such a policy, which does not take account of the cultural and social circumstances within which individuals make health choices. Breastfeeding is a choice that women and their families make, but whilst the health benefits described below make breastfeeding an obvious imperative, the choice to formula feed is often based on other considerations. This issue of choice is discussed later in the chapter.

Health gains of breastfeeding for infants

As already indicated, there has been much research conducted into the ways in which babies can benefit from breast milk; not all of which is conclusive. However,

238

two published reports of a prospective study conducted in Dundee have found some convincing findings about the public health benefits of breastfeeding for infants. The first of these was published in 1990 (Howie et al 1990) and reported on the relation between breastfeeding and infant illness in the first 2 years of life, with particular reference to gastroenteritis. The study was based on a prospective, observational design of 750 pairs of mothers and infants of whom 618 were followed up for 24 months after birth. The infants were observed in detail at 2 weeks and at 1, 2, 3, 4, 5, 6, 9, 12, 15, 18, 21 and 24 months by health visitors. This regularity of surveillance minimised detection bias, as did rigorous definitions of the diseases being observed for and the ways in which the health visitors were instructed to ask parents questions. Gastrointestinal illness, for example, was defined as vomiting or diarrhoea or both lasting as a discrete illness for 48 hours or more. The main outcome measure was the prevalence of gastrointestinal disease in infants during the follow-up. Women were categorised for the purposes of the study by their breastfeeding behaviour at 13 weeks as either full breastfeeders ($n=97$), partial breastfeeders ($n=130$), early weaners ($n=180$) or bottle feeders ($n=257$). This was a helpful distinction as several previous studies had not made any attempt to define breastfeeding. The results showed that there were 50 episodes of gastrointestinal illness among bottle fed babies compared to two among fully breastfed babies. When these data was adjusted for variables such as social class and parental smoking, it was found that there was a significant difference in the prevalence of gastrointestinal illness at 13 weeks between babies who were either fully or partially breastfed and those who were bottle fed. There was also evidence that other illnesses were less prevalent among the breastfed babies, for example, respiratory illness was also less common. These benefits were observed to persist up to the first year of life, with fewer babies who were breastfed requiring admission to hospital with gastrointestinal illness. The authors point out that nothing in their study undermines the view that babies should be fully breastfed for 4–6 months. However, they do emphasise that some mothers either decide to bottle feed from the outset or give up breastfeeding prematurely because of the pressures of returning to work. They urge that women should be enabled to breastfeed for a minimum of 3 months through statutory maternity rights and crèche facilities at work. This recommendation is significant in the light of the historical overview at the beginning of this chapter. Interestingly, the Green Paper *Our healthier nation* (DH, 1998) did refer to the idea of the healthy workplace and enjoined employers to consider a contract for health, which included issues such as child-care facilities. It is a matter of some considerable interest that this did not feature strongly in either of the subsequent policy documents *Saving lives* (DH 1999a) or *Choosing health* (DH 2004a) and, therefore, there is no real policy incentive for employers to consider child-friendly environments that include time out to breastfeed or express milk. It is on such important matters for women that health visitors, midwives and other community nurses should be commenting and lobbying government, using the evidence provided by research, such as Howie et al's, to support their arguments.

The importance for public health of Howie et al's (1990) paper lies in its methodological rigour and significance of its findings, which clearly have implications for cost evaluation also, although the researchers do not carry out this exercise themselves. Eight years after the publication of this work, the researchers published their findings of the 7-year follow-up of the same cohort of infants (Wilson et al 1998). This type of long-term follow-up is unusual as it is costly, but it provides strong evidence on the benefits of breastfeeding. In this stage of the study the team analysed the relationship between infant feeding practices and childhood respiratory illness, growth, body composition and blood pressure. Of the original 674 children in the cohort, 545 were available for the study, the mean age of whom was 7.3 years. Outcome measures were prevalence of respiratory illness, height, body mass index, percentage body fat and blood pressure. Parents of the children were asked to complete a questionnaire about childhood illnesses and family history of allergy (545 or 81% of the original cohort) at around the age of 7 years and anthropometric measures including blood pressure, body composition, percentage body fat, skinfold thickness, weight and body mass index and height were completed by 412 or 61% of the original cohort. The same definitions of breastfeeding and the data were used as for the original study. The main findings from this study have important implications for child health, as they confirm that breastfeeding infants exclusively up to at least 15 weeks does confer health benefits into later childhood. For example, there is a significant reduction in respiratory illness during the first 7 years of life for exclusively breastfed infants and exclusive formula feeding is associated with higher blood pressure (mean difference 3 mmHg systolic blood pressure) at the age of 7 and the early introduction of solids is associated with increased weight, percentage body fat and risk of wheezing in childhood. As the authors point out, the observed effects on body composition and blood pressure of bottle feeding and early solids may be magnified over time and become important antecedents of adult health. This again is significant in the light of the policy plans to reduce childhood obesity and the risks of diseases associated with obesity. The findings from Wilson et al's (1998) study do confirm the advice of the WHO (2001) to continue breastfeeding for up to 6 months. It would, therefore, be appropriate for practitioners to utilise the evidence from Wilson et al's (1998) study to support their own arguments to promote, audit and evaluate breastfeeding practice within their own localities. Since the publication of Wilson's study, further evidence has emerged regarding the protective effects of breastfeeding against obesity and the cost benefits to the health care system of such an effect. Examples of such evidence are presented in Table 10.3 for ease of reference. Whilst the evidence presented here meets the criteria for high-quality evidence (Cochrane Collaboration 2006), the reader is advised to follow-up the cit-ations for full access to the individual studies.

It can be seen from Table 10.3 that the evidence on overweight and obesity is equivocal, although there is a definite tendency towards longer-term breastfeeding being protective against overweight and obesity. One of the problems with the evidence, to date, is that trials use different samples, outcome measures and different definitions of breastfeeding and duration, thus it is difficult to be absolute about the conclusion. For example, the Gilman (2001) study was based on a sample of over 15 000 young people up to the age of 14 whereas the Hediger (2001) study was based on a sample of 2685 children between 3 and 5 years who were more ethnically diverse. Perhaps Hediger's study did not find such a strong relationship between breastfeeding duration and obesity because the sample was too small to show such an effect, or the effects do not become apparent until later childhood. However, the published systematic reviews would suggest that there is a benefit and the larger surveys, such as the Czech survey (Toschke et al 2002), certainly demonstrate that breastfeeding is worth promoting to protect children against obesity. This should be sufficient evidence in itself for health policy makers to consider ways in which breastfeeding could be promoted given the global public health problems that are arising from overweight and obesity in childhood. The cost benefit of breastfeeding to a health system would be significant if all the consequences of obesity, such as the treatment of type 2 diabetes and coronary heart disease, could be costed and shown to be off-set by breastfeeding. An American study (Weimer 2001) has estimated that $3.6 billion (bn) would be saved if current breastfeeding rates could be raised from 64% in hospital to 75%, and from 29% at 6 months to 50%. This is based on cost savings from the treatment of three childhood diseases: otitis media, gastroenteritis and necrotising enterocolitis. Whilst obesity is not included in this analysis, it can be seen that the cost benefits might be huge if this were also evaluated in this way.

The overall cost of obesity to the NHS is currently around £1bn, with a further £2.3bn to £2.6bn for the economy as a whole, it is proposed. Current

Table 10.3 ● Summary of evidence of the protective effects of breastfeeding against obesity in childhood

	Author	Year	Title	Journal	Type	Outcome	Sample	Result	Notes
1	Burke et al	2005	Breastfeeding and overweight: longitudinal analysis in an Australian birth cohort	Journal of Pediatrics	Cohort study	95th centile overweight	2087		Babies breastfed for at least 1 year are leaner than those weaned earlier Breastfeeding < 4 months has no protective effect
2	Hardy et al	2005	Duration of breastfeeding and risk of overweight	American Journal of Epidemiology	Meta-analysis	Odds ratio (OR) and 95% confidence interval (CI) of overweight associated with breastfeeding	17 studies		Strongly supports a dose-dependent association between longer duration of breastfeeding and decrease in risk of overweight (> 9 months: OR=0.68, 95% CI: 0.50, 0.91)
3	Toschke et al	2002	Overweight and obesity in 6- to 14-year-old Czech children in 1991	Journal of Pediatrics	Cross-sectional survey	Body mass index (BMI) > 90th centile (overweight) BMI > 97th centile (obese)	33 768 children aged 6–14 years old in 1991		Prevalence of over-weight/obesity was lower in breastfed children and did not diminish with age The effect could not be explained by other factors such as parental education, birth weight or smoking

Table 10.3 (Continued)

	Author	Year	Title	Journal	Type	Outcome	Sample	Result	Notes
4	Hediger et al	2001	Association between infant breastfeeding and overweight in young children	Journal of the American Medical Association	Cross-sectional survey	BMI between 85th and 94th centile at risk of overweight, BMI > 95th centile, overweight	2685 US children between 3 and 5 years	Risk of being overweight was reduced by being ever breastfed (OR = 0.63, 95% CI 0.41–0.96) but obesity was not reduced and the strongest correlator of this was maternal weight and obesity	Breastfeeding should be recommended but may not be as effective as moderating familial effects such as dietary habits and physical activity
5	Gillman et al	2001	Risk of overweight among adolescents who were breastfed as infants	Journal of the American Medical Association	Survey	BMI > 95th centile for age and sex = overwieght	8186 girls, 7155 boys between 9 and 14 years	Only or mostly breastfed were less likely to be overweight than those mostly formula fed (OR = 0.78, 95% CI 0.66–0.91)	

The search was defined by studies that included the effectiveness of breastfeeding on overweight or obesity in childhood since 2000. Searches included PubMed, Cochrane database of reviews, MIDRS and citations from studies and reviews. It is not presented here as a systematic review, but as indicative of the evidence available.

UK breastfeeding rates (see Tables 10.1 and 10.2) remain below the US Surgeon General's recommended rates (above) if the full cost benefit to public health is to be realised.

Health benefits for women

The evaluation of the health benefits of breastfeeding have tended to focus almost exclusively on the health gains for infants and children. However, lactation is a naturally occurring physiological phenomenon that may confer health benefits to those women in whom the natural course of events takes place. Clearly, there are many women who do not lactate either because they have never been pregnant or because they suppress lactation after birth. For those women who are feeding an infant, it is not possible to assign them to an intervention or control group as the choice to breastfeed has to be personal. Epidemiological studies can, therefore, only be observational of the different feeding behaviours. Heinig and Dewey (1997) have conducted one of the few rigorous reviews of the health benefits of breastfeeding for women. It provides further evidence of the longer-term public health gains for the adult female population, which can be conferred through breastfeeding and should be seen alongside the evidence on health gains for infants and children.

In their review, Heinig and Dewey use Baucher's (1986) standards for including studies in the review. These are:

- avoidance of detection bias through prospective study design and active surveillance of subjects
- adequate control of confounding variables
- clearly defined outcome events
- clear definition of breastfeeding.

A total of 144 studies, in which at least three out of the above four standards applied, were reviewed. These papers fell into various categories that included recovery from childbirth, maternal postpartum weight loss, metabolism of lipids and glucose, suppression of fertility, cancer risk (breast, ovarian and endometrial), and bone density. The reader is referred to the original review for a full report on the findings, but for the purposes of discussing the public health issues related to breastfeeding this part of the chapter will address those factors that are relevant to the health targets set out by the government.

In *Saving lives* (DH 1999a) the targets proposed by the DH that could be affected by increasing the number of women who breastfeed are:

- To reduce the number of deaths from cancer amongst people aged under 65 by at least a further one-fifth (20%) by 2010 (Baseline 1996).
- To reduce the death rate from heart disease and strokes and related illnesses amongst people under 65 years by at least a further one-third (33%) by 2010 (Baseline 1996, DH 1999a).

Choosing health (DH 2004a) has put a different complexion on these targets, which were proposed in 1999 (but notably had a target date of 2010) because the areas for focusing public health activity in *Choosing health* are smoking, obesity, exercise, alcohol misuse, sexual health and mental health. The emphasis here is on health related behaviours rather than disease prevention *per se* and, therefore, the evidence that supports the policies can be used in a number of different ways. For example, the evidence on obesity and exercise can be used to support targets on cardiovascular health whilst the evidence on sexual health can be used to support targets on teenage pregnancy and sexually transmitted diseases. These are very different populations with complex health needs and health services, and health professionals would need to consider strategies that support diverse needs in order to deliver on these targets.

The promotion of breastfeeding can be seen to be one strategy for improving health based on the PSA of a 2% year on year increase in breastfeeding rates. Breastfeeding could contribute to targets on cancer and heart disease in women, as the evidence from Heinig and Dewey (1997) suggests.

The evidence on cancer and breastfeeding as presented by Heinig and Dewey (1997) does suggest that there may be significant benefits of breastfeeding, which are mainly conferred to premenopausal women and are also dependent on patterns of breastfeeding and duration. In the case of breast cancer, they reviewed 20 studies, all of which were equivocal in their findings that lactation does not *increase* the risk of breast cancer. The studies were mixed in their conclusions about the risk reduction for pre- and postmenopausal women, although most suggest that the cumulative duration of breastfeeding is important, especially beyond 9 months. One study suggested that a lifetime total of 24 months or longer of breastfeeding could reduce the incidence of breast cancer by as much as 25% (Newcombe et al 1994). This study involved more than 14 000 pre- and postmenopausal women. A UK study by Chilvers (1993) suggested that there was a lower risk of breast cancer associated with the number of children breastfed for at least 3 months. Heinig and Dewey are careful to point out that it is difficult to make comparisons between the 20 studies, as factors such as tumour type, patterns of breastfeeding behaviour and menopausal status are not always taken into account. They recommend that further studies should be undertaken which control for these variables. However, the evidence appears to be robust enough for organisations such as UNICEF to use it in their promotional material for the Baby Friendly Initiative (UNICEF 1996).

In relation to ovarian and endometrial cancer, the authors remain somewhat cautious in their conclusions, as the few studies that have been conducted in this area do tend to conflict. In a meta-analysis of 12 case-control studies in the USA it was found that breastfeeding for 6 months or more was associated with reduced risk of ovarian cancer (Whittemore et al 1992). Some studies of ovarian cancer (e.g. Gwinn et al 1990) suggest that it is lactational anovulation that exerts the protective effect against ovarian cancer, as circulating gonadotrophins are reduced and it is these hormones that have been associated with ovarian malignancy. Other studies have shown no relationship between lactation and reduction in ovarian cancer risk (e.g. Cramer et al 1983, Hartge 1989).

Breastfeeding provides a theoretical protection against endometrial cancer as the risk of this cancer is said to increase in response to circulating oestrogens unopposed by progesterone. During lactation, oestrogen is reduced more than is progesterone. However, the evidence for this protective effect is conflicting. One study (Brinton et al 1992) found no difference in risk for endometrial cancer amongst those women who had ever breastfed and those who had never breastfed, whilst a study by Rosenblatt and Thomas (1995) found a significant decreasing trend in risk of endometrial cancer with increasing cumulative duration of breastfeeding. Again, one of the factors that may explain the difference in these findings is the extent to which the researchers define the pattern of breastfeeding. For example, 'ever breastfed' is a very different definition to total length of duration of breastfeeding. Neither study appears to report on exclusive breastfeeders.

To conclude on the effect of breastfeeding in reduction of cancer risk, it would seem that there is no reason *not* to encourage breastfeeding , especially of sustained duration, and that it is likely that there is some protection for premenopausal women against the risk of cancer of the breast and possibly ovaries if they breastfeed.

In relation to coronary heart disease and strokes, the prospective study by Wilson et al 1998 on children at 7 years of age has already been discussed in some detail and shown that breastfeeding for at least 15 weeks does have a potential beneficial effect on blood pressure and body fat in adult life, both of which are risk factors in coronary heart disease and stroke. However, this study is relevant to the breastfed child – does the mother also share any reduction in risk for these diseases? Heinig and Dewey's review reports on one main study that has investigated cholesterol metabolism and lactation and has some implications for heart disease risk. Raised cholesterol and triglyceride serum levels are recognised risk factors in the development of atherosclerosis and atherothrombosis, leading to coronary events such as angina and heart attack. During pregnancy, serum cholesterol levels rise above the prepregnancy levels, but during lactation this is secreted into the milk at a rate similar to that of cholesterol-lowering medication (Kallio et al 1992). It is thought that this is promoted by an enzyme in the mammary gland that is activated by prolactin (Kallio et al 1992). Kallio et al (1992) studied cholesterol metabolism in women who exclusively breastfed their infants for up to 12 months. These researchers found that total cholesterol, low-density lipoproteins and triglycerides declined to levels significantly lower than the prepregnant state during lactation and returned to normal values after lactation ceased. It is hypothesised that repeated periods of lactation may help to reduce atherosclerotic damage over time, thus reducing the overall risk of coronary heart disease. Heinig and Dewey (1997) recommend that more research be done in this area.

In terms of overweight and obesity, there is very little good quality evidence that breastfeeding might be protective for women as well as babies, which in turn might be protective against coronary heart disease and type 2 diabetes. Despite health professionals' advice to women that breastfeeding will help them to regain their prepregnancy weight, studies indicate that breastfeeding might in fact be related to weight gain (Sichieri et al 2003). This finding was based on a prospective assessment of 1538 nulliparous and 2810 primiparous women in 1989, who gave birth to no more than one child between 1990 and 1991. After adjusting for age, physical activity and BMI in 1989, lactation was associated with a weight gain from 1989 to 1993 of approximately 1 kg, comparing women who breastfed with those who did not.

To conclude on women's health in relation to government targets, it seems that there is some evidence to suggest that breastfeeding protects against some cancers and possibly reduces coronary heart disease risk factors. This is valuable evidence in public health terms but does need further confirmation. There is very little evidence of protection for mothers against overweight or obesity.

It is also important to bear in mind that for many women across the world, especially in developing countries, breastfeeding acts as the only way of spacing families because of lactational anovulation. One systematic review (Van der Wijden et al 2003) has found the evidence for this inconclusive but a prospective Australian study (Short 1991) did find sufficiently convincing evidence that so long as breastfeeding women remained amenorrhoeic, breastfeeding could protect against conception for up to 12 months. Spacing of families is known to reduce maternal and infant morbidity and mortality. In the Western world, breastfeeding does not have such a significant contraceptive effect because the pattern of breastfeeding does not sustain the hormone levels required to prevent ovulation. For example, Western mothers reduce night feeding and frequent feeding after the first 2–3 months. In 1988, researchers from around the world met in Italy and stated that: 'Breastfeeding provides 98% protection from pregnancy in the first six months post-partum if the mother is fully or nearly fully breastfeeding and has not experienced vaginal bleeding after the 56th day postpartum. Additional contraception is required in lactating women who are partially breastfeeding, who have started menstruating or have been breastfeeding for more than 6 months' (Kennedy et al 1989). This was an important statement for women whose only access to contraception is through breastfeeding, as long as women are informed of the need to feed often and frequently during the night. For many traditional communities this is the normal pattern of feeding, but aggressive marketing by formula producers has resulted in changes in these patterns with the subsequent loss of the contraceptive effect (Palmer 1993). Maher (1995) comments on communities in West Africa where feeding up to 3 years of age is the cultural norm and that, as a consequence, women bear between six to eight children during their fertile lifetime as opposed to their potential for around 17. This must bring health benefits to both mother and children, as repeated pregnancies and childbirth are in themselves risk factors for maternal and child mortality. The implications for Western women of lactational ammenorhoea have to be viewed cautiously, whilst breastfeeding practice tends to be up to six feeds a day as opposed to 12 or more feeds amongst traditional communities.

When breastfeeding is contraindicated

There are rarely public health reasons when breastfeeding should not be supported and promoted, but the evidence is now sufficient to suggest that women who are HIV positive should be cautious about breastfeeding. WHO 2001 has published the available evidence on transmission of HIV and breastfeeding. This has shown that the risk of an untreated HIV-positive mother transmitting HIV to her unborn baby is 15–25%, breastfeeding increases this by 5–20% giving an overall risk of up to 45%. This can be reduced by the use of anti-retroviral drugs given prophylactically to as little as 2% but trials are still underway. Overall, breastfeeding probably accounts for up to half of HIV-infected babies. Current WHO guidance is that where mothers can be sure of safe, affordable and acceptable, feasible replacements for breast milk, including formula and heated breast milk, then they should avoid breastfeeding. Where safe replacements cannot be ensured, then the advice is to exclusively breastfeed for 3 months and wean gradually. This is based on observation in sub-Saharan Africa that babies exclusively breastfed for the first 3 months carried lower risk of infection than those who were mixed fed, research is still underway to understand more about the mechanism of protection. Research is also underway to establish the mode of transmission and any protective effects against later HIV infection that breastfeeding may offer to children.

This remains a public health dilemma for many countries of the world where HIV is a known risk and the facilities for preparing safe breast milk replacements are restricted. HIV-infected mothers in the UK are advised not to breastfeed and health professionals are provided with guidance on how to discuss risk with women who are known to be HIV positive (DH 2004b).

Women's perspectives on the benefits of breastfeeding

Typically, when women are asked about the benefits of breastfeeding for them, they do not focus on risk factors for disease. It seems that, whilst social scientists grapple for concepts that can adequately describe and explain health as opposed to disease, women are natural 'postmodernists' in their own explanations of health, wellbeing and breastfeeding. For example, Hauck and Reinbold (1996) conducted a study to determine the criteria Western Australian women used to decide whether breastfeeding was successful. A series of 183 telephone interviews was followed by 19 in-depth interviews with 10 unsuccessful and nine successful breastfeeders. Success or failure was a personally defined experience, not necessarily based on conventional notions of duration. The four major categories that emerged from a content analysis of the data were giving, persistence, meeting expectations and accomplishing personal goals. Such criteria are not consistent with medical orthodoxy related to health outcomes, being scientifically immeasurable, but nevertheless are authentic outcomes for the women themselves. Dignam (1995) explored the concept of intimacy with breastfeeding mothers and associated intimacy with reciprocity, mutual joy, harmony, concern for others, trust and closeness. Whilst none of these characteristics could either be measured or defined as conventional outcomes, they, nevertheless, could be conceptually associated with theories on mental health. For example, Antonovsky's (1984) theory of the sense of coherence is interesting in the light of the characteristics women associate with breastfeeding.

Antonovsky (1984, p. 10) defines sense of coherence as:

'...a global orientation that expresses the extent to which one has a pervasive, enduring though dynamic feeling of confidence that one's internal and external environments are predictable and that there is a high probability that things will work out as well as can reasonably be expected.'

When we consider characteristics such as harmony and mutual joy, it becomes feasible that, if Antonovsky's theory that the sense coherence is central to mental wellbeing holds true, then breastfeeding could contribute to mental health in a positive way. This aspect of breastfeeding should be explored in more detail and valued more highly by the more conventional health analysts. Currently, these aspects of breastfeeding remain 'hidden' behind the cloak of qualitative research, which is itself is not highly valued in the medical domain. Of course, a postmodernist would pose the question why is breastfeeding in the medical domain in the first place? This is perhaps the most enduring question in the analysis of public health and breastfeeding, as it becomes more evident that the contrast between the private experience of breastfeeding and the epidemiologically defined public health benefits are quite disparate.

Why don't more women breastfeed?

Despite all the evidence on the positive benefits for health that breastfeeding can confer, it is clear from the UK evidence on incidence and prevalence (Bolling 2006) that whilst about two-thirds of women may breastfeed at birth, this rapidly declines over the first 6 weeks and beyond, and about one-quarter of all babies in the UK never have the opportunity to be nurtured by human milk (Hamlyn et al 2002). The ONS/IC survey identified some of the variables associated with breastfeeding and breastfeeding patterns, these being: age, social class, age of leaving school and region. Whilst it is useful for public health purposes to know that breastfeeding incidence and prevalence decreases among the manual socio-economic groups, it is also important to understand the explanations for the differences in behaviour towards infant feeding found among various social groupings in the UK. It is equally important to acknowledge that, because, statistically, women from one socio-economic group are less likely to breastfeed than women from another, this does not in itself indicate lack of intention or motiv-ation, and may be indicative of cultural or social barriers to breastfeeding, rather than an active decision not to breastfeed.

It would seem that if age, education, class and region are important statistical variables then one explanation underlying these may be culture. Culture here could refer to the infant feeding or social culture within which women exist, or the wider cultural context of the Western medicalised environment in which women are expected to breastfeed. It has been argued in a previous paper

(Kendall 1995) that practitioners should acknowledge and explore cultural norms and expect-ations before exhorting women to breastfeed, it is particularly necessary to appreciate that for some families the notion of healthiness is not a priority and neither is it ascribed to behaviours such as breastfeeding, which may be regarded as unacceptable or even obscene. For example, Gordon (1998) found in her work in Northern Ireland that the partners of breastfeeding mothers were often of the view that only wayward women did that sort of thing, equating breastfeeding with sexual promiscuity. Under this type of cultural pressure within a strongly patriarchal society, a woman must probably respect the wishes of her husband before anything else and would not want her family or husband's family to think she was 'loose'. In contrast, the evidence from the study conducted by the Institute of Education (2005) showing that more women from black and ethnic minority groups are likely to breastfeed than white women would suggest a cultural influence in a positive direction towards breastfeeding that may not yet be fully understood.

Professional discourse on this topic often refers to the 'failure' to breastfeed. For example, Wylie and Verber (1994) report on women's breastfeeding behaviour at 28 days post-partum, commenting that: 'failing to breastfeed this cohort of babies will inevitably mean increased artificial feeding for the next cohort – we only have one chance to get it right' (p. 118) . This implies that women are weak and uncaring and somehow failing in their responsibility to nurture their babies appropriately. Clearly, from the evidence already cited the public health view is that breastfeeding should both be initiated by more women and continued for longer. However, the barriers to breastfeeding may be more societal than individual. Hoddinott and Pill (1999) conducted a qualitative study amongst working-class women in East London and found that the decision to breastfeed was more influenced by 'embodied knowledge' (that is, having first-hand experience of observing friends and relatives breastfeeding) than theoretical knowledge related to health benefits. The implication of this study is that it is important to find ways of exposing more women to positive experiences of breastfeeding than to provide information about how much healthier their babies will be in the future.

A study by Buckell and Thompson (1995) of two contrasting social areas in an outer London borough found that women in the less affluent area had equally strong intentions to breastfeed as women in an area of higher affluence (house ownership, employment, professional occupations) and that initiation of breast-feeding for both groups was even higher than the national average (82.8% and 85.3% respectively). However, women from the less affluent area were less likely to maintain breastfeeding up to the 3 month point. Given high motivation and initiation, it is disappointing from a public health perspective that in the group in which other indicators of poor health (e.g. smoking, depression) are also high, breastfeeding is not continued regularly beyond 3 months. The study suggests that some of the explanations for this may be that they come from a 'bottle feeding culture', although this is not explored in any detail.

In a study of breastfeeding promotion among low-income women (Entwistle et al 2005) it was found that women on low incomes were positive towards breast-feeding, but do not always receive the support they need from health professionals or family, which perhaps contributes to the bottle-feeding culture. Where midwives were provided with an educational intervention based on Successful Steps to Breastfeeding (UNICEF 1998), low-income women were more satisfied with their care, were able to ask for support when they needed it and reported more practical help from the midwives. However, the culture in which the women lived influenced their long-term breastfeeding behaviour; for example, one mother breastfed for 4 days and then gave her baby breast milk via a bottle for a further 2 weeks to give the baby the health benefits, but after that she had to do the school run and saw bottle feeding as an easier option to fit in with her lifestyle needs. This mother lived in a bottle-feeding environment, but she knew that if she gave her baby some breast milk it would improve the child's health outcomes; it was not, however, culturally acceptable for her to breastfeed for longer than the first week.

The way in which we disseminate information about breastfeeding may also be an important factor, since it is apparent that information alone does not significantly change behaviour. Britton (1998) has discussed the ways in which antenatal information influences women's breastfeeding experiences. From a series of qualitative focus groups, with a total of 30 mothers aged between 20 and 39 years, the majority of whom were primigravidae and had breastfed for upwards of 5 days and were continuing at the time of the study (up to 20 weeks), Britton found that there were three main sources of influence antenatally. These were the media construction of breastfeeding, professional influence through antenatal classes and information from other women. The participants commented on how the media construction was often falsely rosy in its perspective and did not portray the realities of night time and the exhaustion associated with a crying baby and sore nipples. Antenatal classes were criticised for putting too much emphasis on labour and the physiological aspects of breastfeeding rather than the emotional and social aspects. Most supportive and relevant to the needs of this group of women was the information they received from other women who had previously breastfed, including other women in the focus groups. This information is supportive of the idea of role modelling and that if health professionals explored women's concepts of successful breastfeeding, rather than the medically determined outcomes, then their 'success' rate at helping women to breastfeed might be improved. Britton concludes that midwives and health visitors should probably do more to facilitate peer learning and peer support for breastfeeding, this is supported by Dennis's (2002) study, which found that women had positive perceptions of peer support and found it beneficial in continuation of breastfeeding.

Community practitioners and the promotion of public health through breastfeeding

The forgoing discussion has raised a dilemma for the community practitioner and midwife: having collated the evidence for health improvement through breast-feeding, how are culturally and socially acceptable methods of promoting the incidence, prevalence and duration of breastfeeding to be achieved? Is breastfeeding a public health issue or is it simply a matter of personal preference? Should breastfeeding be part of healthy public policy, for example, in terms of the workplace, public places, health service policy? There are, embedded in these deliberately rhetorical questions, three levels of public health action to be addressed – the individual/community, the professional sphere and the policy making process.

Each of these will be addressed in terms of the contribution they could make separately and collectively to improving public health through breast-feeding and, also, it will be concluded how a concerted action could facilitate a shift from a bottle-feeding to a breastfeeding culture.

Individual/community

Britton's (1998) study has raised the question of support for breastfeeding women coming primarily from other, experienced breastfeeders rather than through a professionally led route, such as antenatal classes. This is not a novel idea and studies have been conducted to review the effectiveness of mother-to-mother programmes. We argue that if the evidence from a range of qualitative studies on breastfeeding is analysed concurrently, then a theoretical position emerges that proposes that *women gain more support for breastfeeding from other women than they do from health professionals, because other experienced breastfeeders promote the outcomes as defined by women, rather than medically determined outcomes.* These outcomes could be significant for the mental wellbeing of both mother and baby, which have been largely overlooked in the medical literature. For example, Locklin (1995) focused on 17 low-income, culturally diverse women in a qualitative study that involved peer counsellors to support breastfeeding. Through the constant comparative analytic approach, five themes emerged from her data that indicated the empowering effect that this type of support had on the breastfeeding experience. The five themes were: making the discovery, seeking a connection, comforting each other, becoming empowered and telling the world. As suggested in relation to Dignam's (1995) study, these themes are highly suggestive of the sense of coherence Anotnovsky (1984) has described.

In Tarkka and Paunonen's (1996) study of social support to 200 new mothers, they found that the support they received least of in hospital was emotional. Locklin's study would suggest that this could be provided through the peer support system and this would also support Britton's (1998) conclusions. A study in Glasgow was reported by Gribble in 1996. At that time the breastfeeding rate in the Easterhouse district of Glasgow was 12%, one of the lowest in Europe. A 'breastfeeding helper' scheme was set up and organised by midwives as it was understood that the culturally embedded and negative attitudes towards breastfeeding on the estate would be more likely to respond to local women who 'spoke their language' than to health professionals. The six trained helpers involved found that they were able to encourage other women to breastfeed, or to at least give it serious consideration, and that an additional bonus was their own self-esteem and self-confidence increased, enabling them to become spokeswomen on behalf of breastfeeding in the community. The outcomes on breastfeeding rates were unreported, but these qualitative effects of peer support are relevant to public health initiatives.

One of the recent initiatives of the DH in England has been to set up Sure Start initiatives. Specified areas of the country where health indicators such as housing tenure, unemployment, ethnic mix and population trends, high teenage pregnancy rates, morbidity and mortality rates are suggestive of inequalities in health compared with more affluent areas have been identified. The Sure Start areas provide the opportunity for primary health care organisations to work in partnership with other agencies to support children and parents to improve health and social outcomes. One of the aims of Sure Start Plus was to improve the health of young mothers and their children through the promotion of breastfeeding. However, the national evaluation of Sure Start Plus (Wiggins et al 2004) describes the difficulties in identifying improvements in breastfeeding through the Sure Start work. This was explained by a lack of breastfeeding data in many local areas, difficulty for Sure Start workers in making breastfeeding a priority and a persistent culture of formula feeding, even when young mothers intended to breastfeed. The evaluators conclude that it might be more beneficial to focus on aspects of Sure Start that increase young women's emotional wellbeing and self-esteem, and that, in turn, might enable them to be supportive of breastfeeding in the longer term. This finding makes theoretical sense when considered in the light of Antonovsky's work, discussed above, and should be subjected to more prospective evaluation.

Professional sphere

The professional scope for contributing to public health through the promotion of breastfeeding focuses on the way in which professional groups can be trained to improve their support of breastfeeding families and the effectiveness of professional advice and support (NICE 2005). It has already been noted that

Britton (1998) implies that the women in her study found that the information received in antenatal classes was over medicalised and did little to prepare them for the experience of breastfeeding.

It is not unusual to find examples of women in the literature who give up breastfeeding either because professional support was indifferent or because advice was conflicting from different professional groups. Approaches to assess the level of professional attitude, knowledge and skill in relation to breastfeeding have been reported, as well as studies on effectiveness of professional advice and training initiatives. One of the methodological problems for all of these studies is the difficulty in demonstrating long-term changes in breastfeeding rates, partly because randomised controlled trials are ethically difficult to design and also because long-term observational studies, like the Wilson et al (1998) study discussed above, are very costly to run.

The most recent evidence on what works in the promotion of breastfeeding, particularly in relation to disadvantaged women, is the report of the systematic review published by the National Institute for Health and Clinical Excellence in 2005. The review included 80 eligible studies, only 17 of which reported the needs of women from disadvantaged groups. Ten of these were conducted in the UK. The review provides evidence from studies that supports the need for skilled breastfeeding support from professionals or peers as well as a range of other factors, such as professional training, unrestricted feeding after birth, unrestricted skin-to-skin contact after birth, positioning and attachment education and *tailored* antenatal education. Overall, the review concludes that to enable women to breastfeed the following changes are needed:

'Co-ordination of national with local policy so that department (of health) policy is funded, enabled and monitored at the level of, for example, PCTs, Sure Starts and acute trusts, with a two way flow of information to enable both a bottom-up and top-down approach

Ongoing monitoring of rates of variation in infant feeding, with agreed definitions and timing of follow-up, combined with socio-demographic data.'
(NICE 2005, p. 3)

This review is highly relevant to the approach that might be taken to promoting breastfeeding through professional support – it is important not only to ensure that professionals have an evidence-based knowledge about breastfeeding, but it also it draws on the peer-support concept in the context of professional support, as it would seem that the likelihood of giving confident and appropriate advice is enhanced if the professional has a positive approach to breastfeeding and is able to draw upon those client-determined outcomes referred to earlier, such as mutual joy and closeness, as well as medically defined outcomes. In this respect, the professional and the individual spheres become intertwined as the professional comes to understand support for breastfeeding within the cultural and social context of women's lives. However, as the NICE review indicates in its conclusions, this will only be effective if the practice is 'joined up' with national policy and all key stakeholders are supportive of this.

Public health and breastfeeding policy

The orthodox approaches to public health rely heavily on an individualist model of public health in which women are assigned a responsibility to do what is best for their infants. They retain a taint of the victim blaming culture of the pre-1980s, when women who did not breastfeed were said to bring their problems on themselves and their babies. The new public health (Ashton & Seymour 1990) argued for a more structuralist approach in which policies addressing the complexities of culture, social variation, multi-agency involvement and consumer involvement were developed. There is evidence that such policies have emerged in the UK: Sure Start is an initiative that is responsive to structural issues related to inequality in health as well as to conceptual issues around health promotion and health improvement, such as consumer involvement. Healthy public policy integrates concepts of health, environment, economics, social milieu and work so that people can expect to be as safe and well as possible in all aspects of their lives. In England, the Acheson report (DH 1999b) reported on inequalities in health and highlighted the need to improve the health of women and children through nutrition. It particularly referred to much of the evidence cited here on the benefits of breastfeeding:

'We recommend policies which increase the prevalence of breastfeeding.'

(p. 71, para 22.1)

The integration of public policy to meet this recommendation is vital, and the full and proper evaluation of initiatives such as Sure Start is central to the future success and survival of such policy. So whilst it is a significant achievement that the importance of breastfeeding has been recognised through the PSA target of 2% per year increase in breastfeeding, the structural and cultural issues that affect women's decisions to breastfeed need to be addressed through healthy public policy that is supportive of women and children in their communities.

In England and other countries in the UK, public policy has started to emerge that is supportive of breastfeeding and directs health professionals to promote breastfeeding. However, this is often seen in isolation of a more global approach to public health. For example, the European Commission report on the *Protection, promotion and support of breastfeeding in Europe* (EC 2004) provides a blue print for action across Europe in support of breastfeeding and public health. The cross-cutting document calls for actions that have been initiated in the UK, such as training of health professionals and the setting and monitoring of targets. But it also calls for more controversial action such as the development of the International Code on the Marketing of Breast Milk Substitutes (WHO 1981) and its implementation across Europe in such a way as to make it a legal requirement not to contravene the Code. This is an action that, for most governments, is fraught with economic sensitivity in relation to the manufacture and marketing of baby milks and the industries that profit from formula feeds and related products. The UK charity Baby Milk Action (http://www.babymilkaction.org) monitors the behaviour of the companies to observe to what extent the Code is violated, every month there are new reports of companies unethically promoting their products across the world. This year (2006) is the 25th anniversary of the formulation of the Code by the WHO, but unless European countries develop a policy framework that supports the Code there will be a significant gap in the public health jigsaw.

Other interesting policy initiatives have emerged, although, as with other matters discussed, most are under-evaluated in the traditional sense. For example, women around the world have been campaigning for the right to breastfeed in public places and at work. In Scotland, the Scottish Parliament has been instrumental in developing strategies to change the culture of breastfeeding and has invested resources to support converting policy into practice; for example, television campaigns and a Breastfeeding Bill making it an offence to prevent any woman from breastfeeding in a public place.

At the beginning of this chapter, we referred to how, historically, women have been driven into working away from the home and to the inherent difficulties of maintaining breastfeeding in an environment that may be male dominated, lacks childcare facilities and is suffused with negative attitudes towards breastfeeding. In 1993, a campaign in Australia tried to address some of these problems by introducing the 'Mother-friendly workplace initiative', in association with world breastfeeding week (World Alliance for Breastfeeding Action, 1993). This was predicated on the Innocenti Declaration referred to on p. 233.

The Declaration calls on all governments by 1995 to 'enact imaginative legislation protecting the breastfeeding rights of working women'. The Australian initiative can be seen as an example of healthy public policy in the making because of the way in which it integrates the physical and emotional health benefits to infants and mothers with employment, environmental and economic benefits. For example, it was argued in the document that breastfeeding women are less likely to be absent from work as their children are healthier and the morale of the women is better as they feel more able to meet their family responsibilities. This, the argument continues, leads to higher productivity. Breastfeeding is environmentally friendly, leading to only biodegradable waste, and, as more women breastfeed at work this would probably have the effect of the workplace becoming a cleaner and safer place for everyone to work in. Economically, as more women breastfeed, there would be savings on the health service budget.

The initiative also provides a strategy for employers to provide a workplace environment that supports breastfeeding women. The strategy is built on three tenets: time, space/proximity and support. Time refers to paid maternity leave as well as time out at work to breastfeed, including flexible working hours. Space and proximity refers to childcare facilities that are based on or near the workplace, comfortable and private facilities for breastfeeding or expressing, and a clean work environment that is safe from hazardous waste or chemicals. Support should be in terms of ensuring women are aware of their maternity rights, full job secur-ity, ensuring a positive attitude towards breastfeeding at work and encouraging women to establish their own support networks. Considering the positive benefits this strategy could bring to the work environment, it is interesting to reflect on the extent to which employers in the UK have adopted it. The World Alliance for Breastfeeding Action website (http://www.waba.org.my) provides interesting comparative data on national strategies and polices that might be enabling for women to combine breastfeeding with employment. Interestingly, the UK compares well with the USA, but not so well with developing countries, such as Vietnam and Venezuela, which both provide longer maternity leave and 100% maternity pay. Both these countries have also been proportionally more successful than the UK or USA in establishing Baby Friendly Hospitals.

In 1996, Britten reported on workplace initiatives that have developed in the UK largely as result of individual pressure rather than integrated policy. She explores a number of case studies within the context of Health and Safety legislation (Health and Safety Executive 1994), which gives some guidance to employers on the rights of expectant and new mothers at work but, Britten argues, is a long way from the 'imaginative legislation' agreed in the Innocenti Declaration. Nevertheless, the case studies do provide examples of the way in which employers could address some of the issues inherent in the 'Healthy Workplace' initiative that was proposed by the DH (1998), although this is not prominent in the subsequent *Choosing health* (DH 2004a). For example, one employer negotiated with Liz that her return to work could be on a flexible basis while she was breastfeeding, she was allowed time out to express milk and storage arrangements were available in the staff kitchen. Morag had to negotiate with her personnel department to provide expressing facilities, which were eventually found in the occupational health department. She had an informal agreement to take time out to express. Davina's return to work was more difficult. Her request to take time out to breastfeed her 4-month-old baby was turned down by a committee. Davina had to make arrangements to leave her son with her mother and then to take a 25-minute walk there during her break to feed him. It was Davina's health visitor who lobbied the committee on her behalf and eventually the decision was overturned by a minority vote. This case study provides a good example of the way in which practitioners can support and raise awareness of policy within the existing legislative framework. The three case studies described go some way towards meeting the strategic objectives of the 1993 Australian initiative: time, space/proximity and support. However, it is clear that there is still a great deal more to be done in relation to the workplace and the development of healthy public policy.

Conclusions

This chapter has taken the theme of breastfeeding and public health as its focus. The underlying thesis of the discussion has been the way in which the orthodox discourse on public health interacts with a 'postmodern' agenda of health improvement. Breastfeeding represents an aspect of public health that impacts on traditional public health issues such as morbidity and mortality, but also raises questions about public perceptions of health and health outcomes.

There is ample evidence that breastfeeding is an effective way of reducing the risk of disease among infants and mothers. There is evidence that breastfeeding can contribute to significant public health improvements, such as childhood obesity and cancer risk in women. But there should be caution in relation to breastfeeding where the woman is HIV positive. A small percentage of that evidence has been discussed here. The IC (Bolling 2006) data that demonstrate an increasing trend in breastfeeding are encouraging, but the continuing variations in breastfeeding across regions and social class and income remain a concern. There are still many women in the UK who choose either not to breastfeed or give up in the very early weeks, despite all the health benefits it can bring. However, synthesis of trends within the evidence would seem to suggest that recognition of client determined outcomes might be one way of addressing the reluctance to breastfeed among some groups of women. This can possibly be achieved through drawing on the recent public health strategy (DH 2004a) to develop new ways of enabling women to breastfeed. This should include using mother-to-mother support programmes, introducing practitioner training programmes that challenge beliefs and attitudes as well as improving knowledge and by development of healthy public policy such as employment conditions, which enable women to continue to breastfeed.

The primary care organisations will need to provide evidence of effective interventions that enable 2% increases in breastfeeding year on year. This will need to be achieved within an organisational framework for assessing local health need, developing approaches that contribute towards health improvement and, integral to this, quality improvement techniques such as teamwork and clinical audit, which will monitor and evaluate the effectiveness of interventions. Community practitioners, especially health visitors and midwives, must ensure that they are making a constructive and well-argued contribution to the needs of breastfeeding women in their population, so that the public health benefits can be realised at all levels. However, any public health policy has to be integrated sufficiently to enable individuals, practitioners, employers and health care providers to be able to implement the policy and realise the health benefits that breastfeeding can bring. Integration should be the key to establishing a warm chain for breastfeeding.

DISCUSSION QUESTIONS

- Do women in the 21st century have a choice about breastfeeding?
- How would you advise a woman who was undecided about breastfeeding?
- What are the issues facing women from low income/low socio-economic groups in relation to breastfeeding?

- What are the issues in society which we need to address to improve breastfeeding rates?
- Do health professionals have a public health responsibility to promote breastfeeding?

References

Akobeng A, Ramanan A, Buchan I, Heller R 2006 Effect of breast feeding on risk of coeliac disease: a systematic review and meta-analysis of observational studies. Archives of Disease in Childhood 9 1: 39–43

Antonovsky A 1984 The sense of coherence as a determinant of health. Advances 1: 37–50

Ashton J, Seymour H 1990 The new public health. Open University Press, Buckingham, UK

Baby Milk Action 2006 Citing WHO, http://www.babymilkaction.org. Baby Milk Action, Cambridge

Bauchner H, Leventhal J, Shapiro E 1986 Studies of breastfeeding and infections: How good is the evidence? Journal of American Medical Association 256: 887–892

Bolling K 2006 Infant Feeding Survey 2006 – Early Results. NSO, London

Brinton L, Berman M, Mortel R et al 1992 reproductive, menstrual and medical risk factors for endometrial cancer: results from case control study. American Journal of Obstetrics and Gynaecology 167: 1317–1325

Britten J 1996 Employers and breastfeeding. New Generation, March 1996, 26–27

Britton C 1998 The influence of ante-natal information on breastfeeding experiences. British Journal of Midwifery 6(5): 312–315

Buckell M, Thompson R 1995 A comparative breastfeeding study in two contrasting areas. Health Visitor 68(2): 63–65

Chilvers C 1993 Breastfeeding and risk of breast cancer in young women. British Medical Journal 307: 17–20

Cochrane Collaboration 2006 Cochrane Handbook of Systematic Reviews of Interventions Cochrane Collaborations, Oxford

Cramer D, Hutchinson G, Welch W, Scully R, Ryan K 1983 Determinants of ovarian cancer risk. Journal of the National Cancer Institute 71: 711–716

Dennis C, Hodnett E, Gallop R, Chalmers B 2002 The effect of peer support on breastfeeding duration among primiparous women: a randomized controlled trial. Canadian Medical Association Journal 166(1): 21–28

Department for Education and Skills 2004 National healthy schools programme: briefing for directors of public health. Health Development Agency, London

Department of Health (DH) 1998 Our healthier nation. HMSO, London

Department of Health (DH) 1999a Saving Lives: Our Healthier Nation. HMSO, London

Department of Health (DH) 1999b Independent inquiry into inequalities in health, chair Sir Donald Acheson. HMSO, London

Department of Health (DH) 2004a Choosing health. HMSO, London

Department of Health (DH) 2004b HIV and infant feeding: guidance from the UK Chief Medical Officers' Expert Advisory Group on AIDS. DH, London

Department of Health/NHS 2005 Delivering Healthy Start, a guide for professionals. DH, London

Department of Health/Treasury 2002 Tackling inequalities in health: a cross cutting review. HMSO, London

Dex S, Joshi H 2005 Children of the 21st century: from birth to nine months. Policy Press, London

Dignam D 1995 Understanding intimacy as experienced by breastfeeding women. Health Care for Women International 16(5): 477–485

Entwistle F 2005 An evaluation of the effect of training on midwives' ability to promote breastfeeding among low income women. MSc by Research Thesis. University of Hertfordshire

European Commission 2004 Protection, promotion and support of breastfeeding in Europe: a blueprint for action. European Commission, Luxembourg

Gillman MW, Rifas-Shiman SL, Camargo CA et al 2001 Risk of overweight among adolescents who are breastfed as infants. Journal of the American Medical Association 285: 2461–2467

Gordon M 1998 Empowerment and breastfeeding. In: Kendall S (ed.) Health and empowerment: research and practice. Arnold, London

Gribble J 1996 An alternative approach. New Generation, March 1996, 12–13

Gwinn M, Lee N, Rhodes P, Layde P, Rubin G 1990 Pregnancy, breastfeeding and oral contraceptives and the risk of epithelial ovarian cancer. Journal of Clinical Epidemiology 43: 559–568

Hamlyn B, Brooker S, Oleinikova K, Wands S 2002 Infant feeding 2000. ONS, London

Hartge P, Schiffman M, Hoover R, McGowan L, Lesher L, Norris H 1989 A case-control study of epithelial ovarian cancer. American Journal of Obstetrics and Gynaecology 161: 10–16

Hauck Y, Reinbold J 1996 Criteria for successful breastfeeding: mother's perceptions. Journal of the Australian College of Midwives 9(1): 21–27

Health and Social Care Information Centre (HSCIC) 2005 Health survey for England. HSCIC, London

Health and Safety Executive 1994 New and expectant mothers at work – a guide for employers. HS(G) 122. HMSO, London

Hediger ML, Overpeck MD, Kuczmarski RI, Ruan WJ 2001 Association between infant breastfeeding and overweight in young children. Journal of the American Medical Association 285: 2453–2460

Heinig M, Dewey K 1997 Health effects of breastfeeding for mothers: a critical review. Nutrition Research Review 10: 35–56

Hoddinott P, Pill R 1999 Qualitative study of decisions about infant feeding among women in the East End of London. British Medical Journal 318: 30–34

Howie P, Forsyth J, Ogston S, Clark A, du Florey C 1990 Protective effect of breastfeeding against infection. British Medical Journal 300: 11–16

Kallio M, Simes M, Perheentupa J, Salmenpera L, Miettinen T 1992 Serum cholesterol and lipoprotein concentrations in mothers during and after prolonged exclusive lactation. Metabolism 41: 1327–1330

Kendall S 1995 Cross cultural aspects and breastfeeding promotion. Health Visitor 68(11): 450–451

Kennedy K, Rivera R, NcNeilly A 1989 Consensus statement on the use of breastfeeding as a family planning method. Contraception 39: 477–496

Kolezko S, Sherman P, Corey M et al 1989 Role of infant feeding practices in development of Crohn's disease in childhood. British Medical Journal 298: 1617–1618

Lancet 1994 A warm chain for breastfeeding. Lancet 344: 1239–1241

Locklin M 1995 Telling the world: low income women and their breastfeeding experiences. Journal of Human Lactation 11(4): 285–291

Maher V (ed.) 1992 The anthropology of breastfeeding. Berg, Oxford

Metcalf M, Baum J 1992 Family characteristics and insulin dependent diabetes. Archives of Disease in Childhood 67(6): 731–736

National Institute for Health and Clinical Excellence (NICE) 2005 The effectiveness of public health interventions to promote the duration of breastfeeding. NICE, London

Newcombe P, Storer B, Longnecker M et al 1994 Lactation and a reduced risk of premenopausal breast cancer. New England Journal of Medicine 330: 81–87

Palmer G 1993 The politics of breastfeeding. Pandora Press, London

Rosenblatt K, Thomas D 1995 Prolonged lactation and endometrial cancer. WHO collaborative study of neoplasia and steroid contraceptives. International Journal of Epidemiology 24: 499–503

Savage F 1992 Breastfeeding – SIDS. Midirs Midwifery Digest 2(1): 3–5

Short R, Lewis P, Renfree M, Shaw G 1991 Contraceptive effects of extended lactational amenorrhoea: beyond the Bellagio Concensus. Lancet 337(8751): 1232–1233

Sichieri R, Field A, Rich-Edwards J, Willett W 2003 Prospective assessment of exclusive breastfeeding in relation to weight change in women. International Journal of Obesity 27(7): 815–820

Tarkka M, Paunonen M 1996 Social support provided by nurses to recent mothers on a maternity ward. Journal of Advanced Nursing 23(6): 1202–1206

Toschke AM, Vignerova J, Lhotska L, Osancova K, Koletzko B, von Kries R 2002 Overweight and obesity in 6- to 14-year-old Czech children in 1991: protective effect of breast-feeding. Journal of Pediatrics 141: 764–769

UNICEF 1996 The Baby Friendly Initiative. UK Committee for UNICEF, London

UNICEF 1998 Implementing the Ten Steps to Successful Breastfeeding. UNICEF London

Van der Wijden C, Kleijnen J, Van der Berk T 2003 Lactational amenorrhoea for family planning. Cochrane database systematic review, 4, CD001329

256

Weimer J 2001 The economic benefits of breastfeeding. Food review. Washington DC, US Department of Agriculture

Whittemore AS, Harris R, Intyre J, Halpern J 1992 Characteristics Relating to Ovarian Cancer Risk. Am J of Epidemiology 136(10): 1175–1183

Wiggins MH 2004, Austerberry M, Rosato M, Sawtell S 2003 Sure Start Plus National Evaluation Service Delivery Study: interim findings. Social Science Research Unit, Institute of Education, London

Wilson A, Forsyth J, Greene S, Irvine L, Hau C, Howie P 1998 Relation of infant diet to childhood health: seven year follow up of cohort of children in Dundee infant feeding study. British Medical Journal 316: 21–25

World Alliance for Breastfeeding Action (WABA) 1993 Women, work and breastfeeding. WABA, Penang

World Health Organization (WHO) 1981 International Code on the Marketing of Breast Milk Substitutes. WHO, Geneva

World Health Organization (WHO) 2002 The optimal duration of exclusive breastfeeding: a systematic review. WHO, Geneva

World Health Organization (WHO) 2001 Breastfeeding and replacement feeding practices in the context of mother-to-child transmission of HIV. WHO, Geneva

Wylie J, Verber I 1994 Why women fail to breastfeed: a prospective study from booking to 28 days post-partum. Journal of Human Nutrition and Dietetics 7: 115–111

Further reading

Heinig M, Dewey K 1997 Health effects of breastfeeding for mothers: a critical review. Nutrition Research Review 10: 35–56

This review brings together much of the research into breastfeeding that has findings that support the health of women. The research is wide-ranging and critically analysed, providing a clear view both of the evidence available and of the strength of this evidence. The authors have also published a second review on the health effects of breastfeeding for infants.

Hoddinott P, Pill R 1999 Qualitative study of decisions about infant feeding among women in the East End of London. British Medical Journal 318: 30–34

This paper provides an interesting insight into women's decisions about breastfeeding. It is of particular relevance as the study was conducted in an inner city area. It is also a good example of how qualitative research can demonstrate sound evidence through a systematic approach.

Maher V (ed.) 1992 The anthropology of breastfeeding. Berg, Oxford

This text draws on the experience and expertise of a collection of anthropologists who have studied breastfeeding in various cultures. It not only provides rich descriptions of cultural variation and practice, but enables the reader to think critically about the ways in which we approach breastfeeding in the UK context.

NICE 2005 The effectiveness of public health interventions to promote the duration of breastfeeding. NICE, London

This systematic review provides evidence from 80 eligible research papers reporting interventions that enable women to continue breastfeeding with special reference to women from disadvantaged groups. Of the 80 studies reviewed, only 17 examined the needs of women from disadvantaged groups, of these only 10 were conducted in the UK. The review concludes with a series of changes that need to take place to enable women to breastfeed for longer that involves policy, professionals, organisations, employers and families.

Palmer G 1993 The politics of breastfeeding. Pandora Press, London

This text details much of the historical context of breastfeeding. It also provides a critical and important insight into the politics that have disabled women from breastfeeding globally and show this affects health, the environment and global economy.

Safeguarding children:
a public health imperative

Jane Appleton and Jill Clemerson-Trew

Key issues

- Refocus of current policy to safeguarding and promoting children's welfare
- Safeguarding children incorporates all aspects of work with vulnerable children, children in need and children who are suffering, or at risk of suffering significant harm
- Adopting a public health approach ensures that potentially vulnerable children can be identified early and receive the support and services that they and their families need to maximise the health and wellbeing of the child and potentially to prevent child maltreatment

Introduction

All children and young people have a right to be safeguarded and their welfare promoted. In its broadest sense 'safeguarding' encompasses a wide spectrum of activity including the prevention of impairment of children's health and development, the maximisation of children's potential through stimulation, play and education, protection from disease via immunisation, prevention of harm from accidents, through to protection from child abuse and maltreatment. The terms 'safeguarding', 'vulnerable children', 'child(ren) in need' and 'child protection' will be used throughout the chapter as these reflect terms used in current practice and encompass most elements of the recently adopted, broad concept of safeguarding children. Identification of child welfare needs, through services that are developed from sound public health principles, is of paramount importance for the wellbeing of all children in our society. Themes will be developed through the chapter to illustrate the public health basis of safeguarding work and its significance to health inequalities and childhood outcomes. These themes will be examined within the context of current policy developments and contemporary community public health practice.

Policy and the discourse pertaining to child welfare have altered over the last two decades (see in particular Parton 2006). The concept of 'protecting children' became a central focus in the 1980s and early 1990s, bringing with it a shift in emphasis to one of protection, from the narrower historical one traditionally associated with child abuse. 'Child protection was not only concerned with protecting children from danger but also protecting the privacy of the family from unwarrantable state interventions' (Parton 2006, p. 36) with an emphasis on State agencies increasingly working in partnership with parents/carers. That central focus on child protection, which was felt by many to be too narrow, has now been superseded by another subtle shift, reflecting changes in law and policy to that of safeguarding and promoting the welfare of children and young people. This new focus on safeguarding reflects a much broader focus and, as well as protection, encompasses prevention and an emphasis on all children's safety, not just those in need and suffering, or at risk of harm.

Safeguarding children and public health

Public health interventions are principally societal and not focused solely on the individual. In safeguarding work, adopting a public health approach ensures that potentially vulnerable children can be identified at an early stage and receive the services and support that they and their families need to maximise the health and wellbeing of the child and potentially to prevent child maltreatment. A wealth of recent policy as part of the Every Child Matters: Change for Children programme (DfES 2004) has reiterated the need for children's interests to be viewed as paramount in our society. Internationally, a failure to safeguard children leads to significant public health problems and long-term individual suffering. Prevention needs to focus at all levels along a continuum of need.

World view

The World Health Organization (WHO) has emphasised that investment in children's health should include the prevention of abuse (WHO 2002). Child abuse does not discriminate against sex, age, social class, community or country, which is illustrated by the international interest in this area and the existence of organisations such as the International Society for the Prevention of Child Abuse and Neglect (ISPCAN). This international society was founded in 1977 with the aim of 'prevent[ing] cruelty to children in every nation, in every form: physical abuse, sexual abuse, neglect, street children, child fatalities, child prostitution, children of war, emotional abuse and child labor. ISPCAN is committed to increasing public awareness of all forms of violence against children, developing activities to prevent such violence, and promoting the rights of children in all regions of the world' (ISPCAN 2006, p. 1).

International organisations promoting children's welfare and supported by world governments, such as UNICEF and the World Health Organization, accept that child protection issues can and do occur in all cultures and countries across the globe and across all social groups (WHO 2002). A number of initiatives emphasise children's rights, such as the adoption in many countries of the United Nations Convention of the Rights of the Child (UN 1989), which was ratified by the UK government in December 1991. This policy document has led to the increasing development of child-friendly and child-focused policies at a national level in many countries. Progress towards implementing the UN Convention varies from some countries where children are viewed as an integral part of society to the other extreme, where children are left to live on the streets or are exploited in war, as slave labour and through child prostitution.

The Wave Trust (Worldwide Alternatives to ViolencE) is an international charity dedicated to raising 'public awareness of the root causes of violence, and the means to prevent and reduce violence in our society' (Hosking & Walsh 2005, p. 4). The organisation was established in 1996. WAVE is particularly concerned with 'reducing child abuse and neglect because these are the major root sources of teenage and adult violence; they underlie much emotional suffering in adults who may never be violent; and violence and abuse are entirely preventable through implementing known, economically viable, and effective programmes to break the cycle of violence' (Hosking & Walsh 2005, p. 4).

Childhood outcomes

Perhaps the most important reason for taking a public health approach to safeguarding children is the impact of unidentified or unresolved children in need or child abuse issues on the individual and society. There is a growing body of evidence which links the failure to address the needs of children to a negative outcome in terms of their social and emotional development and their ability to form positive social relationships (see for example Macdonald 2001). Furthermore, evidence from neurobiological studies is increasingly illustrating that brain development is associated with the quality of the emotional support and environment in which an infant is nurtured (Hosking & Walsh 2005, Lowenhoff 2004, Shonkoff & Phillips 2000). In particular, these studies are providing evidence of the deleterious effects on brain function due to maltreatment and an increase in stress hormones in childhood (Bremner et al 2003, Glaser 2000, Hosking & Walsh 2005, Teicher 2002).

The relationship between problems in child rearing, such as harsh family discipline and 'consequent childhood behaviour problems, later delinquency and criminality' is well recognised in the literature (Buchannan 1996, Farrington 1995, p. 100, Hosking & Walsh 2005). Farrington (1995) and Silverman et al (1996) highlight the possible long-term mental health and behavioural problems associated with childhood physical abuse or neglect.

Research evidence suggests that there may be a correlation between adult mental health problems, a history of past abuse, and subsequent ability to parent successfully and positively rear children (Gibbons et al 1995). Child abuse can result in poor self-esteem or an inability to make social relationships. As a worst-case scenario this may lead to childhood delinquency, offending behaviour, substance misuse and later delinquency, violence and imprisonment. Bifulco and Moran (1998) illustrated through in-depth interviews with over 800 women, that childhood abuse and neglect can increase the probability of women suffering depression in adulthood. Their research evidence also demonstrates how such negative childhood experiences can result in low self-esteem for women and abusive relationships in their adult life. This supports the findings of Mullen et al (1996), who studied the long-term impact of childhood physical, emotional and sexual abuse in a group of women and found that a history of any form of abuse was associated with increased risk of mental health problems, interpersonal problems and sexual difficulties. Lang et al (2006) also report an association between maternal childhood maltreatment and increased depression, anxiety and illicit drug use during pregnancy and the early postnatal period.

A study by Glaser and Prior (1997) indicated links between parental attributes and outcomes for children's emotional health. These parental attributes were mental illness, domestic violence and alcohol or drug misuse, which appeared to impair parenting and affect children's emotional and social development. These researchers raised questions about the appropriateness of professionals' early responses to concerns about children's emotional health. Rather than immediately using formal child protection procedures in the investigation and assessment of suspected emotional abuse, they suggest using alternative strategies, where a multi-disciplinary approach is taken and preventative work with the child and family in the form of planned interventions undertaken over a time-limited period.

> 'This process does, however, depend on the parents' recognition of the concerns about the child, and their willingness to become involved and work with professionals towards change.'
>
> (Glaser & Prior 1997, p. 27)

Messages from research (Department of Health (DH)/Dartington Social Research Unit 1995) described the long-term ill-effect for children of living in a low-warmth/high-criticism environment as far more damaging than a single incident of over-chastisement. Roberts (1996) and Hagell (1998) have also reported the negative impact of children growing up in such low-warmth/high-criticism environments. Roberts (1996) describes how absence of family support interventions during childhood may result in high levels of aggression and risk-taking behaviour in adulthood. Reder and Duncan (1999) suggest that a further effect of childhood distress can be seen in family life-cycles, particularly at times of transition, such as birth, death or loss of a job. Unresolved child in need or child protection issues can affect adults, so their ability to adjust to changes may be prolonged, or result in psychological symptoms or relationship struggles.

Domestic violence is increasingly recognised as having a damaging effect on childhood outcomes (Department of Health 2006, Osofsky 2003, Smith Stover 2005) and, in particular, children's emotional and behavioural development (Edleson 1999). The Department of Health (2002a, p. 16) estimated that 'nearly three-quarters of children [on the child protection register] live in households where domestic violence occurs'. The risks to children are increased when domestic violence occurs alongside parental mental illness, or drug and alcohol abuse (Cleaver et al 1999). Violent childhood experiences have also been linked with intimate partner violence in later adulthood relationships (Coid et al 2001, Whitfield et al 2003).

While the Wave Trust has highlighted the significant economic costs of rising violence in the UK (Hosking & Walsh 2005), it is important to highlight that, in spite of adversity or adverse backgrounds, people can and do rise above past abuse, poverty, loss and relationship difficulties to become mature and balanced individuals (Bifulco & Moran 1998, Heller et al 1999). As yet, though, there is little understanding of the factors that make some children more resilient to maltreatment than others (Macdonald 2001).

Safeguarding children: policy

Key definitions

'Safeguarding children' is a relatively new term; at its simplest, safeguarding is about 'keeping children safe from harm, such as illness, abuse or injury' (Children's Rights Director 2004, p. 3). The term was initially referred to in The Children Act (1989) introduced on 14th October 1991, when a duty was placed on local authorities 'to safeguard and promote the welfare' of children in need (Section 17). This focus was further examined by Sir William Utting in his report *People like us – a review of the care system for children living away from home*, where he described the terms 'safeguard' and 'promote' as 'equal partners in an overall concept of welfare. Safeguards are an indispensable component to the child's security, and should be the first consideration for any body providing or arranging accommodation for children. Safeguards form the basis for ensuring physical and emotional health, good education and sound social development' (Utting 1997, p. 15).

This broadening of focus was reiterated in the *Framework for the assessment of children in need and their families consultation draft* (DH 1999, p. 3), which identified that safeguarding has two dimensions: 'a duty to safeguard children from maltreatment' and 'a duty to prevent impairment'. This assessment framework supported the shift in policy focus from the identification of abuse and significant harm to one that adopted a broader view of children's needs and wellbeing and identified impairment in the context of a child's developmental needs and his/her current and long-term health and wellbeing (Cleaver et al 2004, DH et al 2000b, Gray 2002, Parton 2006).

Despite the Children Act (2004) placing a new duty, in Section 11, on all the key agencies who work with children 'to safeguard and promote the[ir] welfare' (p. 9), and the term 'safeguarding' being used in the titles of several influential child welfare policy documents, such as *Working together to safeguard children* (DH/ Home Office/Department of Education and Employment 1999), *Safeguarding children involved in prostitution* (DH et al 2000a), and Core Standard 5 in the National Service Framework for Children, Young People and Maternity Services (DH & DfES 2004), the term was not defined in government guidance until 2005. Instead, the definition commonly in use in the literature was that offered in the first joint Chief Inspectors' *Report on arrangements to safeguard children* (DH 2002b) and retained in the second Safeguarding Children report published in July 2005 (CSCI 2005).

These reports stated that safeguarding involves:

- 'All agencies working with children, young people and their families take all reasonable measures to ensure that the risks of harm to children's welfare are minimised; and
- Where there are concerns about children and young people's welfare, all agencies take all appropriate actions to address those concerns, working to agreed local policies and procedures in full partnership with other local agencies.'

(CSCI 2005, p. 3)

In 2005, 'safeguarding and promoting the welfare of children' was defined for the first time in statutory guidance on making arrangements to safeguard and promote the welfare of children under section 11 of the Children Act 2004 (HM Government 2005a) and the draft consultation document of *Working together to safeguard children* (HM Government 2005b) guidance as:

- 'protecting children from maltreatment;
- preventing impairment of children's health or development; and
- ensuring that they are growing up in circumstances consistent with the provision of safe and effective care;
- and undertaking that role so as to enable those children to have optimum life chances and to enter adulthood successfully.'

(HM Government 2005b, p. 18)

This definition was maintained when the final document was published in April 2006.

Working together to safeguard children (HM Government 2006a) stresses that these aspects of safeguarding a child's welfare are cumulative, reinforcing their important contribution to the five outcomes identified in *Every child matters* (DfES 2003). These are legally recognised as the components of wellbeing in the Children Act (2004, Section 10(2), pp. 7–8) and the purpose for co-operation between agencies:

- physical and mental health and emotional wellbeing
- protection from harm and neglect
- education, training and recreation
- the contribution made by them to society
- social and economic wellbeing.

Defining child abuse and neglect

Defining child abuse is difficult (DH/Dartington Social Research Unit 1995) and there are many alternatives. The relative nature of the concept is accentuated in Gil's (1975, p. 346) definition:

'Any act of commission or omission by individuals, institutions or society as a whole, and any conditions resulting from such acts or inaction, which deprive children of equal rights and liberties, and/or interfere with their optimal development, constitute by definition abusive or neglectful acts or conditions.'

This broad yet complex definition also emphasises society's responsibilities and children's rights, which are central features of the current safeguarding agenda. In 1999, the World Health Organization's *Consultation on child abuse prevention* drafted the following definition of child abuse:

'Child abuse or maltreatment constitutes all forms of physical and/or emotional ill-treatment, sexual abuse, neglect or negligent treatment or commercial or other exploitation, resulting in actual or potential harm to the child's health, survival, development or dignity in the context of a relationship of responsibility, trust or power.'

The *Working together to safeguard children* (HM Government 2006a, p. xxvii) guidance describes abuse and neglect as 'forms of maltreatment of a child' and outlines the four main categories as: physical abuse, emotional abuse, sexual abuse and neglect.

The WHO has recently illustrated in a typology of violence that child abuse occurs within the broad category of interpersonal violence, which is divided into two subcategories (WHO 2002). Family and intimate partner violence includes child abuse, elderly abuse and intimate partner violence; 'it occurs largely between family members and intimate partners, usually, though not exclusively, taking place in the home.' Community violence occurs 'between individuals who are unrelated, and who may or may not know each other' (WHO 2002, p. 6). This includes youth violence, rape or sexual assault by strangers, and whilst it generally takes place outside the home, it may arise in institutional settings, such as schools, workplaces, nursing homes and prisons. Although family violence is both more prevalent and potentially more damaging than community interpersonal violence, the latter is more frequently the focus of media attention.

Categories of need

The new *Working together to safeguard children* (HM Government 2006a, p. 73) guidance talks about 'working with children about whom there are child welfare concerns' and stresses the need for interagency working as soon as concerns arise about a child's welfare. During an initial assessment of a child referred to the local authority, the local authority children's social care team should determine:

- Is this a child in need? (Section 17 of the Children Act 1989)
- Is there reasonable cause to suspect that this child is suffering, or is likely to suffer, significant harm? (Section 47 of the Children Act 1989).'

(HM Government 2006a, Section 5(43), p. 85)

Over the last 10 years, children in need have been frequently described within the wider population of vulnerable children. 'Vulnerable children are those disadvantaged children who would benefit from extra help from public agencies in order to make the best of their life chances' (DH 1999, p. 4). Terminology is often used interchangeably and in some policy guidance, such as the *Lead professional good practice guidance* (DfES 2005a) and *Common assessment framework (CAF) documentation* (HM Government 2006b, 2006c) vulnerable children and children in need are referred to as 'children with additional needs' or 'complex needs'. However, the Children Act (1989) defined child protection in terms of 'children in need' and 'significant harm'.

A child will be in need (Part III, Section 17(10)) if his/her vulnerability is such that:

'…he is unlikely to achieve or maintain, or have the opportunity of achieving or maintaining a reasonable standard of health or development without the provision for him of services by the local authority'

'…his health or development is likely to be significantly impaired, or further impaired without the provision of such services,'

or

'…he is disabled'.

'The critical factors to be taken into account in deciding whether a child is in need under the Children Act 1989 are what will happen to a child's health or development without services being provided, and the likely effect the services will have on the child's standard of health and development.'

(HM Government 2006a, Section 1(22), p. 5)

When an initial child protection conference is convened:

'… the conference should consider the following question when determining whether the child should be the subject of a child protection plan:

Is the child at continuing risk of significant harm?

The test should be that either:

- the child can be shown to have suffered ill-treatment or impairment of health or development as a result of physical, emotional, or sexual abuse or neglect, and professional judgement is that further ill-treatment or impairment are likely; *or*
- professional judgement, substantiated by the findings of enquiries in this individual case or by research evidence, is that the child is likely to suffer ill-treatment or the impairment of health or development as a result of physical, emotional, or sexual abuse or neglect.'

(HM Government 2006a, Section 5(102–103), p. 101)

Over the last two decades, various theories and models have been debated in an attempt to understand the causal factors involved in child abuse; the 'integrated' model is now widely accepted. This theoretical model takes an eclectic viewpoint by combining the individual, social, environmental and interactive models and supports the view that child abuse and neglect is multi-factorial; it also recognises the potential complexity of family life. This model has been described by Browne (2002) and encompasses four elements that mitigate for or against the child's present situation. These include:

1. The range of differing relationships and potential disputes between caregivers, which may impact on the children.
2. The relationships with and between the children, including the size and spacing of the family, attachments to and expectations of the child(ren).

3. Stress caused by the child, for example, a child who is not wanted, one who is difficult to discipline, demanding or temperamental, or a child who is often ill or has physical or learning disabilities.
4. Structural stress. Environmental and sociological stresses, such as housing issues, social isolation, unemployment, and 'threats to the care-giver's authority, values and self-esteem' (Browne 2002, p. 58).

'Significant harm' is the threshold beyond which 'children in need' are also regarded as 'children in need of protection' and child protection procedures are instigated. A child is in need of protection where there is likely or actual 'significant harm' to him/her or he/she is at risk. However, the Children Act 1989 does not give a definitive interpretation of the concept of 'significant harm'. Furthermore *Working together to safeguard children* recognises that 'there are no absolute criteria on which to rely when judging what constitutes significant harm.' It states:

> 'Sometimes a single traumatic event may constitute significant harm, e.g. a violent assault, suffocation or poisoning. More often, significant harm is a compilation of significant events, both acute and longstanding which interrupt, change or damage the child's physical and psychological development.'

(HM Government 2006a, Section 1(25), p. 6)

It also draws attention to existing research on sources of stress for children and families that may have an adverse effect on a child's health, development, and wellbeing, which should be taken into account when assessing children and families needs. These sources of stress include social exclusion, domestic violence, mental illness of a parent or carer, parental learning disability and drug and alcohol misuse (HM Government 2006a, Section 9(11–25), pp. 158–162).

Policy focus: understanding the definitions

From the definitions outlined above, a broad picture of safeguarding emerges, which encompasses not only protection but a broader, more positive emphasis on prevention and ensuring children's safety. Furthermore, the new *Working together to safeguard children* (HM Government 2006a) guidance describes child protection as 'a part of safeguarding and promoting welfare' (HM Government 2006a, p. 5) and states that it refers specifically to the activity undertaken to protect any child who is at risk of, or is suffering, significant harm. The document maintains that 'effective child protection is essential as part of wider work to safeguard and promote the welfare of children' (HM Government 2006a, p. 5).

The term 'safeguarding children' is, therefore, an umbrella term (or spectrum) incorporating all aspects of work with vulnerable children, children in need and children who are suffering, or at risk of significant harm.

Since the mid-1990s there has been a change of focus for much of the work that in the late 1980s and early 1990s would have been considered to be child protection work. Since the publication of *Messages from research* (DH/Dartington Social Research Unit 1995) and the subsequent 're-focusing debate' it has been widely accepted that child protection must be viewed as a broad concept, which includes all elements of 'children in need' and 'significant harm'. This is further substantiated by the recent policy move to focus on safeguarding children. Safeguarding also includes the need for early interventions to proactively identify children and their families who need professional input and support.

Local Safeguarding Children Boards are largely in agreement that initial responses to referrals should be seen as being about child welfare concerns. Following an initial assessment, this may indicate that a child is a 'child in need' as defined by Section 17 of the Children Act 1989, while the child protection focus (where it is suspected that a child is suffering or is likely to suffer significant harm) is retained for the more serious or chronic cases (DH/Dartington Social Research Unit 1995, HM Government 2006a, Thorpe & Bilson 1998).

This reframing of the issues in current policy to safeguarding and promoting children's welfare (DH et al 1999) was further supported by the introduction of a new approach to assessment (Parton 2006). In recognition of the fact that there was no standardised approach to the assessment of children in need, the Department of Health produced a consultation document in 1999 aimed at clarifying such processes (DH 1999). *The framework for the assessment of children in need and their families* (DH et al 2000b) was developed as part of the Quality Protects Programme and introduced as a structured model for assessing children in need. It was produced primarily for social work practitioners; however, the assessment framework has been widely adopted as a framework for assessing all children and their families, across not only social care but health and education agencies. The assessment framework offers a core foundation and interagency model for a systematic approach to assessing children and families' needs, emphasising the importance of safeguarding and promoting children's welfare. It acknowledges the importance of combining evidence-based practice and professional judgement and incorporates three key areas:

1. The child's developmental needs.
2. The capacity of parents or caregivers to respond appropriately to those needs.
3. The impact of wider family and environmental factors on parenting capacity and the child (DH et al 2000b).

The assessment framework supported the shift in policy focus from one that centred on the identification of abuse to an assessment that focuses on the whole child and impairment in terms of his/her developmental needs, current and long-term health and wellbeing. Most recently the Common Assessment Framework for Children and Young People (CAF) developed from the underlying model of *The framework for the assessment of children in need and their families* (DH et al 2000b) has been launched by the Department for Education and Skills (DfES) to assist practitioners in all agencies in making assessments of children with additional needs. The DfES website states that the CAF 'has been developed for practitioners in all agencies so that they can communicate and work together more effectively. It is particularly suitable for use in universal services, to tackle problems before they become serious. It helps practitioners identify the issues facing a child or young person who may have additional needs, in order to take appropriate action to provide them with the right kind of support.' A number of local authorities piloted the CAF and the lead professional role in 2005–6. The CAF is discussed further in Chapter 1. It was rolled out across the UK in 2006, with social care taking the lead; however, it remains to be seen how agencies who have already integrated the assessment framework in their local procedures and assessment documentation take forward the CAF in practice.

Impact on public health: statistics

Burden of disease

The World Health Organization usually describes the global burden of disease in two ways; first through the numbers of deaths from the leading causes of disease and injury and, second, in terms of disability adjusted life years (DALYs) (Peden et al. 2002). One disability adjusted life year is defined as one lost year of healthy life, due either to premature death or disability. Interpersonal violence is the third most common cause of death from injuries amongst 15- to 44-year-olds world wide and the ninth most common cause of burden of disease for all ages. In the UK, injuries account for 3% of annual deaths, being ranked the 14th leading cause of death in 2004, for all ages. Most injury deaths result from unintentional incidents, particulary amongst children and young adults. However, just 76% of fatal injuries to 1- to 4-year-olds, to 83% to 5- to 14-year-olds and 59% to 15- to 24-year-olds are classified as 'unintentional' (Jones & Parry 2005), raising questions of intentionality for a substantial number.

The DALY is a very broad-brush approach to measuring the extent of harm to individual and public health, as it cannot pick up the extent of lost life chances or of mental and emotional harm from a childhood spent in adverse conditions. It does not, either, identify the extent to which inequalities in health, known to stem from early childhood, are mediated through negative patterns of parenting and behaviour towards children in their earliest years. However, one advantage of the DALY, combined with the WHO typology of violence, is that it helps to illustrate the importance of safeguarding children in traditional public health terms. There is a need for more systematic collection and analysis of data about harm to children within their families, to bring this topic more firmly into the public health arena.

Gathering the data

Since 1988 the Department of Health has collated child protection statistics, on an annual basis, on the numbers of children registered on local authority child protection registers, and those subsequently de-registered in England. Prior to this time no national statistics were maintained (Corby 1990). The most recently available statistics demonstrate that the protection of children is a significant public health issue affecting many children in society.

> 'At 31 March 2005 there were 25,900 children and young people on child protection registers in England, 1% fewer than a year earlier. This represents a rate of 23 children per 10,000 in the population aged under 18.'
> (National Statistics & DfES 2006a, p. 10)

These statistics are based on the responses from all local authorities with children's social care services responsibilities. However, caution needs to be maintained when interpreting these statistics as they are not a record of all child abuse (DH 1997a). A recent NSPCC report *Child maltreatment in the family: the experience of a national sample of young people* (Cawson 2002) estimates that 16% of children experienced serious maltreatment by their parents. Corby (1990, p. 305) has stated that child protection statistics reflect 'the tip of the iceberg', as 'they do not show the true extent of violence and ill-treatment towards children in our society'. The statistics 'refer only to abuse which is officially recognised' (Corby 1990, p. 305). Furthermore, the 1999 *Working together* guidance 'raised the threshold for registration by changing the criteria' from having suffered or was likely to suffer significant harm 'to continuing risk of harm' and the requirement to have a child protection plan put in place (National Statistics & DfES 2006a, p. 10).

Another example of the extent of serious injury and death to children is the number of serious case reviews (previously known as Part 8 Reviews or Chapter 8 Reviews) carried out by Local Safeguarding Children Boards (LSCBs), formerly Area Child Protection Committees (ACPCs). Such reviews are conducted 'when a child dies (including death by suicide), and abuse or neglect is known or suspected to be a factor in the child's death' (HM Government 2006a, p. 143). Serious case reviews examine the involvement of agencies and professionals with the child and family to 'establish, whether there are lessons to be learned from the case about the ways in which local professionals and organisations work together to safeguard and promote the welfare of children' (HM Government 2006a, p. 142). However, there are currently no readily available data on the number of serious case reviews that are completed across the country, although recent estimates by the Department of Health suggest that there are about 90 child deaths each year that are the subject of a serious case review (Sinclair & Bullock 2002), while the NSPCC (2000) reports that there may be as many as 100–200 case reviews in the UK each year involving the death or serious injury of a child as a result of abuse or neglect.

The collation of more accurate data may be more likely in future, with the requirement outlined in the new *Working together* (HM Government 2006a) guidance that LSCBs should provide a copy of the overview report, action plan and individual management reports for each serious case review to the CSCI and DfES. This information would then need to be 'systematically collated on a national basis' (NSPCC 2000, p. 8). It is also planned that national overview reports will be commissioned by the DfES every 2 years. In addition, LSCBs are now required to establish child death review panels to collect and analyse information on the deaths of any children (under 18 years) resident in the LSCB area; this function of the LSCB will become compulsory on 1 April 2008.

Reder and Duncan (1999, p. 22–23), commenting on an earlier study of 'Part 8' notification statistics provided by the Department of Health, reported that out of 120 child deaths for the year ending March 1995, '54 were the result of non-accidental injuries', or required further investigation. These researchers also describe the inherent difficulties in estimating child abuse fatalities because of, 'problems of definition, recognition, misdiagnosis and data collection' (Reder & Duncan 1999, p. 2). They put forward three arguments for why 'Part 8' reviews do not provide an accurate indicator of non-accidental injury. Reder and Duncan (1999, pp. 22–23) state: 'Child abuse is not a precise diagnosis and parameters for concluding whether maltreatment caused or contributed to a death are ambiguous. It is possible that pathologists and coroners are cautious about recording a death as being the result of non-accidental injuries. Second, criteria for setting up the reviews leave room for flexibility and local circumstances may lead one (LSCB) to review a particular case, which, if it occurred elsewhere, would not be considered necessary. Third, the quality of the information available may not allow a reviewer to form an opinion as to the likely contribution of maltreatment to the child's death.'

In 1999, new guidance on serious case reviews was issued in *Working together to safeguard children* (DH et al 1999); 'It altered the focus from compliance with procedures to lessons for collaboration and remedial action locally' (Sinclair & Bullock 2002, p. 60). Yet in their more recent review of serious case reviews, Sinclair and Bullock (2002) highlighted marked variation in the way that these reviews are carried out and pointed to the difficulties in ensuring that evidence from such cases was used to its best potential to inform local and national practice.

Obtaining accurate details about child homicide figures in the UK is also extremely difficult. The central problem seems to be that accurate figures are not currently recorded for all fatal child abuse. Indeed, the National Society for the Prevention of Cruelty to Children, in what is described as 'a very conservative estimate' of child homicide, suggests that each week at least one–two children die following abuse and neglect (NSPCC 2000). This organisation is continuing to push for more accurate and reliable official figures. The NSPCC is currently compiling a factfile of the various official government statistics relating to children and child protection into a single publication, which it intends to update on an annual basis to review child protection trends. As the NSPCC (2000, p. 8) point out, as well as 'a lack of clear statistical data on child deaths … there is a real difficulty in determining the cause of death because of the legal difficulty of proof of homicide; the loss or lack of identification of a child's body; misdiag-nosed "sudden infant death syndrome"; and problems where maltreatment is not the immediate cause of death and the child is diagnosed as dying of "natural causes", including accidents, even though maltreatment has occurred'. Wilczynski (1994) and Creighton (1995, 2000) also maintain that the official homicide statistics grossly underestimate the actual incidence of fatal child abuse.

Since February 2000, data have also been collected from local authorities on children in need, through the Children in Need (CiN) census, which is 'a biennial census of all children receiving a service from a social services department during the nominated census week' (National Statistics & DfES 2006a, p. 6). This census has been undertaken on four occasions and child-related social services activity is classified into three areas of work: (1) intake and referral, (2) initial assessment work, and (3) ongoing work (but not children having core assessments or entering the child protection system) (National Statistics & DfES 2006a). In February 2005 it was calculated that there were 385 300 children in need in England. At 31 March 2005, 'out of a total of 552,000 referrals to social services departments, 121,800 (22%) were repeat referrals that had previously been made within the last year' (National Statistics & DfES 2006a, p. 5).

The statistics for children looked after by local authorities also provide an indicator of the numbers of children in need. Children looked after include: '(i) children who are accommodated under a voluntary agreement with their parents, (ii) children who are the subject of a care order and (iii) children who are compulsorily accommodated. This includes children on remand and those subject to short-term emergency orders or the protection of the child' (DH 1997b, p. 9). In England on 31 March 2005, it was estimated that 60 900 children were being looked after by local authorities, with 3000 of these on child protection registers (National Statistics & DfES 2006a, 2006b).

Table 11.1 illustrates the numbers of children looked after by local authorities since March 1995 and demonstrates the increasing numbers of looked-after children; there has been with only a slight fall in 2006. Parents may, while recognising the needs of their children and themselves, agree to the use of support by a foster family to augment their parenting ability and/or energies. Indeed, at 31 March 2005, 18 800 (31%) children accommodated by local authorities were placed, with the agreement of their parents, under Section 20 of the Children Act 1989 (National Statistics & DfES 2006b). Such placements may be time-limited to cover a period of family or parental stress.

Clearly, the above statistics do not offer a complete picture of the numbers of children in need, however, they do go some way towards demonstrating that safeguarding children is a significant public health issue affecting the child population. Furthermore, the Wave Trust (Hosking & Walsh 2005, p. 91) also draws attention to the many public inquiries following child abuse deaths '24 in the 1970s, 25 in the 1980s, and 22 in the 1990s' with 'no visible reduction in levels of child abuse', as such public inquiries tend to address 'the symptoms of child abuse, not its root causes'.

Safeguarding and promoting the welfare of children

Safeguarding children – the continuum of need

Over the last decade the concept of the 'child in need' has been conceptualised as a continuum. This viewpoint emerged from publication of *Messages from research* (DH/Dartington Social Research Unit 1995), leading to the 'refocusing debate'. Professionals related to this viewpoint, which centred around the need to identify areas in which more multi-agency work could be undertaken preventatively with

Table 11.1 ● Children Looked after by local authorities at 31 March in England by gender and age (numbers and rate per 10000 children under 18 years)[1,2]

Age at 31 March	1995[3]	1996[3]	1997[3]	1998[4]	1999[4]	2000[4]	2001[4]	2002[4]	2003[4]	2004[3]	2005[3]
All Children[1]	49 900	50 800	51 500	53 300	55 500	58 100	58 900	59 700	60 800	61 100	60 900
Rates per 10 000	45	46	46	48	49	52	53	54	55	55	55
Male	26 800	27 600	28 200	29 200	30 200	31 900	32 600	33 200	33 600	33 900	33 700
Under 1	830	890	900	940	1100	1200	1200	1200	1300	1400	1400
1–4	3600	3900	4300	4600	4900	5100	4900	5000	4900	4700	4600
5–9	5700	6000	6100	6500	6800	7100	7200	7300	7200	7100	6700
10–15	11 800	12 000	12 200	12 400	12 700	13 500	14 100	14 500	14 800	14 900	14 900
16 and over	4800	4800	4700	4800	4700	5100	5200	5200	5400	5800	6100
Female	23 200	23 200	23 300	24 200	25 300	26 200	26 300	26 500	27 200	27 200	27 200
Under 1	770	750	830	870	1100	1000	1100	1100	1300	1200	1400
1–4	3200	3400	3800	4200	4400	4500	4400	4300	4300	4200	4100
5–9	4600	4800	4900	5300	5900	6200	6100	6100	6000	5600	5500
10–15	10 000	9800	9500	9600	9800	10 400	10 600	10 800	11 300	11 600	11 600
16 and over	4600	4500	4300	4200	4100	4000	4100	4200	4200	4500	4700

(Source: Adapted from Table A. National Statistics and DfES 2006b)

1 Figures exclude children looked after under an agreed series of short-term placements

2 Historical data may differ from older publications. This is mainly due to the implementation of amendments and corrections sent by some local authorities after the publication date of previous materials

3 Figures are taken from the SSDA903 return

4 Figures are taken from the CLA100 return

5 Rounding and suppression: To ensure that no individual child can be identified from statistical tables we have used the following conventions throughout this publication – national figures have been rounded to the nearest 100 if they exceed 1000 and to the nearest 10 otherwise.

(Crown copyright material is produced with the permission of the Controller of her Majesty's Stationery Office).

'children in need', rather than waiting until children are 'in need of protection'. This is further supported by the broadening policy emphasis on safeguarding children. *Messages from research* also highlighted the dilemmas in practice between working preventatively with children in need of services as opposed to children in need of protection. The research evidence presented in this document suggested that the focus on child protection investigation does not result in support to children and families in many cases. It highlighted that in practice there are good systems in place for the assessment and inquiry into child protection concerns. Yet research has demonstrated that much time and energy from social workers is put into this aspect of practice, rather than intervening and working preventatively at an early stage to prevent a higher level of family breakdown (Gibbons et al 1995, Thorpe & Bilson 1998).

However, Parton (2006, p. 82) has argued that with the arrival of New Labour 'the government was keen to broaden the "refocusing initiative" beyond simply rebalancing family support and child protection, to embrace concerns about parenting, early intervention, supporting the family and regenerating the community more generally.' Yet in the case of Victoria Climbié there appeared to be a total breakdown of effective children in need/child welfare work. This point was highlighted by Lord Laming in the inquiry report:

> '…it is not possible to separate the protection of children from wider support to families. Indeed, often the best protection for a child is achieved by the timely intervention of family support services. The wholly unsatisfactory practice, demonstrated so often in this Inquiry of determining the needs of a child before an assessment has been completed, reinforces me in the belief that "referrals" should not be labelled "child protection" without good reason. The needs of the child and his or her family are often inseparable.'
>
> (DH/Home Office 2003, Section 1.30)

Lord Laming also criticised the use of eligibility criteria to restrict access to services and resources. He stressed the importance of undertaking a thorough professional assessment, before making a judgement about determining the suitability of a referral, degree of risk to the child and the urgency of response required (DH/Home Office 2003, Section 1.53). Indeed, Parton (2006, p. 115) draws attention to how the inquiry report strongly argued that it was because Victoria's 'case was defined as a "child in need", as opposed to a "child protection" case [that it] was taken less seriously as a result' and was 'a major factor contributing to her tragic death'.

Working together to safeguard children (HM Government 2006a) emphasises the need for 'initial' and 'core' assessments, to consider the welfare needs of children. These assessments are the response to a referral whether or not significant harm is likely to have occurred or to continue. This guidance encourages local authority children's social care staff to make assessments with other agencies to prevent further breakdown of the child's situation.

Figure 11.1 illustrates the 'continuum of need' and the range of family-centred interventions and targeted support that public health specialists/workers might undertake with families. In the UK, 'children in need' identification is addressed through public health values and concepts, principally universal access to professionals through the Child Health Promotion Programme (Department of Health & DfES 2004, Hall & Elliman 2003), which includes the whole population and ensures targeted follow-up of children and their families who do not initially take up the service. Individual work with a child and family would only take place once a health or development need has been identified, and this individual focus is not reached unless the whole population has access to child health promotion review services.

271

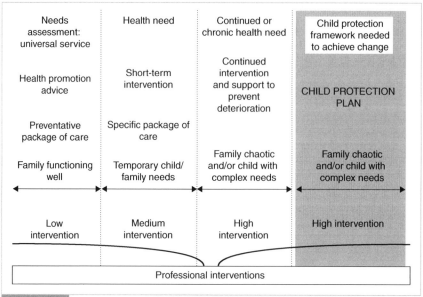

Needs assessment: universal service	Health need	Continued or chronic health need	Child protection framework needed to achieve change
Health promotion advice	Short-term intervention	Continued intervention and support to prevent deterioration	CHILD PROTECTION PLAN
Preventative package of care	Specific package of care		
Family functioning well	Temporary child/ family needs	Family chaotic and/or child with complex needs	Family chaotic and/or child with complex needs
Low intervention	Medium intervention	High intervention	High intervention

Professional interventions

Figure 11.1 ● Safeguarding children – the continuum of need (from Appleton & Clemerson 1999)

At one end of the continuum (low professional intervention, or early intervention) a parent might seek professional guidance or reassurance which would constitute the beginning of base-line preventative work. For example, a mother seeking advice on a feeding difficulty may lead to the professional suggesting ways of managing a difficulty and supporting a change in parenting pattern, or referring a child in need and their family for specialist assessment and input. Further along the continuum, at the medium intervention level, programmes promoting the development of parenting skills may be offered through children's centres or Sure Start projects. Still further along, day or respite care for children might be offered and the provision of services for 'looked-after children' (Children Act 1989, Part III, Section 22(1), p. 17). At the other end of the continuum, the high level of intervention will include children who are at continuing risk of significant harm and are the subject of a formal child protection plan, and the minority of cases that culminate in court proceedings (HM Government 2006a). It is important to recognise that multi-disciplinary and multi-agency assessment and care planning could occur at any point along the continuum, reinforced recently through the implementation of the *Framework for the assessment of children in need and their families* (DH et al 2000b) and the CAF (HM Government 2006b, 2006c).

In safeguarding children work, this shift from child abuse to concepts on a continuum is analogous to the 'individual vs community discussion' in public health.

Population-based safeguarding work

The structural and organisational efforts of society and communities to support positive outcomes for children, and provide advice and guidance for parents/carers, must be based on whole-population approaches as reinforced by the Every Child Matters: Change for Children programme (DfES 2004) and the National Service Framework for Children, Young People and Maternity Services (DH & DfES 2004). Such collective approaches are required, at least initially, to ensure those vulnerable children who are in need (and their families) are reached and offered services. These approaches to service provision fit closely with the expanding public health agenda proposed in *Choosing health* (DH 2004a), the Wanless report (DH 2004b), *National standards, local action* (DH 2004c) and *Our health care, our say* (HM Government/DH 2006). Government policy is increasingly recognising the importance of supporting children and their families, while emphasising the need for professionals and their organisations, families, local communities and the voluntary sector to work more closely together to improve outcomes for children and young people, and the health outcomes of society as a whole (HM Government 2005a, DfES 2005b).

There are additional key themes in safeguarding children and public health working to identify child welfare issues and those children who are in need of protection. These include partnership with both children and their parents and between professionals and their agencies to ensure the needs of these children are met (DH et al 1999, HM Government 2005a, 2006a). It is generally recognised that improved outcomes are more likely to be achieved if the child or young person is focused on as a whole, if services are child centred and if people work together (DH & DfES 2004, HM Government 2005e). 'Team working and partnership is an essential prerequisite to effective public health work' (Royal College of Nursing 1994, p. 1). This theme of partnership is of central importance in recent government policy documents, which continually emphasise the need for effective interagency strategies and professionals to work openly together and with children, young people and their families (HM Government 2005a, 2006a). There is an increasing emphasis on integrated service planning and delivery to provide needs-based services relevant to the local community, for example, through the Children and Young People's Plan (CYPP) (HM Government 2005d).

Joint assessment is another central feature of public health working and research evidence indicates that interagency collaboration during the assessment process of a child referred to local authority social care departments has improved since the implementation of the National Assessment Framework (Cleaver et al 2004) and may continue to lead to improvements in joint working as the CAF is rolled out. This is important in the area of safeguarding work where analysis of serious case review evidence continues to provide evidence of poor assessments and recording, inadequate information sharing amongst professionals and a lack of interagency working (Sinclair & Bullock 2002). In England, it is also planned that ContactPoint (previously know as the Information Sharing (IS) Index) will enable practitioners working with children to find and contact each other easily and to share information when children need services and support (DfES 2006).

A further theme is that of 'equity of access', which is a cornerstone of public health work and supported by the professions who provide universal services for children and their families (Burke 1998). Similarly, the concept of the 'organised efforts of society' Acheson (1988) is reflected in two ways. First, there is a reliance on the community to identify children and families in need of professional support. Government policy following the murder of school girls Holly Wells and Jessica Chapman in Soham in 2003 emphasised that safeguarding children is everybody's business (DfES/DH 2005). Second, collective societal efforts/action are also reflected in the systems set up by individual agencies and through integrated services to ensure children are growing, developing and being educated appropriately.

Child Health Promotion Programme

The Child Health Promotion Programme, implemented primarily through the work of primary care providers (PCPs) but also offered in other settings, such as children's centres, early years provision and extended schools, ensures that some regular contacts are offered by members of the primary health care team to families with young children (although, arguably, this 'regular contact' is becoming increasingly limited). This programme provides the gateway to health needs assessment and increased levels of preventative intervention by public health workers (Appleton & Clemerson 1999). It covers:

- the assessment of the child's and family's needs (including physical, emotional social and environmental health needs)
- childhood screening and targeted developmental review
- immunisations
- health promotion
- early interventions to address identified needs
- safeguarding children from harm (DfES & DH 2004).

The Child Health Promotion Programme should enable professionals to reach all children and identify those who, with their families, are potentially in need of advice, support and guidance, including those children who are potentially vulnerable to significant harm.

Figure 11.2 illustrates a public health framework for safeguarding and promoting the welfare of children in local communities. It highlights the variety of services available to children and their families, ranging from universal services to those specifically for vulnerable children, 'children in need' and 'children in need of protection'. Interagency working is extremely important to ensure the effectiveness of these services as public health practitioners increasingly work across professional and organisational boundaries (DH 2004d, HM Government 2005a). It is this universal contact with all children in our communities that ensures equity of access to Child Health Promotion Programme services. Thus, a broad picture of safeguarding emerges, which encompasses a spectrum ranging from protection from abuse, to protection from disease (immunisation), protection from harm (accidents in the roads and home) through to maximising children's

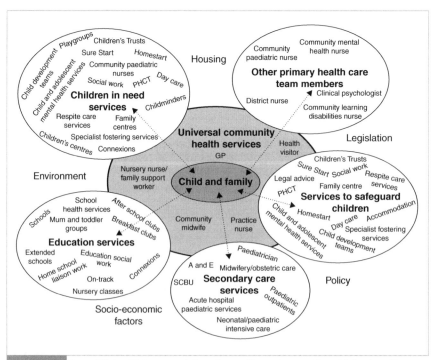

Figure 11.2 ● The public health framework for safeguarding and promoting children's welfare

welfare and development. It should encourage supported, responsible parenting leading to children reaching their maximum potential socially, emotionally and educationally.

Individual and organisational responsibilities

Section 11 of the Children Act 2004 emphasised that 'safeguarding children is everyone's responsibility' (HM Government 2005a, p. 9) and placed a statutory duty on key agencies to safeguard and promote the welfare of children. Practitioners implementing the Child Health Promotion Programme and having contact with children, young people and their parents, are potentially in a unique position to identify families experiencing stress (Appleton 1996). It is important to stress that all public health practitioners working with children, and their families, have a potentially important public health role in the identification of vulnerable children and 'children at risk of significant harm'. Safeguarding children is everyone's responsibility and all staff working with children and young people must be trained and aware of the signs of child maltreatment. *Every child matters* (DfES 2003) recommended that all people working with children, young people and their families should have a common core of skills and knowledge. As a result, and in recognition of the increasingly multi-disciplinary workforce, the DfES has published a document outlining the common core of skills and knowledge for the children's workforce (HM Government 2005c). One of the six areas of expertise outlined is the required knowledge and skills to practice at a basic level in safeguarding and promoting the welfare of children (HM Government 2005c).

National standards, local action (DH 2004c, p. 28) set out in Core Standard C2 the responsibilities of health care organisations in safeguarding work. This standard states that 'Health care organisations protect children by following national child protection guidance within their own activities and in their dealings with other organisations.' Standard 5 in the National Service Framework for Children, Young People and Maternity Services (DH & DfES 2004) outlines eight markers of good practice in how to achieve this. All organisations providing children's services must ensure that they have clear policies and procedures for employees about how to safeguard and promote the welfare of children (HM Government 2006a). In addition, many specialist community public health nurses will have access to practice guidelines and protocols, as well as focused training, and child protection supervision, which will aid in the identification of children and families who may be experiencing stress or vulnerability. They will also be supported by named and designated child protection professionals.

Working together to safeguard children (HM Government 2006a) has detailed the role expected of all health professionals who work with children and families in terms of safeguarding and promoting the welfare of children (see Box 11.1). It is expected that staff will adhere to the Department of Health (2003) guidance *What to do if you're worried a child is being abused*, Local Safeguarding Children's Board (LSCB) procedures and *Responding to domestic abuse: a handbook for health professionals* (DH 2006). Furthermore, public health practitioners should be using the *Framework for the assessment of children in need and their families* (DH et al 2000b, p. 3) for assessing children in need and their families. Indeed, many PCTs have adapted their health records to incorporate this framework and are planning implementation of the CAF locally to avoid duplication and repeated assessments of children and families. It is also likely that some public health practitioners will take on the 'lead professional role' with some children and young people who have significant or complex needs, to avoid overlap of and reduce inconsistency of services (DfES 2005a).

Box 11.1

Working together to safeguard children (2006) Section 2(34)

'All health professionals who work with children and families should be able to:

- Understand the risk factors and recognise children in need of support and/or safeguarding
- Recognise the needs of parents who may need extra help in bringing up their children, and know where to refer for help
- Recognise the risks of abuse to an unborn child
- Contribute to enquiries from other professionals about a child and their family or carers
- Liaise closely with other agencies, including other health professionals
- Assess the needs of children and the capacity of parents/carers to meet their children's needs including the needs of children who display sexually harmful behaviours
- Plan and respond to the needs of children and their families, particularly those who are vulnerable
- Contribute to child protection conferences, family group conferences and strategy discussions
- Contribute to planning support for children at risk of significant harm, e.g. children living in households with domestic violence, parental substance misuse
- Help ensure that children who have been abused and parents under stress (e.g. who have mental health problems) have access to services to support them
- Play an active part, through the child protection plan, in safeguarding children from significant harm
- As part of generally safeguarding children and young people provide ongoing promotional and preventative support through proactive work with children, families and expectant parents
- Contribute to serious case reviews and their implementation'

(Source: HM Government 2006 Working together to safeguard children – a guide to inter-agency working to safeguard and promote the welfare of children. DfES, London, Section 2(34): p. 17–18).

High professional intervention – targeted support and integrated working

High intervention cases will involve working jointly with another agency or agencies or another section of the health service. A key feature of this level of working is that the professional who identifies the need for this level of intervention will remain proactively engaged with the family. This will include ongoing work and the assessment/monitoring of progress with the other agencies or professional groups who are involved. It is not a case of referring the family and being able to withdraw after a short period of support. Indeed, in many situations, if services are adequately resourced public health professionals such as health visitors and school nurses are in an ideal position to take on the lead professional role, co-ordinating support for children and their families.

Box 11.2 offers a case history example of high intervention work. In this case history, if the family refuses to co-operate or just continues to avoid contacts and appointments, then the agencies would need to discuss whether the children are suffering or at risk of significant harm, and whether a Section 47 enquiry and child protection procedures were needed. Work with families

Box 11.2

Case history

The family has three children aged 5-and-a-half, 3 and 15 months, and the mother is 6 months pregnant. Mother's first partner left when she was pregnant with her second child and she met her present partner soon after the birth of that baby. Both the mother and her partner have stormy relationships with their families and spent periods in care as children when their parents were going through difficult times. The 5-year-old is not in school regularly, is difficult to manage in class, has a poor concentration span and appears to have difficulty in co-ordination. The class teacher and the school's head have met mother once to discuss this, but she has now failed to attend two arranged meetings. The school nurse has carried out school entry screening of vision, hearing and growth and, because of the school's concerns, has referred for a specialist school medical.

The 3-year-old is shy and quiet with delayed speech; she has a place in the local day nursery and has had appointments arranged with the speech therapist. She has not been taken to the day nursery regularly and is in danger of losing the place, and she failed to attend her last appointment with the speech therapist. The 15-month-old baby girl gained weight erratically between the ages of 4 and 10 months and the heath visitor wondered if she was being fed regularly. Mother has been to the GP to confirm her pregnancy and was booked in to see the midwife at the next antenatal session. As she had diabetes of pregnancy with her last baby, her health assessment is particularly important, however, she has not attended any appointments.

The family seemed initially to cope well, but as successive children have come along a pattern of lurching from crisis to crisis has developed. They regularly seek financial support from social services and have difficulty paying the rent and the debts from the last time they were nearly evicted.

Following assessment, the identification of health needs and agreement of care plans the family has already had a number of offers of support for the issues relating to each of the children, but has not been able to consistently take up that support. The pattern of their difficulty in coping is affecting the children and the school teachers, the school nurse and the health visitor are concerned that the parents need to be confronted with the effects on the children and offered a comprehensive care programme including support for their parenting skills.

The health visitor has tried to work with the family, as agreed with them in a care plan, to enable them to take up the services that would support their parenting with less and less success. She has offered to work with them on stimulating and playing with the children and on the programme outlined by the speech therapist. The midwife has tried to visit at home as well as inviting the mother to clinics; however, contact has not yet been established. The health visitor and school teacher/head teacher make a joint 'child in need' referral to social services, suggesting a meeting to share information about their professional assessments and to agree a joint agency approach to the family that would aim to result in their co-operation with a support package. This package or plan would include some of the issues and plans that the single agencies have been working on. Its strength comes from the joint approach to the family by the agencies and the negotiation with the parents about the seriousness of the needs of the children and the support on offer for them to change.

There is usually a time lag between referral to LA Children's Social Care and a meeting with the family to agree a care plan. LA Children's Social Care having received the referral has the responsibility for collating the assessment data from all the professionals who have been working with the family to varying degrees of success. During this time, the midwife and school health service would continue to try to establish contact. The health visitor would be the most appropriate person to support the family while reiterating the need for change and that professionals are there to help.

277

whose parenting difficulties or vulnerabilities are long lasting or chronic in nature is often perceived by health and other professionals as particularly difficult and challenging. Although an individual practitioner may not have very many families who need this level of intervention, the workload is widely acknowledged as being high and sometimes stressful (Appleton 1996).

The identification of children in need of protection flows from single agency work with 'children in need' and their families. Where single agency 'children in need' work has not resulted in improvement for the children there will be a need to discuss the child and family's situation with an agency that has statutory responsibility under The Children Act (2004). The Act identifies the local authority (LA) Children's Social Care as the agency statutorily responsible for carrying out assessments to ascertain if this is a 'child in need' (Section 17 of the Children Act 1989) or if there is 'reasonable cause to suspect that this child is suffering or likely to suffer, significant harm' and therefore 'in need of protection' (Section 47 of the Children Act 1989).

The above case history (see Box 11.2) illustrates how health professionals regularly identify the need for social work intervention and support in such fam-ilies. However, research evidence indicates that social work intervention has often only been accessible if a referral is couched as a child protection issue (Gibbons et al 1995, Hallett 1995). It is important to clarify at this point that the majority of cases fall within 'child(ren) in need' referral criteria and only in complex, chronic or very severe cases will a strategy discussion involving the relevant agencies and a core assessment under Section 47 of the Children Act 1989 be conducted.

Working together to safeguard children (HM Government 2006a) emphasises the need for 'initial' and 'core' assessments to consider the welfare needs of children. These assessments are the response to a referral whether or not significant harm is likely to have occurred or to continue. This guidance encourages LA Children's Social Care staff to make assessments with other agencies to prevent further breakdown of the child's situation. As already outlined, although social services are the responsible statutory agency for such inquiries, many professionals who are in contact with the family will have undertaken a recent needs assessment or CAF and can provide that information for the Children's Social Care team. Thus, the initial assessment constitutes a brief assessment of each child referred to Children's Social Care to determine 'whether the child is in need, the nature of any services required, and whether a further, more detailed core assessment should be undertaken' (DH et al 2000b, paragraph 3.9). Following this initial assessment a meeting is held between the professionals and the family, the focus of which should be the parent's perception of the child(ren)'s needs and what would enable those needs to be met. This meeting should result in a plan that is agreed between all parties to address the child(ren)'s and parent's needs. This form of joint working has been outlined as part of the refocusing debate and falls within children in need legislation in The Children Act (Section 17, 1989).

Working together to safeguard children (HM Government 2006a) guidance reiterates the need for LA Children's Social Care services to co-ordinate the multi-agency children in need assessments that should result in welfare support for the child and family. The joint agency care plan agreed with the parents should include practical steps that the parents agree to carry out to achieve change in their parenting with the support of appropriate professionals. Some activities may be jointly undertaken, for example, a children's centre worker, and speech and language therapist might work with the parents on a child's language development. The extended family may also be included in the care plan, for example, to give regular breaks for the parents.

After a relatively short period of intensive work with a family on a joint agency 'child in need' care plan, it will be clear whether the family is able and willing to change, with support, the patterns that resulted in the original concerns for the children. The reasons for a lack of improvement are usually multi-factorial and may be due to the family's inability to change or due to its avoidance of profession-als who are offering support and intervention. Other reasons might include situ-ations where a family or parents do not agree with the professionals' assessment and do not perceive the need to change their parenting patterns and behaviours. It is important to recognise that a minority of parents may not be able to put their children's needs before their own and this is usually due to other influences in their lives such as the use of drugs or alcohol, mental health difficulties or being in a relationship that makes a parent very vulnerable (Glaser & Prior 1997). In these cases it will be of vital importance to formally consider whether the children are 'at risk of significant harm'. This will usually be addressed through child protection procedures, including a strategy discussion, a local authority Section 47 enquiry and a child protection conference.

If the child protection conference participants decide that the child is at continuing risk of significant harm, a formal child protection plan will be prepared outlining the interagency help and interventions that will be delivered by the various agencies. The conference chair must also determine which category of abuse or neglect the child has suffered, or is at risk of suffering (HM Government 2006a). The resulting child protection plan may not differ significantly to the 'child in need' care plan that may have preceded it. This reflects that the changes needed for the physical, emotional and social health of the child(ren) and family are not different, but that the context of the work is more formal and potentially 'serious'. It is only after this progression from 'child in need' work through child protection procedures that professionals can demonstrate that a court case for the protection of the children should be considered. A court case will only be appropriate when the preventative 'child in need' work and the formal child protection plan have not resulted in major improvements for the children and their family. In the majority of cases, the identification of a 'child in need of protection' flows from 'child in need' work. The assessment of risk and subsequent framework for work with the family will usually be related to the omissions or commissions of parents and their ability or willingness to change. Within a framework of good quality needs-based public health practice, all those working with children need to respond to child welfare or safeguarding concerns as a progression from normal working practices.

Conclusion

There is a continuing debate within health and social care policy about the extent to which services generally, and not only in terms of 'child(ren) in need', should be targeted at the level of the individual or the community. This chapter has argued that safeguarding children work based on the principles of public health must adopt a combination of both whole-population and individual approaches. In order to view safeguarding children as part of their public health work, practitioners will need to be familiar with the continuum of need and the concepts of universality and targeted services. Universal services will be necessary at an initial contact or assessment level to identify the 'needs' of a given population, which can then be targeted and met through group and community work or individual interventions, such as support to parents. Vulnerable children and 'child(ren) in need' can only be targeted by ensuring universal contact with all children in our communities.

In addition, public health practitioners will need to be knowledgeable about the new legislative and multi-agency practice issues surrounding safeguarding children work. This chapter has described how the Child Health Promotion Programme is the universal service offered to all families with children. This programme ensures contacts at key child developmental stages and provides the gateway to family health needs assessment from which targeted family-based interventions may ensue. Policy has clearly acknowledged the public health relevance of safeguarding children at both a national and international level. The challenge is getting that put into practice and getting recognition for the time and skills required of staff working at grassroots level with children, young people and their families as part of that universal provision.

It is in children's best interests for society to ensure that effective steps are taken to identify the needs of children, as research evidence continually demonstrates that a failure to address these needs may lead to negative outcomes in terms of a child's social development, emotional growth and ability to form positive social relationships. The public health importance of safeguarding children work to ensure that all children have optimum life chances and enter adulthood successfully cannot be underestimated.

DISCUSSION QUESTIONS

- How can you safeguard and promote children's welfare in your professional practice?
- Why are universal services important in safeguarding and promoting children's welfare?
- What factors would you take in to account in recognising that a child is in need of support and/or safeguarding?
- How do you assess the needs of children and the capacity of parents/carers to meet their children's needs?
- Why does 'the continuum of need' in safeguarding children work benefit multi-agency working?

References

Acheson C 1988 Public Health in England. HMSO, London

Appleton JV 1996 Working with vulnerable families: a health visiting perspective. Journal of Advanced Nursing 23: 912–918

Appleton JV, Clemerson J 1999 Family-based interventions with children in need. Community Practitioner 72(5): 134–136

Bifulco A, Moran P 1998 Wednesday's child. London. Routledge

Bremner JD, Vythilingham M, Vermetten E et al 2003 MRI and PET study of deficits in hippocampal structure and function in women with childhood sexual abuse and posttraumatic stress disorder. American Journal of Psychiatry 160(5): 924–932

Browne K 2002 Child abuse: defining, understanding and intervening. In: Wilson K, James A (eds) The child protection handbook. Baillière Tindall, London

Buchannan A 1996 Cycles of child maltreatment: facts, fallacies and interventions. Wiley, Chichester

Burke W 1998 Letter to members of the RCN health visitor forum. Royal College of Nursing, London

Cawson P 2002 Child maltreatment on the family: the experience of national sample of young people. NSPCC, London

The Children Act 2004. Chapter 31. The Stationery Office, London

Children's Rights Director 2004 Safe from harm: children's views report. Commission for Social Care Inspection, London

Cleaver H, Unell I, Aldgate J 1999 Children's needs – parental capacity: the impact of parental mental illness, problem alcohol and drug use, and domestic violence on children's development. HMSO, London

Cleaver H, Walker S, Meadows P 2004 Assessing children's needs and circumstances. The impact of the assessment framework. Jessica Kingsley Publishers, London

Coid J, Petruckevitch A, Feder G, Chung WS, Richardson J, Moorey S 2001 Relation between childhood sexual and physical abuse and risk of revictimization in women: a cross-sectional survey. The Lancet 358: 450–454

Corby B 1990 Making use of child protection statistics. Children and Society 4(3): 304–314

Creighton SJ 1995 Fatal child abuse – how preventable is it? Child Abuse Review 4: 318–328

Creighton SJ 2000 Government statistics on child deaths where abuse or neglect may be implicated. In: NSPCC Out of sight. NSPCC, London

Commission for Social Care Inspection (CSCI) 2005 safeguarding children. The second joint Chief Inspectors' report on arrangements to safeguard children. CSCI, London

Department for Education and Skills (DfES) 2003 Every child matters. HMSO, London

Department for Education and Skills (DfES) 2004 Every child matters: change for children. DfES Publications, Nottingham

Department for Education and Skills (DfES) 2005a Lead professional good practice guidance. DfES, London

Department for Education and Skills (DfES) 2005b Engaging the voluntary and community sectors in Children's Trusts. DfES Publications, Nottingham

Department for Education and Skills (DfES) 2006 Fact sheet. Information sharing (IS) Online. Available: http://Index. www.ecm.gov.uk/index

Department for Education and Skills (DfES)/Department of Health (DH) 2004 National Service Framework for Children, Young People and Maternity Services. Core Standards. DH, London.

Department for Education and Skills (DfES)/Department of Health (DH) 2005 Making safeguarding everybody's business: a post-Bichard vetting scheme. A consultation. DfES, London

Department of Health (DH) 1989 An introduction to the Children Act 1989. HMSO, London

Department of Health (DH) 1997a Statistics of children and young people on child protection registers. Year ending 31 March 1997, England. Government Statistical Service, London

Department of Health (DH) 1997b Children looked after by local authorities. Year ending 31 March 1996, England. Government Statistical Service, London

Department of Health (DH) 1999 Framework for the assessment of children in need and their families. Consultation draft. DH, London

Department of Health (DH) 2002a Women's mental health: into the mainstream. Startegic development of mental health care for women. DH, London

Department of Health (DH) 2002b Safeguarding children. A joint Chief Inspectors' report on arrangements to safeguard children. DH, London

Department of Health (DH) 2003 What to do if you're worried a child is being abused. DH, London

Department of Health (DH) 2004a Choosing health. Making healthier choices easier. DH, London

Department of Health (DH) 2004b Securing good health for the whole population. Final report. Derek Wanless. HMSO, London

Department of Health (DH) 2004c National standards: local action. Health and social care standards and planning framework 2005/06–2007/08. DH, London

Department of Health (DH) 2004d The Chief Nursing Officer's review of the nursing, midwifery and health visiting contribution to vulnerable children and young people. DH, London

Department of Health (DH) 2006 Responding to domestic abuse. A handbook for health professionals. DH, London

Department of Health (DH)/Dartington Social Research Unit 1995 Child protection: messages from research. HMSO, London

Department of Health (DH)/Department for Education and Employment/Home Office 2000b Framework for the assessment of children in need and their Families. HMSO, London.

Department of Health (DH)/Department for Education and Skills (DfES) 2004 National service framework for children Young people and maternity services. Core standards. DH, London

Department of Health/Home Office 2003 The Victoria Climbié inquiry. Report of an inquiry by Lord Laming. HMSO, London

Department of Health (DH), Home Office and Department for Education and Employment 1999 Working together to safeguard children: a guide for inter-agency working to safeguard and promote the welfare of children. DH, London

Department of Health (DH)/Home Office/Department for Education and Employment/National Assessmbly for Wales 2000a Safeguarding children involved in prostitution. Supplementary guidance to working together to safeguard children. DH, London

Edleson JL 1999 Children's witnessing of adult domestic violence. Journal of Interpersonal Violence 14: 839–970

Farrington D 1995 Intensive health visiting and the prevention of juvenile crime. Health Visitor 68(3): 100–102

Gibbons J, Conroy S, Bell C 1995 Operating the child protection system: a study of child protection practices in English local authorities. HMSO, London

Gil D 1975 Unravelling child abuse. American Journal of Orthopsychiatry 45: 346–354

Glaser D, Prior V 1997 Is the term child protection applicable to emotional abuse? Child Abuse Review 6: 315–329

Glaser D 2000 Child abuse and neglect and the brain – a review. Journal of Child Psychology and Psychiatry and Allied Professions 41(1): 97–116

Gray J 2002 National policy on the assessment of children in need and their families. Chapter 8 In: Ward H, Rose W (eds) Approaches to needs assessment in children's services. Jessica Kingsley Publishers, London

Hall DMB, Elliman D 2003 Health for all children, 4th edn. Oxford University Press, Oxford

Hallett C 1995 Interagency co-ordination in child protection. HMSO, London

Heller SS, Larrieu JA, D'Imperio R, Boris NW 1999 Research on resilience to child maltreatment: empirical considerations. Child Abuse and Neglect 23(4): 321–338

Hosking G, Walsh I 2005 The WAVE Report 2005. Violence and what to do about it. Wave Trust, Croydon, Surrey

HM Government 2005a Statutory guidance on making arrangements to safeguard and promote the welfare of children under section 11 of the Children Act 2004. DfES Publications, London

HM Government 2005b Working together to safeguard children. Draft for public consultation. DFES Publications, London

HM Government 2005c Common core of skills and knowledge for the children's workforce. DfES Publications, Nottingham

HM Government 2005d Guidance on the children and young people's plan. DfES Publications, Nottingham

HM Government 2005e Statutory guidance on inter-agency co-operation to improve the wellbeing of children: children's trusts. DfES Publications, Nottingham

HM Government 2006a Working together to safeguard children. A guide to inter-agency working to safeguard and promote the welfare of children. Online. Available at: http://www.everychildmatters.gov.uk/socialcare/safeguarding/workingtogether/

HM Government 2006b The common assessment framework for children & young people: practitioners' guide. Integrated working to improve outcomes for children and young people. DfES Publications, Nottingham

HM Government 2006c Common assessment framework for children and young people: managers' guide. Integrated working to improve outcomes for children and young people. DfES Publications, Nottingham

HM Government/Department of Health (DH) 2006 Our health care, our say: a new direction for community services. DH, London

International Society for the Prevention of Child Abuse and Neglect 2006 ISPCAN: our mission. Online. Available at: http://www.ispcan.org/aboutISPCAN.htm

Jones S, Parry S 2005 Burden of disease – injuries. An overview. Report commissioned from the Department of Epidemiology, Statistics and Public Health (Cardiff University) on behalf of the Health Protection Agency, Cardiff

Lang AJ, Rodgers CS, Lebeck MM 2006 Associations between maternal childhood maltreatment and psychopathology and aggression during pregnancy and post-partum. Child Abuse & Neglect 30: 17–25

Lowenhoff C 2004 Have talents: need liberating! Community Practitioner 77(1): 23–25

Mcdonald G 2001 Effective interventions for child abuse and neglect. An evidence-based approach to planning and evaluating interventions. John Wiley and Sons Ltd, Chichester

Mullen PE, Martin JL, Anderson JC, Romans SE, Herbison GP 1996 The long term impact of the physical, emotional and sexual abuse of children: a community study. Child Abuse & Neglect 20(1): 7–21

National Statistics/Department for Education and Skills (DfES) 2006a Statistics of education: referrals, assessments and children and young people on child protection registers: year ending 31 March 2005. National Statistics, London

National Statistics/Department for Education and Skills (DfES) 2006b Statistics of education: children looked after by local authorities year ending 31 March 2005, volume 1: national tables March. National statistics, London

NSPCC 2000 Out of Sight. NSPCC, London

Osofsky J 2003 Prevalence of children's exposure to domestic violence and child maltreatment: implications for prevention and intervention. Clinical Child and Family Psychology Review 6: 161–170

Parton N 2006 Safeguarding childhood: early intervention and surveillance in a late modern society. Palgrave Macmillan, Basingstoke

Peden M, McGee K, Krug E 2002 Injury: a leading cause of the global burden of disease, 2000. World Health Organization, Geneva

Reder P, Duncan S 1999 Lost innocents. A follow-up study of fatal child abuse. Routledge, London

Roberts I 1996 Family support and the health of children. Children and Society 10: 217–224

Royal College of Nursing 1994 Public health: nursing rises to the challenge. Royal College of Nursing, London

Shonkoff JP, Phillips DA (eds) 2000 From neurones to neighbourhood: the science of early childhood development. National Research Council Institute of Medicine. Washington DC, National Academy Press

Silverman A, Reinherz HZ, Giaconia RM 1996 The long-term sequelae of child and adolescent abuse: a longitudinal study. Child Abuse and Neglect 20(8): 709–723

Sinclair R, Bullock R 2002 Learning from past experience – a review of serious case reviews. Department of Health, London

Smith Stover C 2005 Domestic violence research what have we learned and where do we go from here? Journal of Interpersonal Violence 20(4): 448–454

Teicher MH 2002 Scars that won't heal: the neurobiology of child abuse. Scientific American. 286(3): 68–75

Thorpe D, Bilson A 1998 From protection to concern: child protection careers without apologies. Children and Society 12: 373–386

United Nations 1989 United Nations convention on the rights of the child. Office of the United Nations High Commissioner for Human Rights, Geneva

Utting W, Baines C, Stuart M, Rowlands J, Vialva R 1997 People like us – the report of the review of the safeguards for children living away from home. HMSO, London

Whitfield CL, Anda RF, Dube SR, Felitti VJ 2003 Violent childhood experiences and the risk of intimate partner violence in adults: assessment in a large health maintenance organization. Journal of Interpersonal Violence 18: 166–185

Wilczynski A 1994 The incidence of child homicide: how accurate are the official statistics? Journal of Clinical Forensic Medicine 1: 61–66

World Health Organization 2002 World report on violence and health. WHO, Geneva

Further reading

Appleton J 2006 Safeguarding children. Community Practitioner 79(6): 176–177

Department of Health (DH) 2006 Responding to domestic abuse. A handbook for health professionals. DH, London

Department of Health (DH)/Department for Education and Employment/Home Office 2000 Framework f0or the assessment of children in need and their families. HMSO, London

HM Government 2006a Working together to safeguard children. A guide to inter-agency working to safeguard and promote the welfare of children. Online. Available at: http://www.everychildmatters.gov.uk/socialcare/safeguarding/workingtogether/

HM Government 2006b The common assessment framework for children and young people: practitioners' guide. Integrated working to improve outcomes for children and young people. DfES Publications, Nottingham

The Children Act 2004. HMSO, London

12 Leadership through alongsideness

Robyn Pound and Ruth Grant

Key issues

- Development of leadership for relationship-centred public health and community development.
- Shared power for influencing change towards agreed aims.
- 'Practice-as-enquiry' with families, communities and agencies.
- Action research for improving and explaining practice.

Introduction

We are two health visitors who independently undertook higher degrees to understand and respond to changing expectations informing new public health activity, family visiting and children's health in communities and came together to share experiences. Our individual journeys of discovery involved researching and learning while practising as we each endeavoured to improve what we were doing to influence the health of our communities. Ruth, in a large rural village and Robyn, in an inner city practice, independently reached similar conclusions about 'ways of being' with people that promote the wellbeing of those with greatest health need. We will describe our separate learning experiences to show how we arrived at our current understanding of leadership in working with individual families, community groups, colleagues and other agencies. Although our experiences are drawn from health visiting, leadership in public health practice is not discipline specific. Our learning is influenced by a range of professional and academic disciplines in the field. For this reason we believe the key messages are transferable.

Our intention is not to produce a model of good leadership practice for others to follow, but to share our experiences in the hope it is valuable to you in your reflections. We chose a first person narrative (Connelly & Clandinin 1990) to show the developmental personal nature of our learning and to bear you, the reader, in mind as we write. Leadership qualities appear indistinguishable from effective health visiting relationships and each of us felt clear before we began that leadership is not about being first, best or most powerful. Our enquiring process clarified relationship qualities and skills we now find effective and leadership involves using professional power by acting in ways that influence change towards agreed aims. Sharing power to support change may be the most important feature of the public health practice we find effective. We utilise knowledge available to us from a range of sources, including our own beliefs and values, as we share with you our search for improved understanding in a process we now call practice-as-enquiry. Our leadership styles are guided by personally held interpretations of professional values that we independently developed through practical experience. The similarity of our explanations is of interest to us because we both intend

Box 12.1

Values and skills

Values and skills in leadership by alongsideness

- Respect for people
- Self-determination
- Life as process of becoming
- Connection with people
- Acceptance of differences
- Encouragement
- Containment
- Taking responsibility
- Sustainability
- Embracing contradictions
- Integrity, honesty, openness
- Emotional strength, courage
- Creativity
- Light heartedness and humour
- Reciprocity in partnership
- Empathic listening
- Modelling
- Use of expertise
- Risk taking
- Advice giving and teaching

These values hold individually constructed meanings for each of us

promoting collaborative thinking and action planning with clients, communities and colleagues for improving how we all work together. This chapter explains how and why we arrived at our leadership styles and improved our effectiveness. We will tell our stories separately before integrating themes. Box 12.1 introduces the values and skills that we now recognise are individually constructed in our alongside leadership styles.

Ruth's story: practice development

My interest in community development in a large rural village emerged from an MSc in Health Studies (Grant 2001). I used interviews, a focus group and questionnaires to understand lay perspectives of health and for identifying service requirements for those in greatest need. Here, I explain my learning through reflection on community development activity following the MSc. I now call it 'micro' public health. I will show how my understanding of leadership for promoting social inclusion developed.

Although the reflective journey is mine, I would like to acknowledge my colleague Annie Saberwal, who was a source of excellence and unselfish inspiration to me. The journey began when health visiting was required to change from universal child- and family-focused public health work to targeting those with greatest health needs (Department of Health (DH) 1998a). Health visitors were encouraged to adopt population-based public health roles in order to address the needs of their communities. At the time there was little information on methods for working effectively with populations (Parston & Timmins 1998). Statistical data I had gathered for an area health profile gave little insight into the needs of the population. I was aware I had not worked effectively with families who were poorest, socially excluded and suffered the worst health. Although, like all clients, they were offered a universal service, this group did not call on my support as often as more articulate, affluent members of the community. I believed this indicated they did not feel comfortable with me, although research shows this was the group most likely to suffer ill health in my case load (DH 1998b). For this reason I decided to find a more effective method of improving health in this population. At the same time, the government encouraged practitioners to work towards a range of interventions to improve the nation's health and set primary care trusts (PCTs) a number of targeted objectives (DH 1999, 2000). Until I had a clear picture of the health needs of my local population, I did not know how to begin.

Discoveries

In research for an MSc in Health Studies (Grant 2001), I discovered some of the health needs of the large rural village (5700 population) in which I work. The aim of the study was to determine the unexpressed health need of the population in order to maximise health gains and target health inequalities. Community participatory appraisal (CPA) is frequently used by the World Health Organization to gather information on health needs of a population where little is known (Ong & Humphris 1994). CPA research has shown that professionals are often unaware of community benefits that may be obtained from relatively simple solutions (Sewell & Wade 2000). Obstacles to change are sometimes revealed by the process and communities empowered to act. Furthermore, communities hold knowledge that can influence the development of polices and service provision that are more likely to be effective (Johnston & Mayoux 1998). I undertook a needs analysis to determine lay perspectives of health using CPA methodology (Grant 2005). Semi-structured face-to-face interviews with 11 adults were analysed followed by a focus group with seven adults. A questionnaire was developed based on data generated from interviews, the WHO Quality of Life study (WHO 1998) and Orientation to Life questionnaires (Antonovsky 1993). The amalgamated questionnaire was posted to 350 adults randomly selected from the general medical practice list. I elicited a good response (40%). The predominant feature of the interviews and focus group was that the divided nature of the village impinged on social cohesion and health of the population. Questionnaire respondents suggested a link road to the village, a supermarket, banking facilities, evening doctors' surgeries, a State-run nursery, wrap-around child care and leisure activities. An important finding was the level of psychological distress amongst males, particularly in the 18–25 age group. To the Quality of Life question about anxiety and despair, 12.5% of most male age groups reported feeling severe anxiety and despair 'frequently' and 'always'. This increased to 42% in the 18- to 25-year age group.

Other findings pertinent to the poorest population in the social housing area, was rural isolation (8 miles from the nearest town) and lower educational achievement and life expectancy. This group showed a 'sense of coherence' profile similar to more affluent owner occupiers in the new estate, but with more respondents in the highest and lowest scoring categories (Antonovsky 1998). Plotted on a graph, a parabola emerged demonstrating normal distribution of the 'sense of coherence' scores across the whole community. My purpose in determining the 'Orientation to Life' of the population by using Antonovsky's 'Sense of Coherence' questionnaire was so that I could discover if there was a group of individuals who would have greater health needs in the future. These data revealed that the 45- to 65-year-old age group has the most 'low' scorers, who have a poorer sense of coherence and are, therefore, less likely to cope well in adversity as they age. This information, plus my knowledge of families, informed my decision to work at addressing the health needs of the poorest population. Many of the low-income families lived in the same social housing estate, thus they also belonged to a geographical or neighbourhood community. I spent time learning all I could about the local voluntary and statutory service provision.

Beginning to reach the socially excluded – sustainability

It was my plan to start a group and, as community leaders merged, train them to continue the group. I was keen to build in this element of sustainability so that I would then be free to address other 'communities of need'. In order to start a group I produced an invitation to a meeting that was delivered to 350 residents in the social housing estate. I was encouraged when around 30 men, women and children came. I recognised they were from amongst the poorer, more socially excluded members of our village. Lots of ideas for a group were offered but they also expressed doubts that it could be sustained. They told me about a group started by the local authority that had collapsed acrimoniously. I provided refreshments and listened. I decided to be client led with this group in the same way as I try to be in my family practice and research. Although this sounds like the opposite of leadership, it was a conscious decision as a strategy for empowering this population to take responsibility for their future health, including social and fiscal health. I needed to provide exactly what they wanted so that they would want to make use of the services. I had to recognise that this may not be what I thought was good for them. Even so I still made errors. At about the same time I learned of the opportunity to join a co-enquiry group Robyn was running. As the project unfolded I decided to use an action research process of critical reflection and action in order to learn and develop effective ways to practice, and thereby influence healthy changes.

In the beginning, what they wanted was a meeting place to enjoy company and have fun. They also wanted computer lessons and free computers to take home. Sixty attended computer courses during the following year and received second-hand computers. I wanted to provide parenting classes. I found other parents attended the classes, not those from the group I was most concerned about. Much later, when they trusted me, I was told that parenting and household duties were the areas in which they felt confident. I acknowledged I had been disrespectful by suggesting that parenting classes were necessary. It reinforced my determination to be led by them. I had to learn how best to do that as I went along. I decided to commit to facilitating the group for one morning a week for a year. I remained confident that by the end of the year, community development techniques would have enabled members to take over the group and run it without my help. It was important to me that the group should sustain itself after I had withdrawn as I recognised some health gains would be slow to evolve. I was to learn that it would take longer than a year to support this community in working together. The reason why previous attempts to develop such a group had not succeeded were complex, but one compelling reason was the withdrawal of the previous local authority community development worker.

Containment, reciprocity, reassurance and encouragement

Initially I was exhausted by group members. Some people shouted at me about what they wanted, some expressed doubt about my ability to help them. Others spoke harshly, were rude and lacked confidence that the group would continue. Every week a traumatic event occurred and members moved from one house to another retelling the story. I surmised that a great deal of energy was spent in anxiety and distress. Perhaps this was why many appeared to struggle emotionally and lack emotional literacy, and the energy to develop their lives. One week the crisis was a domestic violence incident in which a man, armed with a knife, chased his screaming wife around the estate. Another week youths poured petrol onto a cat and set fire to it. Yet another week, a 33-year-old woman in the third trimester of pregnancy died of a heart attack. Her baby was delivered by emergency caesarean and died 3 months later. These examples demonstrate the serious nature of the crises people commonly experienced on the estate. Some of the residents act as 'emotional amplifiers' spreading news that affects other people. Many residents have poor emotional literacy and problem-solving skills and, thus, share in the trauma these experiences generate. My colleague, Annie, and I interpret this emotional cyclone to be the result of poor physical and emotional health. We concluded that in order to help we needed to buttress their emotional health whilst teaching them new emotional literacy skills.

From the start of the group I became aware of using psychotherapeutic skills, particularly 'containment' (Shuttleworth 1999). Containment involves emotionally holding distressed people until they are no longer afraid and can begin to cope. I became conscious of how I listened supported and encouraged people. I also used Brazleton's notion of reciprocity. I realised that by being sensitive and responsive to moods I could enable the members to cope with their problems (Brazelton 1992). Some said they found this helpful. Each meeting a crowd gathered and reported the latest disaster. After Annie and I helped them think it through, they relaxed and started chatting. Some began to think creatively about activities for the group. Gradually, we witnessed people becoming more optimistic. This role became an important part of our work. I now recognise that by using different skills I began to develop a style of leadership useful for this particular depth of need.

Annie and I used our knowledge of local services to arrange exercise classes, yoga, Tai Chi and family fun days. I observed that small children spent most of their time either on their parent's lap or in their pushchairs. Few parents actively played with their children. Older children played amongst themselves. Recently, a play worker has begun introducing young parents and their children to new ways of playing in the group. She also makes visits to their homes. Funding was provided from government Children's Centre money following a successful bid. I notice some parents have begun playing with children during group activities. One young mother, whose first child had been compulsorily adopted, continually berated her 2-year-old, 'Get up, get down, get off'. Lacking language, the child was timid and anxious. By learning to play, he has grown in confidence, increased his use of language and appears a happier little boy. His mother, meantime, has also given up smoking and is considering seeking work. I learned that through our modelling ways of being together, and by teaching parents and children to play, parents now appear to appreciate being with the older children. I recognise that these skills are part of my leadership style. I now know that there may be greater success to be found in working with families to help meet their needs than from pursuing a child protection route.

Slowly, as confidence in Annie and me grew, I found members would run to the surgery and burst in on us when they were worried. I was delighted to realise they had become comfortable with us and sought us out to share their difficulties. It made me aware of the complex, time- and energy-consuming nature of the problems people frequently faced. One day a very fat young man ran sweating into my room to tell me that two men were dealing drugs in a car outside his home. He was angry that they were 'shooting up' and throwing discarded syringes in the gutter in front of his children. These men threatened him and he was afraid.

Not knowing how to handle the situation he ran to the surgery to be comforted and to seek advice. I realised that sometimes I must be prepared to give advice and accept the lack of knowledge in some areas. I identified advice amongst my leadership styles. Some people expected me to know everything and to be able to sort out all their problems. I felt overwhelmed by the burden, but my growing respect for these families made me realise that if they can learn to carry their awesome burdens, then I have helped them in a small way. I observed that as families learn to put down other people's problems they become clearer on how to tackle their own. My understanding grew about the impact of living in rural poverty in an estate where families with multiple problems were housed. I worked at attracting services to the area and in time was joined by the Citizens Advice Bureau outreach worker whose knowledge and help about welfare benefits, debt management and many other topics has been invaluable. Annie has ably demonstrated her wonderful art and drama skills by producing an act for the local community play and running a hugely successful 'POP Idols' competition, as well as continuing to carry a great deal of the daily practice management.

I was amazed at the resilience of group members and began to understand the 'Sense of Coherence' scores from Antonovsky's Orientation to Life questionnaire I had used. They appeared not to lack self-esteem, but to have heightened sensitivity to problems experienced by their neighbours. On the whole, many appear to feel good about themselves, but to have little resilience to cope with emotional challenges. General practitioners reported reduction in frequency of consultations amongst people who attend the group and began recommending it to other patients who frequently attend the surgery. During the last 2 years, six lifelong smokers have given up, with support from a smoking cessation specialist who comes to the group. Other resources and activities are listed in Box 12.2.

Box 12.2

Opportunity project activities

- **Youth centre** opened for community use
- **Coffee mornings** for sharing laughter, problems and fears
- **Lunch** prepared and shared together
- **Computer classes** and second-hand computers given to low-income families (around 60 so far)
- **Keep fit**, weight and dietary discussion
- **Yoga**
- **Tai Chi**
- **Holiday fun days** to encourage parents and children to play
- **Home safety** audit scheme
- **Meetings** with parish councillors, Lord Warner and local PCT Board
- **Day trips** to zoo, pantomime, science museum, safari park, London and Alton Towers (teenagers)
- **Christmas and Halloween parties**
- **Christmas lunch** for 50 older people
- **Community play** and participation in the **Bath Fringe Festival**
- **Welfare Benefits Advisor**
- **Smoking cessation support worker**
- **Pension service, financial audit** and inquiry into social needs of older residents
- **Police** talk for teenagers on personal safety
- **Table top sales** monthly
- **'POP Idols'** singing competition

(Grant 2005)

Understanding my values

I assumed members would gradually be able to run the group themselves. In time, I realised that experiences I regarded as 'normal' in people's development had been missed by these families. For example, to experience the kind of communication that encourages people to express themselves and expect to be heard. I saw little capacity for conversational turn-taking, communication with children, ability to plan, cooperate or share work loads. I frequently saw arguments between people. It took 3 months to form a committee, accept a constitution and open a group bank account. I use my financial skills and knowledge of writing bids to raise charitable funds, because this was, and still appears to be, beyond them. We have had a turnover of officers on the management committee, but as individuals have grown stronger they have taken up the challenge.

I noted that given opportunities to learn about matters of relevance, new ideas are put it into practice. After two family fun days run by the Community Education Department, the committee decided to hold one of their own and was heartened to find their day successfully attended by even more families. Following this they planned Christmas lunch for 50 lonely, older residents. It was a massive challenge and I was afraid of failure because it was so optimistic. Come the day, everyone worked well with no arguing. I noted teenagers putting out tables and chairs, older people decorating the hall and tree, men collecting guests and offering them drinks, whilst women worked in the kitchen. They organised the guest list, transport, duty rota, old-time music hall entertainment and Christmas songs from 60 nursery school children. I was amazed and delighted. I saw great potential and learned that I needed to have faith in them.

The first funds I raised were used for a trip to the pantomime. None of them had ever been to a theatre and one woman, horrified to find herself on the balcony, was too afraid to sit down. Next time we met she asked why I had not bought tickets for the stalls. I explained the difference in cost. Two years on, I am aware of how close we have become. I had been ignorant of their lives. I believe the ability for closeness is evident in the group. When new people attend, members welcome them and demonstrate listening, containment and reciprocity. Those joining are often angry and distressed, but members are patient and demonstrate they know how to help. First, Annie and I modelled relationship techniques and now they have learned how to do it themselves. This is extremely satisfying. I realise we have more to learn and I do not know when we will reach the stage where they can act as confident leaders and sustain the group without our support. When the group first met, one woman sat hunched at the edge with her partner and 4 children. She looked permanently frightened. She had experienced domestic violence from her ex-husband. Her 16-year-old daughter had suffered psychotic episodes, had special educational needs and no longer attended school. This girl now appears well and a capable mother of a little boy. Her mother also appears happier and more confident. She makes and sells lunches to members each week. Recently she spent her own money to buy prizes and went door to door in the estate selling raffle tickets. She was so pleased to make £50 towards group funds and was downcast when she found out a license was needed to sell raffle tickets to the public. I need to use my knowledge of the law to keep them safe.

Members frequently experienced the local police and doubted their neutrality. Early in the life of the group they agreed to invite the community policeman to a meeting. The policeman was ill at ease, and members were angry and shouted at him about all the injustices they had suffered. He was patient, but he did not come again despite repeated invitations. Two years later a family was terrorised by a group of youths who rammed their garden fence with a car and smashed the double glazed windows with baseball bats. When the man opened the door the youths threatened to hit him too. Later, I heard his partner telling another that she was glad a different officer had attended her call, because their community policeman had a bad leg and could have damaged it dealing with the youths. She was full of praise for the officer who attended. I realised that some members seemed to regard police with less suspicion.

On a day trip not all bus seats were booked, so I offered the seats to a large family hoping they would join the group. When the bus came a teenage boy refused to board because he was afraid of one of the women I had invited. He walked away but his mother became incensed, driving him back to the bus by shouting at him. He still refused to get on and lay across the door, whereupon his mother pushed him in the stomach forcing him on the bus. It was quite clear she wanted to go very much. Eventually he capitulated. I thought a great deal about the incident. In most families the mother's behaviour would be thought of as child abuse. According to my values it seemed abusive. During time spent with this woman I understood that she was excitable, erratic, used foul language and fought with other women. I knew she loved her children passionately too. Her behaviour was in conflict with my norms and values. After reflection I decided to watch and wait as I considered my more important target of working to improve her mental health by teaching her to relax in her relationships with her children. The trip and her belonging in the group was an important part of this process. The most important change for this woman is that she contacts us when she feels overwhelmed by her emotions and wants to talk it through. Her changing attitudes towards her children are marked. For the most part she no longer appears to bully them into compliance. She is now a staunch group member and her language is less abusive. She spoke movingly of the meaning the group has for her when Lord Warner, the then Under Secretary of State for Health, visited. She helps run car boot sales each month to generate income for the group. I have come to love her and value her resilience and sense of humour.

Before the car boot sales began, the group invited a tutor to teach them for a food handling and hygiene certificate. The women were amazed that I did not know all the answers. Like them I also had to learn. For them it was a first academic success that they use to serve food at the car boot sales. New-found knowledge led to a dilemma for one woman. She was conscious of keeping the bacon rolls clean. To prevent people breathing on them she stored them underneath the counter. By the end of the morning she had sold so few rolls because they could not be seen, that takings were low. To raise funds she sold them at a bargain price, not realising she would make a loss. Now, she keeps the rolls covered on display and food sales raise around £100 a month.

Whilst facilitating this group I have spent time debating whether what I am doing amounts to cultural hegemony. Despite seeking to work with clients using a bottom-up approach, I realise the norms and values I bring to my work are those of an educated professional and I may be imposing them on the group. I believe I act for the benefit of members. Through reflection with colleagues and group members in an action research process, I am becoming clearer about what we are trying to achieve. I await independent evaluation by students from Bath University and look forward to learning how I can take the group forward. See Box 12.3 for some outcomes.

Strategic work linked to research and the project

I realised I could not meet all needs expressed by the population in my research, especially services to ameliorate male mental ill health. However, I believed appropriate service provision might help. I joined a local strategic partnership looking at children and young people's services and was co-opted onto the board of the Children's Fund, the Children's Centre planning group and interagency groups looking at youth crime, information sharing, domestic violence and others. Through this work I helped create strategies for addressing needs expressed by

Box 12.3

Early results

- 1 member reduced weight by 5 stone
- 6–8 enjoy aerobics
- 40 enjoy Tai Chi
- 6 long-term smokers quit, 1 more makes progess
- 16 year old presented to Princess Royal for Millennium Volunteer work in group
- 2 aged 16 returned to full-time education
- 1 mother trained as childminder, 2 more considering
- 5 teenage mothers regularly attend
- 40 shared lunches changed from fried food to baguettes with salad
- Christmas lunch for older people, knitting blanket squares, drawing pictures together
- Friendship, laughter and less distress

(Grant 2005)

local children through consultation by the Children's Fund. Adult participation has been a feature of local authority service development for some time, but participation of children is more innovative. Children said they needed help forming friendships, reducing bullying, playing and 'hanging about'. It is hoped further services to those in Box 12.2 will be introduced, as a result of ongoing consultation that will promote better emotional and physical health of children and reduce levels of male ill health in the village over time.

I continue working with agencies and my community group members to provide sport and leisure facilities to reduce boredom and the self-destructive behaviour of local teenage youth, such as alcohol and drug misuse, and juvenile crime. This is challenging work because the village divide is not only geographic, but also political, with each faction seeking to reduce the influence of the other. I was invited to join a design group working with the government Department of Education and Skills to create a toolkit to facilitate such work.

Conclusion

So what is leadership in the context of my practice? From experience and reflection I developed a style of leadership that seeks to respond to individuals within the context of their understanding and community. Through the group I discovered that more than client participation is required. Ideas generated by members are essential for the building of acceptable services. Furthermore, the group needed to be built on members' wishes to be inclusive of all family members, both sexes and all ages. Enthusiastic, energised and more confident members have developed the skills to provide local families with new experiences.

I now recognise my values of respect, honesty, integrity and emotional strength are essential for working with socially excluded members of society. My leadership requires that these values be demonstrated in all I do. This includes the courage to speak honestly about my own values and using criticism constructively. A variety of leadership styles including containment and reciprocity, modelling, active listening, teaching, sharing knowledge and advising are utilised. All these I often use within one group meeting. I find I need the ability to move easily between these models whilst speaking with individuals or clusters. As a lead practitioner I must be able to continue retaining both individual and group stories, plus build their confidence whilst pursuing the main group activity for the session.

From believing my public health model of client-led work was substantially different from the alongsideness of Robyn's work, I have been amazed to see emerging similarities. I now recognise that in the alongsideness of my approach, I also use more overt methods of advice giving and teaching. Writing this chapter helped clarify my understanding of what I am doing and I believe my practice has become more robust. By reflecting with Robyn, Annie, the members and in my journal I have been able to evaluate, question and confirm what I am doing.

Robyn's story: from public health action to practical alongsideness

Through an action research process I asked the question 'how can I improve my health visiting support of developing family relationships? ' (Pound 2003). This PhD research explored relationships effective for supporting families, community development and educational public health. I used interviews, videos, questionnaire and critical reflection with clients and others to develop and test a collection of practical values I now call alongsideness in relationships.

During the 5 years leading to my registration for PhD research in 1995, I became passionately committed to raising awareness about rights for children and particularly problems that physical punishment causes for future mental wellbeing. An incident in 1989 alerted my interest in the parenting practices I commonly observed. In a baby clinic a young woman brought her baby for her 6-week check. She also brought her mother to help with the toddler. He was around 15 months old. As they waited, the boy explored the room, preferring things his granny thought he should not touch. Following him she tapped his hand saying 'No!' The child became excited by this game. His eyes sparkled and he giggled while his embarrassed granny appeared frustrated as she chased him. It dawned on me that not only was this ineffective as a way of being with a young child, but her daughter was learning a parenting style from her mother that I could imagine escalating conflict and future behaviour problems.

In another incident, a mother placed her toddler on the scales to be weighed and raised her hand in threat to make the child sit still. I tried not to notice, but I remembered the young woman's anguish at being punched by her partner the week before. I remembered her angry tears followed by her resignation. How could I help her change her future and the future for her child? How could I help the child grow up knowing how to respect herself enough so she did not expect to feel humiliated and powerless in relationships? I wanted to help her become adult knowing how to model something different for her own children. This incident, and my knowledge of the family, raised issues which were fundamental to my work in child protection (physical and emotional abuse), mental ill health (poor self-image, drug abuse and violence), and health promotion (teenage pregnancy, smoking). All were implicated in the parenting demonstrated here. This mother was reproducing the only style she knew.

I noticed these actions by parents at the time because of my increasing interest in children's behaviour and because of a mismatch between my primary preventive remit and the reality of work I actually did. Sometimes I seemed to do little more than watch for parents' actions to be identifiable as abusive, warranting referral to Social Services. I knew how to act when abuse was suspected, and had some skills for responding to parents' complaints about children's behaviour, but felt uncomfortable when I saw unashamed smacking and threatening of children. I found the subject difficult to broach because I had few easy alternatives to offer. I knew solutions lay in warmer relationships and clearer communication, but how could I promote it? How could I act in more preventive ways recognising that some parents never asked for help and that family dynamics required adults to hold different perspectives of children?

Gradually, I came to believe the issue was really one of human rights for children of which physical punishment was just one consideration. From this view, I planned public health action to raise awareness to influence legal reform and joined a London-based pressure group. I began speaking about equity of rights for children and concentrated my energy in searching for evidence to convince people that legal reform with primary preventive action was the way forward. My urgency to act for change seemed to lead to polarisation of people's views in a 'you are either with us or against us' way. It was difficult work. A nationwide movement for children's rights slowly grew and appeared unstoppable in its momentum. Policies for children began to change. I turned to thinking about practical aspects of influencing change in family life so children could experience more nurturing environments. I wanted to understand what healthy family relationships really are and how families can find them?

A new method of enquiry

I enrolled for a PhD research degree expecting to start with knowledge accrued over more than 20 years practice. Using living theory action research (Whitehead 1989) I found I could develop my knowledge, improve my practice and explain it. I could involve all families as co-enquirers in processes of finding what was useful. Living theory educational research leads practitioners to identify values that colour how they interpret situations and plan actions. Practitioners' concerns for clients' health, views about contextual influences on health and about ways to act are all altered by the lens of personal values. Clarification of personal values lies at the heart of building living theories of practice. Concerns identified about what is happening represent contradictions to personally held values. In seeking to understand the gaps between personal/professional values (what is important) and their contradiction in practice (the concerns) opportunities arise to discover more about the guiding values and appropriate actions. I began to see links between my way of being and my practice in leading change in public health. Here, I show how particular values that make up alongsideness became standards for judging the quality of my practice and for explaining my intentions.

Finding a research question began my process of changing practice as I discovered contradictions between my intentions and my actions. I had been so keen to foster respect for children it had not been amongst my concerns that my actions may not be respectful of parents. Yet, I wanted to involve parents in the research so they could both inform and benefit from it. My motivation had been to stop parents hitting their children, but I could not tell them about my intention. By refocusing on myself in the question, 'how can I improve my support of family relationships? ' I could be honest and involve everyone. My work began to shift towards practice-as-enquiry that I called alongsideness. As parents asked questions such as, 'How can I be a better parent? ' I asked, 'How can I be more helpful? ' We were co-learners. After prods from other researchers I also recognised myself as a parent and began to ask, 'How can *we* become better parents? ' A parenting programme based on Adlerian theory (Lew & Bettner 1996) helped me understand more about democratic relationships and how to achieve them.

Human emotional needs

Lew and Bettner's model called the 'Crucial Cs' helped me understand why children and parents behave as they do together. I also began to understand adult relationships in new ways. The model in Figure 12.1 describes the human emotional need to *connect* with others, to feel *capable*, to *count* (matter) and to experience *courage*. These emotional needs explain feelings that trigger the 'mistaken goals of

Human Emotional Needs
CRUCIAL CS

If **I have** the 'Crucial Cs'		If **I don't have** the Crucial Cs
CONNECT		
I feel *secure*	I believe	I feel *insecure*
I can reach out	**I belong**	I'm more susceptible to
and make friends		peer pressure
I cooperate		**I seek attention**
I need *communication skills*		
CAPABLE		
I feel ***competent***	I believe	I feel ***inadequate***
I have self control	**I can do it**	I try to control others or
and self discipline		prove 'you can't make me
I assume responsibility		I become dependent
I am self-reliant		**I seek power**
I need *self discipline*		
COUNT		
I feel ***valuable***	I believe	I feel ***insignificant***
I can make a difference	**I matter**	I may try to hurt back
I contribute		**I seek revenge**
I need to assume *responsibility*		
COURAGE		
I feel ***hopeful***	I believe	I feel ***inferior***
I am willing to try	I can handle	I may give up
I am resilient	what **turns** up	**I use avoidance**
I need *good judgement*		
I AM ENCOURAGED		**I AM DISCOURAGED**

Figure 12.1 ● Human emotional needs (adapted from Lew & Bettner 1996)

behaviour' described by Dreikurs and Soltz (1964) that are frequently recognisable in human relationships. 'Mistaken goals' attempt to meet human emotional needs to belong, feel competent, significant and resilient in ways that may actually make things worse. Our social nature leads to our need to belong by connecting with others. Willingness to co-operate with each other increases in the warmth and security of closeness between us. Children *seek attention* if they feel left out or isolated. Self-reliance and self-control is promoted by feeling capable. Feelings of inadequacy, dependence or that other people are in control lead people to seek *power*. Belief in one's personal significance in relationships (that one counts) can lead to effort to contribute. On the other hand, feeling insignificant and worthless can motivate *revenge* to get even with others.

Life's experience shows us that it is not always possible to connect with others, to feel capable or believe one counts all of the time. What is necessary to cope with life's ups and downs is to have the courage to keep trying. Hopefulness promotes resilience to persist while inferiority and hopelessness lead to feelings of inadequacy and *avoidance* of situations where failure could result. Encouragement is central to relationships that help promote resilience to overcome adversity and retain openness to learning. Understanding unmet emotional needs that lead to mistaken goals and challenging behaviour can prompt responses more likely to help children experience their significance. As I explored these ideas in working with parents, I realised that an early requirement of problem-solving is the restoration of connectedness between everyone involved and the fostering of hopefulness (Pound 2003, pp. 152–154).

As parents worked to adopt democratic principles at home, I found I needed to help them explain what they were doing to teachers in nurseries and schools. This resulted in whole-school discussions with teaching and playground staff. It lead to training with groups of frontline professionals in health, education and social services (Pound 2003, pp. 100–107).

Developing values of alongsideness

Practice values have most meaning when experienced in a relationship; however, for the purpose of sharing my thinking I introduce my values here. As an umbrella value, alongsideness for me is:

- founded on human worth, in that *all* people are valuable, have useful knowledge and are worth my respectful effort
- belief that people live in a process of becoming who they want to be
- belief in a life-affirming energy from connecting with people
- belief in the importance of self-determination and individual significance for developing personal responsibility
- encouragement helps people cope with discouraging feelings of inadequacy
- belief in the creativity of people who search for solutions.

Alongsideness has emerged as the motivating value I try to live in all of my relationships. It relies on my respect for people living a 'process of becoming', as I am myself. As I try to foster connections, often relying on light heartedness, I also need to accept that people may hold different views. My endeavour to ensure that individuals experience self-determination calls for my encouragement. Sometimes decision making is clouded by complex situations and I balance my responsibilities, for example, in acting with parents or for their children. I shall explain each of these points more fully.

Values emerging from different explorative phases of research led me to understand more about myself as a practitioner and to ask questions about times when my values were not recognisable in my actions. As I focused on how I was with families, I noticed similarities between the properties of parenting, effective relationships in health visiting and collaborative researching. Together, in effect, we can be side by side asking how we might begin to understand our concerns for the benefit of everyone. The Adlerian model and the collaborative research process contributed to my growing understanding of relationships.

Looking back at the public health campaigning, when my intention was to produce a convincing case to influence people, I began to understand why it was so stressful. Energy channelled into defending my views from opposing arguments sometimes severed warmth with people and interfered with openness to hear alternative ideas. Thinking about my need to believe in my own competence and the frustrated attempts I made to achieve it, helped me see the importance of encouraging self-determination in people. I could move from an oppositional stance that relied on more powerful arguments, to seeing us as trying to understand and work the problem out together. For me, alongsideness now represents reduction in the power inherent in professional relationships. By asking how *we* can learn and effect change together, our relationships become more reciprocal and responsive to all of our needs. I no longer feel I have to be the one who knows with certainty. A weight lifts because often there are few clear answers, but merit in shared searching for understanding. A contradiction is thrown up in that through practice enquiry I have developed expertise and clarity about how and why I do things. How do I balance clarity with uncertainty?

Respect for people

The shift towards collaborative enquiry relevant to the circumstances of individual families required me to trust parents to strive for better things for their children and themselves. I needed to become more responsive to needs parents identified rather than concentrating on my preoccupation with rights for children. My view of rights began to inform rather than lead our work. Respect for parents became as important as the respect I desired for their children. It became clearer when I saw *myself* as also worthy of respect because of my inherent human worth, as much as having it granted to me as a professional. I became aware of the enabling qualities of the warm, encouraging climate I experienced in an academic research group. Members boosted my confidence by showing me I had important knowledge. I wanted to replicate this climate for families.

I believe the growth of *respect* as a value is evident in my work with very discouraged families. I saw that people living with complex disadvantages do not need respect and self-determination less, as may result from some professional surveillance and interventions. They need to experience it *more* so they begin to respect themselves and, in turn, offer the same for their children. How could the mother above begin to respect herself and those around her when she rarely experienced respectful relationships herself? I saw that families may need support to enhance their self-worth before they begin to question their relationships. A history of disadvantages, including emotional isolation in family relationships, at school and under the gaze of health and social services as parents, may compound feelings of incompetence, alienation and discouragement. The remits of statutory services to promote health, protect children and educate might unintentionally undermine people's basic need for connection, personal significance and self-determination (Pound 2003, pp. 179–180).

Self-determination, containment and encouragement

I now recognise the importance of believing in one's own competence. After exploring a childhood experience of my own I concluded that I work well when I am self-directed and can see good sense in what I am doing. This helped me clarify the importance of helping others to feel in control and self-reliant in taking responsibility for their actions (Pound 2000, p. 368). I now see self-determination as another central tenet of alongsideness, if I am to enhance parents' belief in their ability to improve their lives and nurture the same for their children. Encouragement, as a way of engendering hope for the future, increasing self-worth and social connectedness grew in my awareness. Critique by other researchers and my own uncomfortable feelings showed where my values were denied in practice. Searching for contradictions is effective when held in contrast with espoused values. Identifying what is already useful practice is energising and increases understanding of relationship qualities that are valuable for encouraging each other's process. I believe that feeling encouraged and having a great deal of autonomy in my work and research enables my optimism and passion to endure in the face of uncertainty.

A questionnaire to my caseload of families in 1999 confirmed that, on the whole, I encourage parents and foster their self-determination. Some parents, however, declared frustration that I encouraged them to make their own decisions when they looked to be told what to do. These comments prompted my awareness that during certain times parents may want more advice from me. This call for direction is similar to a need to be physically or emotionally 'held' during periods of uncertainty (Shuttleworth 1999). When giving advice or 'containing' a client in this way I must avoid taking over and be sensitive to opportunities for sharing decisions when possible. This mirrors relationships that work with children as they cope with disappointment, tackle challenges and believe in themselves.

Power of connection and humour

Looking at videos of myself with families I recall the energy, willingness to co-operate and hope generated from our connectedness. We appear relaxed and open to exploring ideas in a process where everyone, including children, is included. Far from complacency or stasis of ideas, I see us willing to take risks because we feel safe together. The power of connection itself, therefore, appears educational and health enhancing. I find parents who are struggling with tortured personal histories can be less defensive and more open to new ideas and challenges when they experience and can trust the security between us. I noticed that our enquiring made warmer communication the desirable option for families and punishments less necessary.

My inclination towards light heartedness and humour stimulated questions and new awareness about how I am with people (Pound 2000, p. 373). I now recognise life-affirming energy from laughing together. I recall an incident with my small son when we had enjoyed belly laughter over nonsense. When finally we could not laugh any more he said, 'say it again, then we can laugh again'. I see this as a magic moment of shared togetherness, a brief at-oneness and under-standing of two equals in a sea of possible misunderstandings between two inher-ently unequal people (Pound 2003, p. 157). I recognised parents transcending despair and finding hope and renewed energy in the face of crisis by seeing the funny side of something (Pound 2000, p. 363).

Summarising literature about humour, du Pré reports psychological benefits, particularly that people who laugh together usually feel comfortable together (du Pré 1998, p. 26). Humour, she says, appears to invite greater social intimacy and serves as a buffer to emotions such as anxiety, anger, fear and embarrassment (1998, p. 22). Kuiper and Martin (1993) suggest that people who use humour as a coping mechanism are quick to laugh in common-place situations and tend to enjoy a more stable and positive sense of self. High humour users are said to judge themselves by less harsh and rigid standards, and regard themselves as more social and less given to depression. This suggests it is health enhancing to laugh and it may itself be a *sign* of wellbeing. I find laughing builds connection by reducing my power as we share silliness.

Process of becoming: offers a kind of evaluation

I came to appreciate Rogers' idea that as people we live in a process becoming more fully ourselves (1961). Research moved me through many stages of discovery to reach understanding of myself and my practice that I offer here. Much of my learn-ing was not through giant leaps but involved nuances of perspective or tiny addi-tions to my knowing in dialogue with families, research groups and critical friends. Commenting on the thesis a critical friend wrote, 'This is why the narrative process, which self-study entails, is so crucially important. Capturing microcosmic details entails 'macrocosmic' patterns to be perceived over time' (Pound 2003, p. 194).

Sometimes, leaps in understanding were bigger. For example, my move from blaming parents for their actions towards children, to searching for alongside re-lationships in co-learning processes of discovery. Being there for parents I now see as similar to effective parenting. We are all becoming more fully ourselves, clarifying and living our values. The wellbeing of one is dependent on the wellbe-ing and growth of others and I recognise our learning is entwined. This interde-pendence of self-enquiry has parallels with learning processes in psychotherapy (Rogers 1961), living educational action research (Whitehead 1989), and con-sciousness-raising for community action (Freire 1972).

I see three levels of evidence when family relationships change:

- what they learn from contact with me (e.g. 'Something you said made me think…')
- behaviour change ('I decided to try…')
- positive outcome ('It's better now…').

Often, parents describe greater harmony without attributing it to their increased empathy and changed behaviour. It is up to me to help them reflect on why it is better and help consolidate their learning so that it will sustain. I am now conscious of intuitively moving between reciprocity and professional responsibility.

Taking responsibility

Working with families with multiple intractable problems I asked how I balance priorities when acting to improve wellbeing of parents for children's benefit. In focusing my energy on supporting parents, the interests of children risked being overshadowed by the family's depth of need. A contradiction emerged when I needed to think about how alongside I could be with a mother involved in child-protection proceedings. Priority balancing requires me to consider the professional remit and my obligations to children while remembering parents' emotional needs. I became clearer that my purpose is to balance my intentions for all the family with wellbeing of children held as priority. In some situations I may use my professional power in acting on behalf of children. This professional action is similar to responsibility parents take in acting for their children. I invite parents into decision making as appropriate and return to more fully sharing power with them as soon as possible. Like children, parents usually see fairness even when struggling to contain their emotions. In these circumstances alongsideness is about maintaining connection and recognising their human worth no matter what has happened. Added value comes from talking about relationship qualities that calm and the benefits for children in their learning how to calm themselves. I notice meanings of the 'Crucial C' words *connect, capable, count* and *courage* are forming a common language with families and colleagues.

I found my actions may be interpreted by other practitioners as colluding with parents when viewed from different perspectives. When this has happened, I realised that each practitioner judges the engagement they can offer according to emotional confidence learned through life experiences. Practitioners seem to know the boundaries they need for keeping themselves and their clients safe. It is up to me to account for my actions and manage risk. I now see that health visitor training, supervision and practical resources, do not take full cognisance of the needs of families, their children or the professionals tackling such emotionally laden work. Families with long-term complex needs require psychotherapeutic awareness amongst professionals they meet; if beyond surveillance and practical help, the task is improving family relationships for wellbeing of the next generation. Critical reflective practice feels essential for clarifying why experiences awaken our personal histories and what represents empathy for clients. A colleague reminded me that it might be easier to act on professional surveillance protocols than therapeutic engagement. Leadership qualities and underlying values differ in these contradictory ways of working. Surveillance assumes professional power for identifying problems; therapeutic engagement is concerned with using relationship to support client's growth.

With regards to social workers, Banks noticed that some showed radical commitment to equality for meeting clients' need while others used organisational rules and procedures to define their expertise (1995, p. 129). Health-need profiling, like other acts of surveillance, does not easily lead into useful activity because of the competing requirements of effective practice. Ruth's story shows how she balances both.

The gap emerging between knowledge about early emotional development of children (Gerhardt 2004) and current criteria for assessing children in need (child protection policy) leaves a gulf of unmet need and a legacy of mental ill health for the future. Children and parents need long-term availability of support from professionals who offer unconditional regard, containment, information and encouragement in their journey to fruitful lives. In this way parents are supported in coping with challenges they may be ill-equipped to face, because of their early learning about relationships. In reality, such support may not be readily available to families. Because child protection intentions make health visiting relationships more complex, I believed long-term befriending might be better provided outside health, education or social service agendas. To this end, with parents I set up an independent family support group and crèche 'held' by a paid facilitator with psychotherapeutic training. It brings together disadvantaged, isolated families in a small city-centre estate. Parents respond to each other and their children in the respectful climate and carry their new friendships into the estate, but I notice they do not seek responsibility for running the group in the way Ruth and Annie have achieved. I am in awe of the breadth of activities they undertake so successfully. My learning from them comes from considering the balance of responsibility-taking with engagement and about working with other agencies.

Accepting differences

As my enquiry progressed I considered the influence of assumptions acquired in my New Zealand childhood and others formed during campaigning experiences. Questions emerged about prejudice and discrimination. I scrutinised some beliefs and became aware that I needed to be tentative in my assumptions about how others may interpret their beliefs in actions towards children (Pound 2003, p. 44). By remaining open to learn and accepting that people hold different beliefs, I could ask how my understanding influences my practice. Researcher Eden Charles questioned my explanation of alongsideness for tackling social inclusion by wondering if it was a way of manipulating people to comply with the social order that caused their exploitation and oppression in the first place. He showed how alongsideness for promoting acceptance into the dominant cultural view would miss opportunities to change or enrich our society qualitatively by challenging its ordering. He wrote, 'I want to work alongside others in creating new, fairer human relationships characterised by equity, justice and love more than uniformity. For me, this can only happen if the emphasis is not on including me within the existing order but working alongside me in evolving another one. This would involve all of us changing some. ' I wholeheartedly agree with Eden (email discussion: May 2004).

Alongsideness as reflective practice

Living theory action research provided a model for health visitors to reflect on their practice in our PCT from 2003 to 2004 (McNiff 2002). I found alongsideness equally rele-vant for enquiring with colleagues. As community practitioners we value our autonomy and need to recognise our competence and self-worth (Pound 2005). Moving our collaborative enquiries from problem-solving to valuing and building practice knowledge, proved energising. Ruth and I met in one of the groups and recognised similarities in our understanding of relationships for tackling social inclusion. I am grateful to her and Annie for expanding the possibilities of community development by fully involving the community whilst working closely with other agencies.

Reflective practice groups are considered for community and hospital clinicians in our Trust. In planning meetings I realised I could not share power with senior colleagues in the same way as with my clients because in this context I did not hold the power. Instead, I needed to establish credibility for what I had to offer and communicate the new methodology to people who inevitably viewed it through their personal lenses of what constitutes action learning, supervision and research. I came to realise that openness to new ideas may be influenced by individual investment in knowledge and power and readiness to embrace truly collaborative processes. I recognise it is common to be oblivious to gaps in our knowledge. Remaining open to possibilities requires continual commitment to learning.

I am fascinated by similarities between this organisational process and the public health campaigning of 10 years before. Now, I am in a climate ready for these ideas. After a hiccup in planning meetings when the others seemed slow to catch on, I realised I should remain conscious of starting where people are and go with them to the agreed new place. Alongsideness moves me from urgency to make others understand by using convincing explanations to a stance where I use my passion and enthusiasm to engender a spirit of enquiry. This means my contribution in the process is not overt. Recent experience is that this kind of influence may not prompt recognition of where ideas are coming from because it is a different kind of expertise in which everyone grows and owns it for themselves. I find it hard to secure paid recognition for such contributions to generating new ideas within the organisation. I took the same enthusiasm to a Department of Health Policy Collaborative for implementing children's policies. Alongsideness for influencing national policies beckons new avenues of reflection. Enquiring with Ruth has encouraged me to consider my alongside expertise and ask how I more overtly take responsibility for using my influence to effect organisational change.

Integrating our insights: leadership by alongsideness

Our excitement grew whilst writing this chapter as we shared our insights and found commonalities in our approaches. Here we integrate our understanding and differences in leadership styles working with families, in community development, awareness-raising public health and in influencing organisations. We agree about starting by valuing the knowledge and beliefs people already have and working with them towards the place they want to be. Leadership by alongsideness involves relationship qualities and skills that use professional power by acting in ways that influence change towards agreed aims. This does not fit easily with Department of Health requirements to provide recognisable outcomes for predefined illness prevention targets that are attributable to costed resources. It clarifies dilemmas for primary prevention that pull practitioners to act in ways that may disempower and further exclude the people we try to help.

Delivering choosing health helpfully builds on previous requirements for agencies to work together by calling for engagement of the public in improving their own health (DH 2005). It promises resources for tackling underlying determinants of ill health such as smoking, obesity and under-18 conception, particularly amongst most disadvantaged people. It does not, however, take into account how inequality and social exclusion come about in the first place and the complexity of what disadvantage really means to people who search for healthier lives. *Delivering choosing health* appears not to recognise that those excluded by disabling, oppressive life histories need a climate change capable of supporting a new inclusional social order underpinned by justice and encouragement. 'Inviting engagement' and 'providing information' calls for thoughtful professional relationships that enable people to be creative in coping with challenges and taking personal responsibility for making healthy choices.

We recognise how much there is to learn from all people we work with, no matter how disadvantaged they seem. Their journey is also our journey as we discover more about ourselves and the impact we make on community health. Together our process generates new ideas, mutually health enhancing and capable of influencing beyond ourselves. Reflective action research is valuable for developing our understanding about how to improve what we do. The value of reflection is enhanced further when shared with clients and colleagues. Collaborative reflection led us to view what we do as practice-as-enquiry as we encourage families and communities to take responsibility in deciding their future. Our alongside relationships hold subtle differences for each of us. This arises because embodied knowledge is built on who we are as people and life experiences contributing to how we see our worlds. We recognise Ruth's tremendous energy for working creatively with communities, other agencies and using local resources. Robyn enjoys working with families, small groups and professional colleagues across disciplines in promoting life as a process of enquiry. Core aspects of being alongside centre on respect for people and connections that engender trust, security and reciprocity. Connecting with others feels health enhancing in itself. We recognise integrity and emotional strength is necessary for withstanding doubt when promoting resilience in people and encouraging their ability to determine their own future. This requires us to show our belief in the personal significance and creative ability of everyone we meet. We each recognise our personal growth in these processes. Aboriginal educator Lilla Watson said:

'If you've come to help me you're wasting your time but if you've come because your liberation is bound up with mine then let's work together.'

(Wadsworth 1997, p. 17)

Dinkmeyer and Eckstein (1993) remind us that 'people need encouragement like plants need water'. Encouragement creates an optimistic climate that bolsters self-esteem, hope and independence. By encouraging reflective self-evaluation rather than reliance on others' opinions, people can experience their personal worth and learn to take responsibility for their actions. This is not to say the opinions of others are of no value, but individuals need to be assured of, and believe in, their own worth before critique is useful to them (Pound 2003). Encouragement turns mistakes into opportunities for learning. Being alongside is complex. We balance different skills and relationship styles for promoting learning through curiosity from empathic listening and encouragement to modelling, teaching, containing crises and using professional power. We recognise ourselves using what may appear to be contradictory skills appropriate to diverse situations, sometimes simultaneously, while keeping a vision of larger aims in mind.

Public health implies focus on the health of populations. We see populations to be consisting of individuals within communities. Our leadership by alongsideness is at the grass roots level of 'micro' public health towards tiny incremental change that is meaningful for families and ultimately their communities (Grant 2001). It recognises the importance of working with individuals, at a pace appropriate to their emerging awareness, as they embody and live new ideas in their actions. Public health targets inform our aims, but we see them as longer-term goals in which wellbeing, fostered by creating and sustaining relationships, is a first priority. Working with all clients and groups in this way begins to influence the wider social order (Whitehead 2004). Ruth's work shows influence on a community group. See also a similar approach by educator Moira Laidlaw as she promotes self-study and community empowerment in educational settings and has influenced significant change in a whole region of central China (http://www.actionresearch.net).

We recognise many public health practitioners work in similar ways in the course of becoming responsive to the populations they serve, but may not be able to explain or fully account for what they are doing. Methods of evaluation and language for explaining tacit knowledge implicit in effective relationships are currently underdeveloped in health research. Rayner et al (2002) recommend developing leadership through action learning. We found living theory action enquiry (Whitehead 1989) gave us confidence to speak in our own voices about the embodied knowledge we each carry and test as we practise. Personal values we independently clarify become standards we use for testing the validity of our claims to know what we are doing. In this way we improve, understand more fully and communicate our practice. Leadership development through critical enquiry feels important for influencing change in organisations and professional practice, especially for ensuring discriminatory practices do not continue (Reid & Phillps 2004). Values we clarified through enquiry align with values declared by our employing authority, however, we recognise that a list of organisational values does not ensure practitioners will embody and live them in their daily practice (Banks 1995). For this reason we are motivated to promote value-led collaborative action enquiry for developing leadership skills across community disciplines.

Conclusion

We are two health visitors who explored our leadership styles as we worked with families and communities, during public health work to raise awareness about health issues, and while trying to influenc organisations. We found leadership involves relationship qualities and skills that use professional power by acting in ways likely to influence change towards agreed aims. Reflective action research, our method of exploration, became integral to collaborative processes in the context of community public health at all levels. Leadership throuh alongsideness has become a way of being that integrates the embodied personal values of us as practitioners with the policy intentions of our employing public health authority in order to generate change. It involves searching for new ways of enriching society by engendering a spirit of collaborative critical enquiry that is inclusive of all the individuals within it. Leadership through alongsideness therefore has implications for practice, education, research and policy.

 ## DISCUSSION QUESTIONS

- What is important to me in how I approach working relationships? Which values motivate my actions?
- What concerns me in my practice? Where are my values not evident?
- What can I do to change it and who can help me?
- What evidence can I produce to show I act as I claim?
- How do I explain my style of working and show it is effective?

Acknowledgements

We feel privileged to learn from communities in these ways. Our gratitude lies with the families, our colleagues and other agencies.

References

Antonovsky A 1993 The structure and properties of the sense of coherence. Journal of Social Science and Medicine 36(6): 725–733

Antonovsky A 1998 Sense of coherence: historical and future perspective. In: McCubbin H, Thompson E, Thompson A, Fromer J (eds) Stress, coping and health in families. Sage, California

Banks S 1995 Ethic and values in social work. BASW/Macmillian, London

Brazelton 1992 Touchpoints: Your child's emotional and behavioural development. Penguin, London

Connelly M, Clandinin J 1990 Stories of experience and narrative enquiry. Educational Researcher 19(5): 2–14

Department of Health (DH) 1998a Independent inquiry into inequalities in health. HMSO, London

Department of Health (DH) 1998b Towards an evidence-base for health services. HMSO, London

Department of Health (DH) 1999 Saving lives: our healthier nation. HMSO, London

Department of Health (DH) 2000 The NHS plan: a plan for investment: a plan for reform. HMSO, London

Department of Health (DH) 2005 Delivering choosing health: making healthier choices easier. Department of Health, London

Dinkmeyer D, Eckstein D 1993 Leadership by encouragement. Kendall/Hunt, Dubuque, USA

Dreikurs R, Soltz V 1964 Children: the challenge. Hawthorn, New York

du Pré A 1998 Humour and the healing arts: a multi-method analysis of humour use in health care. Lawrence Erlbaum Associates, Hove, UK.

Freire P 1972 Pedagogy of the oppressed Penguin, London

Gerhardt S 2004 Why love matters. Brunner-Routledge, Hove, UK

Grant R 2001 A qualitative study to test the hypothesis that the population of Peasedown holds knowledge of their health and health needs for informing services. Unpublished MSc thesis held in CPHVA electronic library

Grant R 2005 Lay perceptions of health and health needs. Community Practitioner 78(4): 133–139

Johnson H, Mayoux L 1998 Investigation as empowerment: using participatory methods. In: Thomas A, Chataway J, Wuyts M (eds.) Finding out fast: investigative skills for policy and development. Sage, London

Kuiper N, Martin R 1993 Humour and self concept. Humour International: Journal of Humour Research 6: 251–270

Lew A, Bettner B 1996 A parents guide to understanding and motivating children. Raising Kids Who Can Series. Connexions Press, Media, Pennsylvania

McNiff J 2002 3rd edition. Action research for professional development: concise advice for new action researchers. Free download available from http://www.jeanmcniff.com/booklet1.html

Ong B, Humphris G 1994 Prioritising needs with communities: rapid appraisal methodologies on health. In: Popay J, Williams G (eds) Researching the people's health. Routledge, London

Parston G, Timmins N 1998 Joined-up management. Public Health Management Foundation, London

Pound R 2000 The significance of personal history in the values and agendas of health visitors. Educational Action Research 8(2): 361–376

Pound R 2003 How can I improve my health visiting support of parenting? The creation of an alongside epistemology through action enquiry. Unpublished PhD. University of the West of England. Online. Available at: http://www.actionresearch.net. Thesis Section

Pound R 2005 How can I/we support the development of family-centred health visiting for improving wellbeing and reducing social exclusion? Collaborative enquiry report. Web link to Robyn's page through http://www.actionresearch.net

Rayner D, Chisholm H, Appleby H 2002 Developing leadership through action learning. Nursing Standard 16(29): 37–39

Reid R, Phillips T 2004 The best intentions? Race, equity and delivering today's NHS. Fabian Society, London

Rogers C 1961 On becoming a person: A therapist's view of psychotherapy. Houghton Mifflin, Boston

Sewell D, Wade N 2000 Quality of life 2: A community participatory appraisal of health perceptions and needs for Thornton Estate Community. Goodwin Centre, Hull

Shuttleworth A 1999 How have we changed? Paper delivered to ACP 50th birthday conference, London

Wadsworth Y 1997 Everyday evaluation on the run. Unwin & Allen, London

Whitehead J 1989 Creating a living theory from questions of the kind, 'How do I improve my practice?' Cambridge Journal of Education 19(1): 137–153

Whitehead J 2004 Can I communicate the educational influence of my embodied values, in self-studies of my own education, in the education of others and in the education of social formations, in a way that contributes to a scholarship of educational enquiry? Presentation for the Fifth international Conference of S-STEP, 27 June–1 July 2004 http://www.actionresearch.net

World Health Organization 1998 The World Health Organization Quality of Life Assessment (WHOQOL). Development and general psychometric properties. Social Science Medical 46(12): 1569–1585

Further reading

http://www.actionresearch.net for links to practitioner action research enquiries

Marmot M, Wilkinson R (eds) 2000 Social determinants of health. Oxford University Press, Oxford

Mosak H, Maniacci M. 1999 A primer of Adlerian psychology: the analytic-behavioral-cognitive psychology of Alfred Adler. Brunner-Routledge, London

Whitehead J, McNiff J 2006 Action Research Living Theory. Sage, London

Quality in a public health service: 13
the 3-5-7 Model

Sinead Hanafin

Key issues

- Understanding service quality in public health services can be difficult because:
  - different stakeholders have different perceptions and priorities
  - different organisational contexts have differing resources
  - outcome measurement, the dominant paradigm in health services, creates difficulties in respect of attribution, longitudinality and the need for change to take place
- This model emerged from a two-phase collective case study of the Irish public health nursing service to families with infants where data were collected from public health nurses, managers and clients
- The model draws on the work of Donabedian and comprises three main parts *viz.* organisational context, process and consequences, all of which are operationalised. Five key concepts, time, knowledge, communication, environment and orientation, are presented as the links between these three parts. Seven steps of process were identified
- Although developed in the Irish public health nursing service, the model can be applied in many other contexts. It can be used, for example, to provide a framework for reviewing existing services, for planning new services, for examining why things went wrong (or why they did not) and for setting standards
- The model presented here provides a mechanism for measuring service quality in a holistic way that takes account of key stakeholder perceptions; the process of the service and the organisational context within which people operate

Introduction

Longman's (1990) definition of quality as 'the degree to which something is excellent; a standard of goodness' (p. 848) assumes that quality is tangible, identifiable and conceptually clear. This may be an appropriate assumption to make in the industrial sector where a clearly identifiable product emerges at the end of a strictly controlled process. In the health care setting, however, where there is infinite demand but finite resources, undemanding clients, complex consumers, a 'high intangible' content and a significant professional component (Øvretveit 1992), this is not the case. It is not surprising, therefore, that, within the heath care literature, the concept of quality has been variously described as slippery and elusive (Pfeffer & Coote 1991), nebulous and lacking consistent definition (Van Maanen 1979) and 'enigmatic and multi-dimensional' (Attree 1993, p. 369) and this has, in turn, led to a proliferation of different understandings of quality.

Quality has been identified, for example, as a political issue (Shaw 1997), a social construct (Redfern & Norman 1990), a philosophy (Øvretveit 1992), professional standards (Dozier 1998), customer satisfaction (Kleinsorge & Koeing 1991), an attribute of a product (Kerrison et al 1994), a system of management (National Standards Authority of Ireland (NSAI 1998) and effectiveness (Katz et al 2004). These differing conceptualisations result in different elements of the service being prioritised over others and this has implications for measurement. While budget holders, for example, will want to include in their assessment a measure of the cost of the service, this may not be the priority for professionals, whose main concern may be that they have adhered to a professional standard. A client who is unable to access the service because it is only available during normal working hours may assess the service as being of poor quality. Other stakeholders, such as the manager or the service provider, however, may evaluate the same service as being of good quality because their main focus may be on the advice given or the user friendliness of the hospital or health centre.

Øvretveit (1992), in the health care context, identifies three key stakeholder perspectives and these are:

- *Client quality* (what clients and carers want from the service).
- *Professional quality* (whether the service meets needs as defined by professional providers and referrers).
- *Management quality* (the most effective and productive use of resources).

In a holistic account of a service, an understanding of each of these perspectives is necessary and further, in the measurement of service quality, this must be operationalised.

Other issues also arise. Donabedian (1988) contends that before quality can be defined, broader principles must be considered, including whether one takes into account only the performance of practitioners or whether the contributions of patients and of the health care system should also be considered. While it is generally accepted that a service has an impact on a client's needs, less attention has been paid to the impact of client's needs on a service and this is particularly the case in community nursing services where even single differences in client group composition, such as social class, can have a significant impact on the work of a public health nurse or health visitor (Reading & Allen 1997, Horrocks et al 1998, Crofts et al 2000).

Other issues also arise, including, for example, how broadly health and responsibility for health are defined; whether maximally or optimally effective care is sought; and, crucially, on whose view that level of care is determined. It is clear, therefore, that quality is a multi-dimensional, multi-faceted concept that can be constructed in a variety of different ways depending on whose perspective or what perspective is dominant and on what elements of the service are taken into account.

While the difficulties outlined above could emerge in respect of almost all services, additional difficulties emerge in respect of public health work where prevention is often a key aim.

Categories of measurement

Two broad categories of measurement have been proposed and these are process measurement and outcome measurement. Judgements of the quality of a service can change depending on where the focus of the measurement is. The example shown in Box 13.1 demonstrates the difference in how the service is judged, depending on whether the focus of the assessment is on the process or outcome.

Box 13.1

Example of difference between process and outcome measurement

In the course of a home visit by the health visitor, a mother of a 4-month-old infant, with whom she has a very good relationship, indicates her intention to give up breastfeeding on her return to work the following month. The health visitor shares her knowledge about the area, communicates it in a non-judgemental way, provides written background material and gives the mother the phone number of a helpline where she can get support. The mother chooses to wean the infant and not continue breastfeeding

If the focus of the assessment is on the process then this service might be judged as very good. If the focus, however, is on the outcome (continuation of breastfeeding) then the process may well be judged as poor.

Outcome measurement has been the dominant paradigm in relation to service quality and an outcome has been defined as:

'… not simply a measure of health, well-being or any other state but rather, a change in status confidently attributable to antecedent care.'

(Donabedian 1988, p. 1745)

Although some authors subscribe fully to this definition (Lohr 1988), others suggest that the predetermination of change as well as a change in status may not be necessary (Bond & Thomas 1991). In the context of public health a sole focus on outcome measurement is very problematic. Public health has been defined as:

'… the science and art of preventing disease, prolonging life and promoting health through organised efforts of society.'

(Acheson 1998, p. 289)

A number of concerns arising from the use of outcomes as measures of service quality in public health have been identified in the literature and these are presented in Box 13.2 below.

A key focus of public health work can be understood to be preventive and this concept has proven very difficult to measure (Barriball & Mackenzie 1993, Campbell et al 1995, Hall 1996, Macleod Clark et al 1997). Factors influencing changes in behaviour have been identified as multi-factorial and, further, changes generally take place over a long period of time (Dines & Cribb 1993, Naidoo & Wills 1994, Tones & Tilford 1994). In these situations, questions arise in respect of longitudinality, attribution and valid outcome measures.

Attribution is considered by a number of authors to be a core element in the measurement of quality outcomes (Donabedian 1988, Redfern & Norman 1990, Schuster et al 1997). The multi-dimensional nature of many public health interventions, means however, that 'outcomes are not predictable, and the lines of attribution are unclear' (Campbell et al 1995, p. 30). Substantial challenges are posed in determining a cause–effect relationship and, indeed, the work of epidemiologists is almost exclusively focused on this area in respect of disease causation (Hennekens & Buring 1987, Mausner & Kramer 1985). In an epidemiological context, it is assumed that unless the principles of Koch's postulates (strength of the association, dose–response, consistency of the association, temporally correct association, specificity of the association, and biological plausibility) can be satisfied, a relationship should not be considered cause-and-effect (Mausner & Kramer 1985). Even where only a single disease with a single intervention is under scrutiny, a considerable body of research is required to establish indicators for all of

307

Box 13.2

Questions arising in respect of outcome measurement

- Is the outcome reflective of some change that takes place?
- Can the change be attributed to a particular intervention?
- Was the outcome predetermined?
- Is a focus on measuring this exerting an influence on the activity?
- Is the measure being interpreted in a way that discriminates in favour of people for whom such gain can be easily achieved?
- What is the cost of collecting the data ?

these postulates. How then can attribution be assigned in interventions that are multi-faceted, multi-disciplinary and multi-sectoral?

Predetermination of outcomes is also a key element of outcome identification. Public health is often focused on the identification of health needs in conjunction with the population itself. The search for, and stimulation of an awareness of health needs means that the specific predetermination of outcome is not possible. There is a paradigmatic gulf between a need for predetermined outcomes and an understanding of the service as one premised on the shared establishment of 'need' (i.e. shared by public health practitioners and the community).

Other difficulties have also been associated with outcome measurement. It has been suggested, for example, that the art of collecting data is not neutral and that, further, it exerts an influence on the activity it is intended to reflect (Cowley 1994). Whitehead (1993) raises concerns about the possibility that health authorities are interpreting health gain in a way that discriminates in favour of those for whom such gain can be easily achieved. Further, the cost of collecting data on outcome measures may be prohibitive in many situations.

The foregoing discussion clearly highlights the difficulties associated with outcome measurement in respect of the quality of a service. Despite these difficulties it is clear that some form of service quality measurement must take place since the maxims 'What gets measured gets done'; and 'If something cannot be measured, it cannot be improved' have some merit in today's health care environment. In an era where many Western countries are developing performance indicators for their health care services, it is simply untenable to suggest that public health work cannot be measured in some way. Issues relating to process are discussed later.

Themes, models, frameworks and dimensions of quality

The conceptual challenges outlined earlier are, in turn, mirrored in the multiplicity of approaches that have been identified, and themes, dimensions, models, frameworks and theories have all been presented as mechanisms through which an understanding of service quality can be facilitated.

The three main 'gurus' of what is known as total quality management (TQM) are Crosby, Demming and Juran. Joss and Kogan (1995) identify a number of common themes emerging from a comparison of aspects from their work:

- staff commitment (especially from management)
- the production of a medium- and long-term organisation-wide corporate plan

- putting structures in place
- process improvement through a commitment to continuous quality improvement
- costs of quality (and also cost of non-conformance)
- quality of information
- empowering and valuing all staff (through bottom-up approaches)
- focusing on the customer
- training and education
- monitoring and evaluation
- achieving a TQM culture.

There is much crossover between these themes and those of clinical governance, introduced in the UK and conceptually underpinned by:

'Doing the right thing, for the right person at the right time and getting it right first time, every time.'

(Donaldson & Muir Gray 1998, p. 28).

Clinical governance focuses on the creation of systems, to ensure safe and effective clinical practice (Huntington 2000, Pringle 2000) as well as individual accountability (Allen 2000). Components include:

- evidence-based practice through the creation of opportunities for staff to undertake professional development (Scally & Donaldson 1998)
- continuous quality improvement (Baker et al 1999)
- cohesion, integration and co-operation at a system level (Malcolm & Mays 1999) and cultural change through the development of technical skills, structural skills and effective leadership (Cambell & Proctor 1999, Huntington 2000).

Others have presented 'models' of quality. In the corporate sector, Haywood-Farmer (1987), for example, proposed a *'conceptual model of service quality'* that takes in to account three types of quality service attributes as follows: physical facilities, processes and procedures; people's behaviour and conviviality; and professional judgement. Itagaki (1997, p. 26) presented a *'hybrid evaluation mode'*, which compared configurations of 'application and adaptation' in industrial settings. Jaros and Dostal (1999, p. 197) describe a model based on teleonics, where rather than being physically bounded, systems are informationally bonded. They report that their theory of teleonics 'arose from a dialectic inter-action between theory and praxis'.

Models of quality have also been presented in the nursing and midwifery literature. Martin-Hirch and Wright (1998), for example, report on a *'quality mode'* to measure effective midwifery services. Their model identifies *client* [constant independent (ethnicity, culture, language and religion) and inconstant specific variables (equity, information, continuity, choice and control, each of equal importance)] and *service provider* elements (tangible and intangible elements). Rantz et al (1999) report on the development of *'a multi-dimensional theoretical model'* to integrate the views of consumers and providers in nursing-home care quality. Here, consumers' and providers' views were integrated around the dimensions of family involvement, communication, environment, staff, care and home. Williams (1998) reports on the use of grounded theory to develop a 'substantive theory' on the delivery of quality nursing care from the perspective of the nurse. This substantive theory included time available, conditions, quality of nursing care and selective focusing.

Yet others argue for different approaches to quality. Pffefer and Coote (1991) propose a democratic approach to quality that acknowledges differences between commerce and welfare as well as drawing on scientific (fitness for purpose), excellence (responsiveness), and consumerist (empowerment) approaches to quality. Maxwell (1984) presents the following dimensions and suggests each needs to be included when considering issues of quality: access to services; relevance to need (for the whole community); effectiveness (for individual patients); equity (fairness); social acceptability; efficiency and economy. Many of these were also presented by Donabedian (1990) in his seven 'pillars' of quality including efficacy, effectiveness, efficiency, optimality, acceptability, legitimacy, and equity.

Any one of the dimensions identified above, however, could form the whole focus for measurement leading to difficulties in prioritisation. Further, different dimensions may be in competition with each other. Equity, for example, may be forfeited in a situation where cost-effectiveness is to the fore, and cost-effectiveness forfeited in a situation where equity is to the fore (Vågerö 1994).

A foucs on process

Process measures have also been suggested, but are also problematic. Process has been defined as:

'…what is actually done in giving and receiving care. It includes the patient's activities in seeking care and carrying it out, as well as the practitioner's activities in making a diagnosis and recommending or implementing treatment.'

(Donabedian 1988, p. 1745)

Many of the processes of the work of public health practitioners remain unexposed, unarticulated and unexplained. The literature on the process of health visiting in the UK demonstrates the complexity of the process when interacting with any individual client (Chalmers 1992, 1993, 1994, Cowley 1991, 1995a, 1995b, 1999, de la Cuesta 1993, 1994, Knott & Latter 1999, Luker & Chalmers 1989, Macleod Clark et al 1997). Cowley (1991, p. 655) writes:

'It has often seemed difficult for health visitors to explain and articulate the deep processes buried within their work; considerable interpersonal skill and receptivity seem to be needed to negotiate the complexities embedded in the process of "stimulating an awareness of health needs". Highly developed professional expertise and non-verbal knowledge may be internalized, thus become "invisible", being recognized only as "intuition".'

The complexity of the process when interacting with one individual is daunting. In a situation where the community or population is the 'client', it is likely that this complexity is magnified. Under the Ottawa Charter (WHO 1986) a number of key public health strategies have been proposed and these include:

- the creation of healthy public policy
- development of supportive environments
- strengthening of community action
- development of personal skills
- re-orientation of health service.

Public health practitioners may have an operational focus on individual elements of any one of these, or they may have a broader, more strategic focus. The processes through which these strategies can be enacted and the circumstances under which they are successfully implemented are likely to be multi-faceted, multi-layered and require many different and complex parallel processes. Most community development work is, by its nature, invisible and requires a strong local understanding of political barriers and needs (Griffiths et al 2003). A focus on social mobilisation, for example, might include community competency, community empowerment, social capital, social connectedness, peer and community norms, public opinion and public mandate for policy action, and community ownership of the programme (Nedham 2000). Any one of these elements, however, might include many different processes and, given the complex and hidden nature of these processes, many questions arise in respect of measurement.

The work of two authors has come to the fore in providing a framework for looking at the process of service delivery. One author focuses on the work of public health nurses (Byrd 1995, 1997, 1998), while the other focuses on the client's journey through the health care system (Øvretveit 1992). The flow-process model presented by Øvretveit (1992) comprises eight components and these are: selection, entry, first contact, assessment, intervention, review, closure and follow-up. The author suggests that by tracing a typical client's career through the service from the client's point of view, it is possible to identify situations and encounters where the client may perceive the service to be poor or where his/her experiences are perceived to be worse than his/her expectations.

The elements of the model are similar to those of the process of home visiting observed by Byrd (1995) from a public health nursing perspective (Table 13.1). Byrd proposes that child-focused home visiting patterns are conducted in three distinct patterns: single, short and long term. The three models presented by Byrd are:

- preliminary process (Byrd 1997)
- child-focused, single home visiting (Byrd 1997)
- long-term maternal–child home visiting (Byrd 1998).

The steps of process outlined in each of Byrd's model highlight differences according to the purpose of the visit. In addition, each of these processes is concerned with home visiting rather than with general interaction between public health practitioner and client. Nevertheless, the steps outlined above provide some explication of the process through which a service is delivered. Both models, however, are deficient in terms of quality because neither provide a mechanism through which the elusive and nebulous concept of quality can be made overt.

Table 13.1 ● Steps of three process models presented by Byrd (Byrd 1995, 1997, 1998)

Preliminary model	Child-focused single home visiting process	Long-term maternal–child home visiting
Identifying medium contacting, going to see, entering, seeing, terminating, telling	Surveying and designating, selling and scheduling, approaching the home, entering the home, gaining permission, making the care-giving judgement, ending the visit, haunting and telling	Responding and scheduling approaching the home, entering the the home, starting with mothers expressed concern, supporting and validating, care-giving, ending the visit, after the visit, maternal consequences, child consequences, environmental consequences

Donabedian

The most referenced framework used in service quality is that proposed by Donabedian: structure, process and outcome (SPO). It has been used in the setting of standards of nursing care (Barker 1991, Maycock 1989, Parsley & Corrigan 1994), ethical principles and health care quality (Huycke & All 2000), the identification of medical outcomes (Tarlov et al 1989), organisational effectiveness (Mark et al 1997), the assessment of palliative day care (Douglas et al 2000), evaluation of discharge planning (Closs & Tierney 1993), a primary health care setting (Coyle 2000), and auditing nursing care (Clarke et al 1998). Others have used Donabedian's SPO as the basis for the development of their own models (Attree 1996, Holzemer 1994, Mitchell et al 1998).

Donabedian's assertion that all three (structure, process and outcome) approaches are necessary suggests a holistic commitment to assessing service quality, see Box 13.3 below.

'For now, all that is needed is to accept provisionally that there are three major approaches to quality assessment: "structure," "process," and "outcome." This three-fold approach is possible because there is a fundamental functional relationship among the three elements, which can be shown schematically.'

(Donabedian 1980, p. 83)

The relationship shown by Donabedian (1980) is as follows:

Structure → Process → Outcome

There have been a number of criticisms of Donabedian's framework. Problems with delineation of the categories of structure, process and outcome have been

---

Box 13.3

Definition of elements of Donabedian's framework

Structure denotes:

'...the attributes of the settings in which care occurs. This includes the attributes of material resources (such as facilities, equipment and money), of human resources (such as the number and qualifications of personnel), and of organisational structure (such as medical staff organisation, methods of peer review and methods of reimbursement.'

(Donabedian 1988, p. 1745)

Process is:

'...what is actually done in giving and receiving care. It includes the patient's activities in seeking care and carrying it out, as well as the practitioner's activities in making a diagnosis and recommending or implementing treatment.'

(Donabedian 1988, p. 1745)

Outcome is:

'The effects of care on the health status of patients and populations. Improvements in the patient's knowledge and salutary changes in the patient's behaviour are included under a broad definition of health status, and so is the degree of the patient's satisfaction with care.'

(Donabedian 1988, p. 1745)

identified by a number of authors (Closs & Tierney 1993, Fihn 2000, Parsley & Corrigan 1994). Fihn, for example, wrote that 'knowledge is the key to good quality care and knowledge is in and of itself neither a structure nor a process' (p. 1741). This is clearly problematic, because delineating concepts, a key element of theoretical development, can be difficult if one item crosses two categories (Davidson Reynolds 1971). Donabedian never dealt satisfactorily with this criticism. The second problem related to the way in which others constructed Donabedian's work and many authors understood Donabedian's work as giving primacy to outcome measurement over process (Badger 1999, Carr-Hill 1994, Coyle 2000, Mitchell et al 1998). Carr-Hill, in making a case for process measures of care, lamented the 'over-indoctrination' of people by Donabedian's focus on outcome. Donabedian himself, however, has made the case many times for the primacy of process over outcome (Donabedian 1968, 1980, 1988, 1993). As recently as 1993, he wrote:

'I place the interaction of patients and practitioners at the centre of the health care universe because I believe that it is there that the processes and decisions most critical to quality take place.'

(Donabedian 1993, p. 33).

Despite these criticisms, the SPO framework proposed by Donabedian has the capacity to take account of services in a holistic way that includes the organisational context within which people work, the process of the service and the consequences of the service. For these reasons, the study on developing a holistic model of service quality was broadly guided by his work.

A holistic model of service quality

The rest of the chapter draws heavily on a holistic model of service quality, which was developed through research about the public health nursing service to families with infants. The study methods are summarised in Box 13.4. The model is 'holistic' because it incorporates multiple stakeholders' views, takes account of the organisational context within which the service is provided and enables both process and consequence to be taken into account.

Overview of 3-5-7 model of service quality

The model of service quality can briefly be understood as having:

- 3 parts (organisational context, process and consequence)
- 5 concepts (time, knowledge, communication, environment and orientation)
- 7 steps of process (initiating, converging, preparing, opening, interacting, closing, follow-up).

Although the model was developed specifically through a study about the organisational context, process and consequences of the Irish public health nursing service delivery to families with infants, the model presented here is both flexible and applicable to a range of other services. The model is presented in Figure 13.1.

Definition and explanation of each component

In this model, the organisational context is broadly similar to Donabedian's structure and refers to the context within which a service is provided. Three constituent parts were identified and these are *people, policy and place*.

Box 13.4

Methodology

A two-phase, collective case study approach was used to research the public health nursing service to families with infants in the Republic of Ireland [a more detailed explanation of the methodology is presented elsewhere (Hanafin 2003, Hanafin & Cowley 2006)]. Phase one involved collecting quantitative and qualitative data, through a national census of public health nurses (PHNs) (response rate 54%; $n = 946$), PHN managers (response rate 75%; $n = 24$) and small group interviews ($n = 5$). In phase two, group ($n = 3$) and individual ($n = 14$) interviews with clients, PHNs and PHN managers were carried out and data emerging from these were supplemented by non-participant observation of the public health nursing service at each of four case study sites.

Analysis of the questionnaire was undertaken using the software package SPSSx and descriptive and inferential techniques. Analysis of individual cases, using concepts, categories and codes was followed by cross-case analysis and triangulation of data, sources and methods. This was facilitated by qualitisation of quantitative data, which was undertaken on completion of the statistical analysis and involved writing the findings in profile documents according to each section of the questionnaire (Tashakkori & Teddlie 1998).

The analysis resulted in a thick description of the structure, process and consequences of the public health nursing service provided along with the identification of five key concepts. These elements form the basis for the model of service quality presented in this chapter.

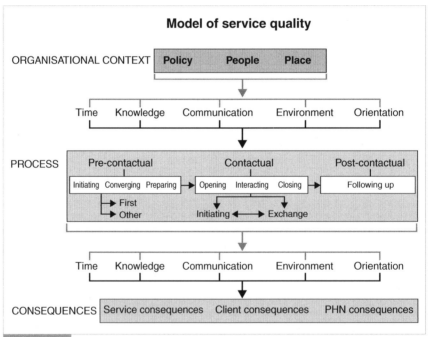

Figure 13.1 ● Model of service quality (Hanafin & Cowley 2006)

Organisational context

POLICY Policy can be understood as a course or principle of action adopted or proposed by a government, party, business or individual (Oxford Dictionary). Policies that influence the organisational context may be related to the service provision, the client group or the overall context within which the service is provided. It can be influenced by local, regional or national policies. Worksheet 13.1 sets out the main elements for consideration.

PEOPLE. Here, all the people who can potentially have an influence on the service should be included. At a minimum this includes the client group, the practitioner and the management team. In addition, other formal and informal service providers to whom, or from whom, referral takes place should be included. Worksheet 13.2 provides an overview of the main elements of this aspect of organisational context, which can be used as a template for assessing your own service.

PLACE. This refers to the where the service takes place and where it is accessed and provided. In respect of the public health nursing service it is this part of the service that differentiates it from other nursing services because the service is provided in the community and also in the person's home, rather than within an institutional setting. Worksheet 13.3 provides you with an opportunity to identify key issues relating to the place of service provision.

Process of service delivery

The process of the service can be broken down into 7 steps,

- 3 of which occur prior to contact
- 3 during the time of contact
- 1 post contact.

PRE-CONTACTUAL PHASE Initating. This is the first step in the process and it includes the rationale for, and mechanisms through which, the process of service delivery takes place. Differences between the first and subsequent steps in how initiation takes place are important to take into account.

Converging. This step is so named because it describes the coming together of stakeholders following the initiation of the process. In order for converging to take place the stakeholders must be available at a mutually suitable time and place, and all parties must have knowledge of these aspects. The step of converging is particularly crucial in situations where client initiation is the norm, such as parent help-lines.

Preparing. Some preparation may need to take place prior to contact. In a situation where, for example, a health visitor is undertaking a home visit, she may read up on previous contacts with the client. It is also important to note, however, that the client may also need to make preparations, including, for example, arranging for a partner to accompany them to the health centre or making arrangements for other children to be cared for. In a situation where a public health practitioner is doing a presentation for a local community group, the practitioner must prepare the presentation. The local community group, however, may need to ensure the venue is available, the necessary equipment is in place and those expected to attend notified.

CONTACTUAL PHASE The time of contact has three steps, which are opening, interacting and closing. During the time of 'interacting' many different issues may be discussed or activities undertaken, such as providing advice on feeding, undertaking a developmental check or weighing the infant. Regardless of the specific activity, an understanding of service quality is constructed on the basis of each one of these three steps.

Opening. This step takes place when stakeholders come in either direct face-to-face, or telephone, contact with each other. In many situations this is a relatively uncomplicated step but in some situations it can be difficult. Where 'cold calling' takes place, for example, it may be difficult to explain the purpose of the contact. Many resources have been invested in recent years in ensuring that telephones are answered in a friendly way.

Interacting. This step forms the substance of the contact between public health nurses (PHN) and client and it is usual for several of these to take place during each time of contact.

Worksheet 13.1 ● Policy

	Description PHN service	Key influences	Description your own service	Key influences
Broad national policy	Welfare state Democratic state Health service executive	Approx. 50% population private health care insurance Approx. 30% population entitled to all health care services free 100% population entitled to free child health services		
Service policy	Single practitioner for multiple client groups Geographically attached Child protection vs. child health Garda (police) vetting of health care workers Number of contacts between client and PHN	Overall population composition Free service to all (in contrast with the GP service) Self referral Non-mandatory reporting of child abuse Children First child protection guidelines		
Client group policies	Maternity leave Parental leave Childcare policies	National Children's Strategy Commission on the Family Child Care legislation		
Other				

Worksheet 13.2 ● People

	Description PHN service	Key influences	Description your own service	Key influences
Client	Families with infants < 1year	Population size Level of deprivation Extent of family support locally Male and female workforce participation rate Perceptions of service		
Practitioner	Public health nurse	Level of basic, post-registration and on-going education Length of time in area Other public health nursing support Importance of this type of work		
Manager	Assistant director of public health nursing Director of public health nursing	Positioning within overall management structure; Management style Ability to seek and get resources Importance attached to this work		
Formal support services	Multi-disciplinary team – speech, therapists, social workers, etc. Other health service agencies Other sectors inc. education, childcare, etc.	Availability of other professionals Contactability Referral and feedback structures Knowability Approaches to working (e.g. partnership)		
Informal support services	Structured funded voluntary services, e.g. St Vincent de Paul; Community mothers; La Leche, Barnardos Unstructured supports, e.g. local breastfeeding support groups; local activists	Availability Contactability Referral and feedback structures Knowability Approaches to working (e.g. partnership)		
Other				

Worksheet 13.3 ● Place

	Description PHN service	Key influences	Description your own service	Key influences
Location of service	Rural/urban Socio-economic status Demographics Institutional	Geographically dispersed or densely population Levels of material or other deprivation Influence of geographic attachment Community		
Setting for contact	Home Community	Choice of setting Suitability and accessibility of health centre		
Other				

The step of interacting can be understood as having two parts:

1. **Initiating** an interaction refers to raising an individual issue or topic and this shares many common features with the initiation of service process in the time before contact. Its importance to service quality lies in stakeholders' willingness and ability to raise any particular issue, question or topic as a focus during the interaction.

2. **Exchange** is so named because each component generally involves 'giving' and 'receiving' by both PHN and client. Each contact usually comprises many different exchanges and in the context of health visiting work may include:
    *   building relationships
    *   support
    *   giving advice and information
    *   assessment and identification of need
    *   general need
    *   maternal need
    *   infant wellbeing, growth, development, neglect and abuse
    *   practical help.

Closing. The contactual phase ends with a step of closing and, as with the step of opening, this may simply be a matter of indicating that the contact has come to an end. Generally, this step does not emerge as having an influence on service quality unless it was ended abruptly or some problem arose.

POST-CONTACTUAL PHASE

Following-up. The final step in the process of service delivery is follow-up and this takes place after completion of the contactual phase. It is so named because, in respect of service quality, stakeholders must act on the findings of the previous phase and what takes place during this phase can influence constructions of service quality. In the development of community services the follow-up may include, for example, making an application for funding or arranging for others to become involved in the development.

In summary, within this model, the process of service quality extends before and after the time of direct contact between client and PHN. Seven steps were identified and three of these take place prior to contact and one following contact. The seven steps are: initiating, converging, preparing, opening, interacting, closing and following-up.

Worksheet 13.4 provides a framework for you to describe your service. Data emerging from the study on the Irish public health nursing service are presented as a guide.

Consequences

The term 'consequences' is used here to describe the effects of the process of the service, because I believe the description provided does not meet the definitional requirements of 'outcome'. Other authors, for example, Byrd (1998), have also used the term 'consequences' to illustrate the effects of the service. The three components of consequences presented here reflect the multiplicity of stakeholders and here they include those of the service, the practitioner and the client.

SERVICE CONSEQUENCES Service consequences are those that occur in respect of the service itself. Within this, issues of availability, contactability, flexibility and knowability all arise. In the corporate sector, 'knowability', or the extent to which people know about the purpose, components and availability of the service, forms the basis for advertising and many companies have significant budgets for this.

CLIENT CONSEQUENCES These may have some commonalities (for example, client satisfaction) irrespective of the service under examination. In the health care sector, however, consequences are likely to include issues relating to accurate and timely diagnosis and improvements in wellbeing.

Worksheet 13.4 ● Process

PHN service to families with infants description of each step	Describe the process of your service
Pre-contactual phase	
Initiation First contact Other provider initiation of contact	Usually PHN initiated in response to statutory obligation Mandatory policy Personal orientation Response to client need identified by client or other agency, organisation, professional
Client initiation (client)	General need to know everything is OK Specific practical, physical Psychological Financial need
Converging	Client and PHN Availability of client and PHN for contact Information about availability and contactability Decision about venue
Preparing	PHN: Identify all known information Bring necessary equipment/literature Make appointment Client: Presenting the house/children at their best Arrange for other children to be cared for during clinic visits Arrangements for getting to
Contactual phase	

Opening

Negotiate entry
Changes depending on whether contact has been pre-arranged and on whether this is the first or subsequent contact

Interacting
Initiation of interaction

Client:
Perceptions of service focus
Prior experience
Preference of PHN service over others
Relationships with PHN
Suitable environment

PHN:
Location
Timing
Topic
Rationale for raising issue

Exchange

Components
Building a relationships
Giving support
Advice and information
Assessment and identification of general (normal vs abnormal) and specific (wellbeing, growth development, abuse, feeding) maternal and infant needs
Broader family health and well-being

Closing

Closing notes
Getting up to leave
Using language to indicate end of interaction
Usually only an issue if a problem

Post-contactual phase
Following-up

PHN follow-up
Client follow-up
Interaction with other services
Wider community development
Organisational follow-up
Client follow-up
Follow up on information given by PHN during contact

PRACTITIONER CONSEQUENCES These would include all those elements that are necessary for the providers to undertake their work to the standard required. It includes having sufficient time, knowledge, environmental supports, communication structures and skills, and being able to enact a service in keeping with the appropriate orientation at the right time.

Links between organisational context, process and consequences

While both structure and process are useful in describing a service and in identifying the elements of the service considered important by stakeholders, they do not in themselves help us to understand service quality, or how a judgement about whether a service is good or not is made. However, such explication is necessary if this model is to provide a basis for service quality. The following five concepts emerged throughout the study and these are now presented as the links between organisational context, process and consequences. Each one of these concepts is taken into consideration in the extent to which the organisational context facilitates (or does not) the enactment of the service and also in the extent to which the process of the service resulted in the consequences.

It can be helpful to view this through the work of Juran and Gryna (1988), who write about the 'internal and external customer'. 'Internal customers' are the recipients of products or services within the organisation while 'external customers' include clients who are not members of the organisation (Juran & Gryna 1988). We can understand the practitioner to be an internal customer of the organisational context within which they operate and it follows from this that a role for management is to ensure that practitioners have the necessary 'products' to ensure it can provide a good quality service. It is then the responsibility of the practitioner to ensure that the consumer (client, other services, etc.) receives the necessary 'products' to receive a good-quality service. The five concepts are summarised in Figure 13.2.

It is important to note that where there is a deficiency in any one of the five conceptual areas, a judgement of poor service quality may be made. These five concepts were found in the study undertaken to emerge from the organisational context within which people work. The questions in Worksheet 13.5 are presented as a guide for you to identify key areas for change within your organisation.

These five concepts also apply to the process of service delivery and Worksheet 13.6 shows how these are applied to the process.

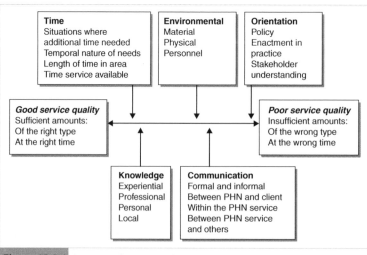

Figure 13.2 ● Concepts of service quality

Worksheet 13.5 ● Organisational context: identification of areas for change using five key concepts

Some key questions	Yes / No	Possible solutions
Time		
Does the composition of the client base or availability of other personnel within the immediate work environment create differences between practitioners in the amount of time available to them? If yes, can this be accommodated by changing the:		
• client base?		
• substance of the work undertaken?		
• getting additional help?		
(In the PHN service in Ireland, for example, this study found that the mean average population size was 3997. The range, however, was from 500 to 16 500 with a standard deviation of 3194. It is very clear that a PHN with a population size twice as high as his/her colleague cannot provide the same service). Does the timing of the availability of the service mirror the client's need and capacity to access it?		
• If no, how can this be accommodated (e.g. out-of-hours service)?		
Are there circumstances where additional time is required (for example, bigger numbers of families with child protection in some areas over others; higher levels of deprivation in some areas over others; very dispersed populations; larger numbers of people with additional needs)?		
• If yes, how can these be overcome so that these additional needs are taken into account in the distribution of resources?		
Is there a temporal aspect to the needs of the client group (for example, if a scheduled contact at 3 months does not take place for a further 3 months, the opportunity for contact is gone)?		
• If yes, how can this be accommodated?		
Does the length of time personnel spend working in a particular setting have a bearing on their work and on choice for providers and clients (the findings from this study suggest that 52% of respondents had been working in the same area for more than 5 years. This has implications for their level of local knowledge but also for their perceptions of families in that area. This can be both beneficial and problematic for families and PHNs alike)?		
• If yes, what are the main problems and benefits emerging and how can these be addressed?		

(Continued)

Worksheet 13.5 ● (Continued)

Some key questions	Yes / No	Possible solutions

Knowledge

What is the professional and experiential knowledge base of the practitioners and is this the most appropriate to meet needs of the client group?

- For example, all PHNS are registered general nurses, midwives and public health nurses. Almost 20% have additional registrations in children's nursing (10%) or in psychiatric care (9%)

What type of on-going education is required by personnel?

- To what extent does it meet the needs of all personnel? (for example, 27% of PHNs had no relevant education in the previous year)

Is there a good knowledge about the service itself among clients, formal and informal providers, managers etc.?

- Is this information easily accessible?

What kind of knowledge is required by the client group?

- Is it available to them in different formats?

Communication

What kind of formal communication structures are in place?

(For example, in this study only one-third of PHN had a personal telephone in their health centre, the remainder shared a telephone with other PHNs or other disciplines.)

Do the communication structures facilitate good communication:

- within the service
- between customer and practitioner
- between practitioner and others?

What kind of informal communication takes place?

How does this influence the formal channels of communication?

Do all providers have the necessary communication skills to communicate with their client group?

Environment

Is the physical environment provider friendly?

Is the physical environment user friendly?

Are there appropriate and sufficient materials (e.g. health promotion material, weighing scales, developmental examination tools, etc.) available to practitioners in order to undertake their work to a high standard?

In what way does the presence or absence of other personnel working within the service influence the provision?

- Is the composition of the service appropriate?

In what way does the presence or absence of other service providers (formal or informal) influence the provision of this service?

- If this is a problem how can changes be made to deal with this?

Orientation

This concept encompasses the general direction of the service in terms of its goals, purpose and focus.

What is the general orientation of the service?

(For example, in the case of the Irish public health nursing service, the service to families with infants was also in competition with other client groups such as terminally ill or clinical nursing care, and this sometimes led to a prioritisation of that work over the child health work. Within the child care remit, the orientation of the service could also be focussed more on child protection issues rather than on more health promotion activities.)

How is that orientation enacted in policy?

How are stakeholders supported in enacting the service in a way that is consistent with that orientation?

- If there is a mismatch between the policy and enactment of the service in terms of the focus and general direction, what are the reasons for this and how can they be addressed?

Worksheet 13.6 ● Key questions about service quality using the five key concepts

Some key questions	Yes / No	Possible solutions

Pre-contactual

General questions

- Is this the right time for this contact and if not why not?
- What information and knowledge is necessary to undertake this contact?
- Where should contact take place and, is it convenient, suitable and accessible?
- What communication needs to take place prior to contact?
- Is there contact I should be having but am not and if yes, why?

Step 1: Initiation

- How soon do you have contact with clients after you receive notification?
- Do you always have contact at the times you are mandated to?
- Is your service available at the times you say it will be?
- Does the availability of the service match the availability of your client?
- To what extent is this work a priority for you
- Do your clients initiate the service?

Step 2: Converging

- Do your clients know where, when and how to contact you?
- Do you know where, when and how to contact your clients?
- How is this information recorded?
- How is this information presented?
- Do you and your client know how, where and when to meet?

Step 3: Preparing

- Do you make appointments with clients prior to contact?
- Do you have appropriate information, materials and tools available for use?
- Does your client undertake significant preparations prior to your contact?
- If yes, is this a requirement of the service; if not how can this be overcome?

(Continued)

Contactual phase

General questions

- Is this contact taking place at an appropriate and convenient time?
- Have you sufficient knowledge of the situation and has the client sufficient knowledge about you?
- Are there any specific communication difficulties (e.g. hearing difficulties, telecommunications problems)?
- Is the environment unsuitable, unfriendly, inappropriate (e.g. lack of privacy, noisy, inaccessible)? Are the materials available to you appropriate (e.g. non-commercial health promotion literature, accurate weighing scales)?
- Is there a shared understanding about the focus of service?

Step 4: Opening

- Do you or your client experience difficulties when you first come in either direct face-to-face or telephone contact with each other?
- If yes, why does this happen?
- What steps can you take to ensure it does not happen?

Step 5: Interaction

Initiation

- Can you or your client always raise issues you think are necessary?
- Can your client always raise issues they think are necessary?
- If not, why not?

Exchange

- Is there enough time to deal with each element of the exchange?
- How much knowledge does the client have and how does this change the way in which the interaction proceeds?
- How well am I able to communicate with this client?
- How well is the client able to communicate with me?
- Is this the best environment to undertake all elements of the exchange?
- What is my main focus in undertaking this interaction?

Worksheet 13.6 ● (Continued)

Some key questions	Yes / No	Possible solutions

Step 6: Closing

· Do I have a set format for ending this interaction?
· Is any part of the way I close an interaction problematic for clients?
· How do I know when the client wants to finish the interaction?
· How do I respond to this?

Post-contactual

Step 7: Following-up

· Do I need to make contact with this client again and if yes when?
· Do I need to contact anybody else arising from this interaction?
· If yes, do I use formal or informal channels?
· What records do I need to keep?
· Does anything I learnt here have implications for the wider community development.

Using the framework to explain judgements of service quality

The material presented to date has demonstrated how this model can be used to describe the service being provided and also to provide a framework for analysis of key issues relating to the service organisation and process. The model can also be used to critique incidents where a good-quality service has not been evident and demonstrate the rationales underpinning the problems.

The incident described in Box 13.5, related by a mother in the course of the study, is used below to guide the analysis. This mother had moved from one area to another and she compares her experiences of the public health nursing service she had received after the birth of her first child (18 months) in the first area with that of her second child (6 months) when she lived in the second area. She had postnatal depression after both births.

In comparing the two experiences identified by this mother, a number of concepts emerged. First, there was the amount of time the PHN spent with the mother and the extent to which contact was initiated by the PHN rather than the client. In the first experience (deemed poor quality) the contact was only at prescribed times whereas in the second the PHN initiated contact many more times than that mandated. This gave the mother a feeling that the PHN was 'very caring'. In terms of communication, the mother did not feel able to initiate an interaction by opening up to the first PHN about how she was feeling. These communication difficulties could have been overcome if the PHN had been knowledgeable about the symptoms of postnatal depression, or if, for example, the Edinburgh Postnatal Depression Scale had been in use.

A key issue arising here relates to the orientation of the service and ways in which this mother made her judgement about that. The mother clearly preferred the orientation of the second service, where the PHN had a focus not only on the infant, but also on how the mother was feeling. In this second service, the PHN was oriented towards the provision of a supportive service and this was enacted in a proactive way by having additional contacts, by identifying broader family issues and making arrangements for their resolution and by the PHN 'wanting to help', and towards an empowerment approach to the interaction. The client had a preference for the latter service, saying later on in the interview that she had felt 'less depressed after this one' because she knew if she 'couldn't get any of the family I could always ring the nurse'. She said that the PHN had 'fixed [name of eighteen-month-old] up with a place in the local crèche' and 'that was great

Box 13.5

Example of service quality in practice

Mother: I find the lady down here very caring and if she was at the house next door she would always pop in. I thought they were very …. friendly and wanting to help. And she would say 'what do you think yourself?. You're the expert here.' Whereas in [name of previous area] they were saying 'oh are you OK?' 'fine bye,' that kind of way … I find them very good down here … When I had [name of first child] and they come to see you after you come home. And so she came in. And I had no family around me so I was totally on my own. And I had a bit of postnatal depression. I was, I was depressed. And it was like 'you know how to make a bottle?.' 'Yeah.' 'OK. Right so how do you make a bottle?.' I told her 'Yes that's right and how are you feeling?' and I didn't want to … so I said 'I'm fine, fine' and I knew I wasn't but … it was just 'OK you're fine. I can see I don't need to come again. I can see you are fine.'

for him and me' and also that the PHN had given her good advice about a family problem that had come up'. It could be argued that this service was oriented towards primary prevention, active support of the mother in parenting, and an empowerment approach to service delivery.

This framework can also be used to illustrate why the service does not provide what is preferred by the client. The following quote from a PHN working in an area with a large population provides some insight into how the organisational context can influence the way in which a service is enacted:

> PHN: I was thinking that for there to be any kind of quality of care for infants in the first year there should be some uniformity of services and there isn't. Say, for instance, one of my colleagues is in an area where sometimes she may have three birth notifications. She gets her babies and she can see them on the day she gets them. She can go back the following day and the following day and she can see them weekly or daily for a week or longer if she thinks they need help and be totally available to them. Whereas, with my numbers ... I see them and unless there's a huge problem I ask them to come to the clinic or to contact me and I think that is unfair like for mums and it's very difficult to explain to people.

This PHN worked with a population of some 12 000 people and within this she had responsibility for clinical nursing care and elderly surveillance as well as her work with families with infants. She had more than 200 infants born in her area each year and in order to meet even the number of contacts mandated, she would have to have some 1000 contacts. This compares with the PHN in the adjoining area (who had on average three new infants born into her area each month) who would need to have less than 200 contacts in order to meet her mandated requirement.

Even without any further analysis it is clear that unless something changed, the PHN with the very large population size would almost never be able to provide the level of contact identified by the client in the example given above as being preferable. The question here is who should be held accountable for the quality of the service provided?

One final example of the model in use is now presented by illustrating how the model can be used to identify key areas for standards development within any given service (Worksheet 13.7).

Conclusion

To summarise, this chapter has presented a model of service quality that was developed for use in public health/preventive care services, and in doing so, provides a framework for measuring service quality in situations where 'change' may not take place, where the lines of attribution are not clear and where short- and medium-term consequences are as important as long-term outcomes. The model, therefore, surmounts the main difficulties raised in respect of outcome measures for services with a focus on prevention. The model also facilitates the inclusion of many different stakeholders in the assessment of quality and, therefore, gets over problems of 'whose quality' should be prioritised within any individual situation. By using the key components described in this model it is possible to reach consensus about the detail of any individual element of the organisational context, process or consequence. In doing so a consensus that values the contribution of each stakeholder can form the basis of the assessment of quality. This partnership-type approach is conceptually and practically appropriate in a public health context. Finally, the organisational context within which a

Worksheet 13.7 ● Potential areas for standard development

	Potential areas for standard development
Initiating	Timing of first visit (e.g. within 24 hours post-notification)
	Shared construction of the need for contact between key stakeholders
	Explicit rationale for initiation
	Contact with client when needed
	Client initiates service
Converging	Mutually convenient client and PHN availability
	Mutually convenient client and PHN contactability
	Accurate and complete information about availability and contactability
	Choice of venue and timing
Preparing	PHN knowledgeable about individual client
	Appointments mutually convenient and timely
	No additional burden on client
Interacting	Initiating:
Initiating	Client able to initiate interaction
Exchange	PHN able to initiate interaction
	Successful follow-on through to exchange
	Exchange:
	Good relationship
	Accurate differentiation of normal from abnormal
	Responsiveness to specific and general client need
	Appropriate up-to-date information and advice
	Client feels supported
Closing	Client does not feel rushed or dismissed
Following-up	Referral process successfully completed
	Involvement in community development
	Comprehensive, complete and accurate record

service is provided has a crucial bearing on how the service takes place. By making explicit the components of organisational context (policy, people, place) and by ensuring that all stakeholders are represented within this explication, it is possible to provide a rich description of the context. This, in turn, can highlight issues that impact either positively or negatively on service quality.

The model was developed using a two-phase collective case study approach that drew on data collected on the Irish public health nursing service to families with infants. Phase one included data from a national questionnaire survey of public health nurses (response rate 54%; $n = 946$) and PHN managers (75%; $n = 24$) and small group interviews. Phase two, focused on four case study sites, theoretically identified from data emerging in the first phase. Data collected in this phase included group and individual interviews with clients (mothers with infants), PHNs and PHN managers, supplemented by non-participant observation. Although the model was developed through a study with this client group, the model, as demonstrated here, is both flexible and applicable to a range of other services.

The 3-5-7 model comprises three main parts (organisational context, process and consequence); five concepts (time, knowledge, communication, environment and orientation); and seven steps of process (initiating, converging, preparing, opening, interacting, closing, follow-up). Within this chapter, the model was applied to three different situations. In applying the model as a tool for analysis of key elements of any individual service, a holistic description can be provided. This, in turn, provides a strong basis for the identification of important elements of organisational context, process and consequences to consider when planning services or when reviewing existing ones. The model was also used within the chapter to provide an explication of why one service was constructed as good and the other as poor. Although the example used was drawn from the Irish public health nursing service to families with infants, the model can, in fact, be successfully applied to many other contexts and situations. While the content of the step of interacting may change according to the service or location under examination, the steps of process as set out in this model do not. These steps can be applied equally to the provision of a service in an institutional setting, the corporate sector or a voluntary context and the provision of a service can be radically altered by changing the way in which a single step of the process is enacted. By changing the 'place' of business from a physical location to a virtual one, the world-wide web, for example, has radically changed the way in the process of service delivery takes place. Such changes have very significant implications for the steps of initiating and converging.

The final application of the model within this chapter was to identify areas for standards development and this is a subject that has been given much attention in the academic and other press, as almost all organisations now have customer service charters.

Heretofore, a holistic understanding of the public health nursing service has not been available and, consequently, where standards have been set they have not taken account of the whole service. This has, in turn, meant that a single aspect of the service is prioritised over all other aspects. People do not construct an understanding of service quality on the basis of one element of the service. Rather, a failure at any individual point of the process due to a deficiency in one of the conceptual areas outlined above leads to a judgement of poor service quality. The correct identification of a hearing problem in an infant does not mitigate the results being given to a parent in an insensitive and poorly communicated way.

To summarise, although developed using the Irish public health nursing service to families with infants, this model has the potential for broader application. The organisational context, comprising policy, people and place coupled with the five concepts of quality, which emerge from the organisational context and influence the seven steps of process, form the basis for the model. The five concepts (time knowledge, communication, environment and orientation) are not in themselves new concepts. Their combined application, however, to any given context or process provides the key to operationalising the 'slippery and elusive' concept of service quality.

DISCUSSION QUESTIONS

- How does the organisational context that I work in facilitate me to deliver a high-quality service?
- Are there steps within the process of service delivery that I could be doing in a different way?
- What are the main outputs from my service?
- How can I give service users a voice in how the service is delivered?

References

Acheson A 1988 Public health in England: the report of the Committee of Inquiry into the future development of the public health function. HMSO, London

Allen P 2000 Accountability for clinical governance: developing collective responsibility for quality in primary care. British Medical Journal 321: 608–611

Attree M 1993 An analysis of the concept "Quality" as it relates to contemporary nursing care. International Journal of Nursing Studies 30(4): 355–369

Attree M 1996 Towards a conceptual model of quality care. International Journal of Nursing Studies 33(1): 13–28

Badger TG 1999 Quality management within a cost-constrained service. Journal of Nursing Management 7(6): 323–329

Baker R, Lakhani M, Fraser R, Cheater F 1999 A model for clinical governance in primary care groups. British Medical Journal 318: 779–783

Barker C 1991 Standard setting in paediatrics. Nursing Standard 5: 32–34

Barriball L, Mackenzie A (1993) Measuring the impact of nursing interventions in the community: a selective review of the literature. Journal of Advanced Nursing 18: 402–497

Bond S, Thomas L 1991 Issues in measuring outcomes of nursing. Journal of Advanced Nursing 16: 1492–1502

Byrd M 1995 A concept analysis of home visiting. Public Health Nursing 12(2): 83–89

Byrd M 1997 Child-focused single home visiting. Public Health Nursing 14(5): 313–322

Byrd M 1998 Long-term maternal-child home visiting. Public Health Nursing 15(4): 235–242

Cambell JL, Proctor SR 1999 Joining up care in London: establishing the North Southwark Primary Care Group. British Medical Journal 318: 850–852.

Campbell F, Cowley S, Buttigieg M (1995) Weights and Measures: Outcomes and Evaluation in Health Visiting. London: Health Visitors' Association.

Carr-Hill RA 1994 Efficiency and equity implications of the health care reforms. Social Science and Medicine 39(9): 1189–1201

Chalmers K 1992 Giving and receiving: an empirically derived theory on health visiting practice. Journal of Advanced Nursing 17: 1317–1325

Chalmers K 1993 Searching for health needs: the work of health visiting. Journal of Advanced Nursing 18: 900–911

Chalmers K 1994 Difficult work: health visitors' work with clients in the community. International Journal of Nursing Studies 31(2): 168–182

Clarke B, Atkinson D, McCarthy C 1998 Clinical audit: meeting a trust's standard for new birth visits. Community Practitioner 71(5): 183–185

Closs SJ, Tierney AJ 1993 The complexities of using a structure, process and outcome framework: the case of an evaluation of discharge planning for elderly patients. Journal of Advanced Nursing 18: 1279–1287

Cowley S 1991 A symbolic awareness context identified through a grounded theory study of health visiting. Journal of Advanced Nursing 16: 648–656

Cowley S 1994 Counting practice: the impact of information systems on community nursing. Journal of Nursing Management 1: 273–278

Cowley S 1995a In health visiting, a routine visit is one that has passed. Journal of Advanced Nursing 22: 276–284

Cowley S 1995b Health-as-process: a health visiting perspective. Journal of Advanced Nursing 22: 433–441

Cowley S 1999 Early interventions: evidence for implementing sure start. Community Practitioner 72(6) 162-165

Coyle Y 2000 Southwestern internal medicine conference: developing theoretical constructs for outcomes research. The American Journal of the Medical Sciences 319(4): 245–249

Crofts DJ, Bowns IR, Williams TS, Rigby AS, Haining RP, Hall DMB 2000 Hitting the target: the equitable distribution of health visitors across caseloads. Journal of Public Health Medicine 22(3): 295–301

Davidson Reynolds P 1971 A primer in theory construction. New York: Macmillan.

de la Cuesta C 1993 Fringe work: peripheral work in health visiting. Sociology of health and illness 15(5): 667–682

de la Cuesta C 1994 Relationships in health visiting: enabling and mediating. International Journal of Nursing Studies 31(5): 451–459

Dines A, Cribb A (1993) Health Promotion: Concepts and Practice. Oxford: Blackwell Science.

Donabedian A 1968 Promoting quality through evaluating the process of patient care. Medical Care VI(3): 181–202

Donabedian A 1980 Explorations in quality assessment and monitoring volume: the definition of quality and approaches to its assessment, MI Health Administration Press, Ann Arbor

Donabedian A 1988 The quality of care. How can it be assessed? Journal of American Medical Association 260(12): 1743–1748

Donabedian A 1990 The seven pillars of quality. Archives of Pathology and Laboratory Medicine 114: 1115–1118

Donabedian A 1993 Quality in health care: Whose responsibility is it? American Journal of Medical Quality 8(2): 32–36

Donaldson LJ, Muir Gray JA 1998 Clinical governance: a quality duty for health organisations. Quality in Health Care 7(Suppl): S37–S44

Douglas H, Higginson I J, Myers K, Normand C 2000 Assessing structure, process and outcome in palliative day care: a pilot study for a multi-centre trial.

Health and Social Care in the Community 8(5): 336–344

Dozier AM 1998 Professional standards: linking care, competence and quality. Journal of Nursing Care quality 12(4): 22–29

Fihn SD 2000 The quest to quantify quality. Journal of American Medical Association 283(13): 1740–1741

Griffiths J, Leemiung A, Bryar T 2003 Evaluating developments in practice. In: Bryar R, Griffiths JM (eds) Practice development in community nursing: principles and processes. Edward Arnold, London

Hall D (ed) 1996 Health for All Children. 3rd Edition. Oxford: Oxford University Press.

Hanafin S 2003 A case study of Irish public health nursing: A model of service quality for families with infants King's College London, unpublished thesis

Hanafin S, Cowley S 2006 Quality in preventive and health-promoting services: constructing an understanding through process. Journal of Nursing Management, Volume 14 (6) September, pp. 472–482

Haywood-Farmer J 1987 A conceptual model of service quality. IJOPM 8(6): 19–29

Hennekens C, Buring SD 1987 Epidemiology in Medicine. Boston: Little, Brown & Company.

Hougaard J 2004 Developing evidence-based interdisciplinary care standards and implications for improving patient safety. International Journal of Medical Informatics 73 (7-8): 615–624

Holzemer WL 1994 The impact of nursing care in Latin America and the Caribbean: a focus on outcomes. Journal of Advanced Nursing 20: 5–12

Horrocks S, Pollock J, Harvey I, Emond A, Shepherd M 1998 Health visitor understanding and rating of 28 health and social factors used as part of a health visitor caseload weighting system. Health and Social Care in the Community 6(5): 343–352

Huntington J 2000 Organisational development for clinical governance. British Medical Journal 321: 679–682

Huycke L, All AC 2000 Quality in health care and ethical principles. Journal of Advanced Nursing 32(3): 562–571

Itagaki H (1997) The Japanese Production System: Hybrid Factories in East Asia Basingstoke, Macmillan Press Ltd.

Jaros GG, Dostal E 1999 A teleonic management framework for organisations. Systemic Practice and Action Research 12(2): 195–217

Joss R, Kogan M 1995 Advancing quality: total quality management in the national health services. Open University Press, Buckingham, UK

Juran J, Gryna P 1988 Juran on planning for quality. The Free Press, New York

Katz DA, Muehlenbruch DR, Brown RL, Fiore MC, Baker TB, AHRQ Smoking Cessation Guideline Study Group 2004 Effectiveness of implementing the agency for healthcare research and quality smoking cessation clinical practice guideline: a randomized, controlled trial. Journal of the National Cancer Institute 96(8): 594–603

Kerrison S, Packwood T, Buxton M 1994 Monitoring medical audit. In: Robinson R, Le Grand J (eds) Evaluating the NHS reforms. King's Fund Institute, Berkshire

Kleinsorge IK, Koeing HF 1991 The silent customers: measuring customer satisfaction in nursing homes. Journal of Health Care Marketing 11(4): 2–13

Knott M, Latter S 1999 Help or hindrance? Single, unsupported mothers' perceptions of health visiting. Journal of Advanced Nursing 30(3): 580–588

Lohr K 1988 Outcome measurement: concepts and questions. Inquiry 25: 37–50

Longman Group Ltd 1987 The Longman Dictionary of Contemporary English 2nd Edition. Essex, England Longman Group Ltd

Luker KA, Chalmers K 1989 The referral process in health visiting. International Journal of Nursing Studies 26(2): 173–185

Macleod Clark J, Francks H, Maben J, Latter S 1997 The developing quality indicators project: health promotion in primary health care nursing. Phase 2 final report. Nightingale Institute, King's College, London.

Malcolm L, Mays N 1999 New Zealand's independent practitioner association: a working model of clinical governance in primary care. British Medical Journal 319(7221): 1340–1342

Mark BA, Salyer J, Geddes N 1997 Outcomes research: clues to quality and organisational effectiveness. Nursing Clinics of North America 32(3): 589–601

Martin-Hirsch J, Wright G 1998 The development of a quality model: measuring effective midwifery services. (MEMS) International Journal of Health Care Quality Assurance 11(2) 50–57.

Mausner J, Kramer A (1985) Epidemiology: an introductory text. Philadelphia: WB Saunders Company.

Maycock J 1989 Standars – let's fly them. Nursing Standard 18(4) 4–5.

Maxwell RJ 1984 Quality assessment in health. British Medical Journal 288: 1470–1473

Mitchell PH, Ferketich S, Jennings B 1998 Quality health outcomes model. Image: Journal of Nursing Scholarship 30(1): 43–46

Naidoo J, Wills J 1994 Health Promotion: Foundations for Practice. London: Baillière Tindall

National Standards Authority of Ireland (NSAI) (!998) NSAI for Health Services: Application of ISO 9002 in a hospital environment Dublin, NSAI/Health services, Joint working group

Needham G. (2000) Research and Practice: Making a difference IN: Gomm R. Needham G. Bullman A. (eds) Evaluating Research in Health and Social Care. London: Sage

Nutbeam D 1998 Evaluating health promotion – progress, problems and solutions. Health Promotion International 13(1): 27–44

Øvretveit J 1992 Health service quality: an introduction to quality methods for health services. Blackwell Science Ltd, Oxford

Parsley K, Corrigan P 1994 Quality improvement in nursing and health care: a practical approach. Chapman & Hall, London

Pfeffer N, Coote A 1991 Is quality good for you? A critical review of quality assurance in welfare services. Institute for Public Policy Research, London

Pringle M 2000 Participating in clinical governance. British Medical Journal 321: 737–740

Rantz MJ, Zwygart-Stauffacher M, Popejoy L et al 1999 Nursing home care quality: a multidimensional theoretical model integrating the views of consumers and providers. Journal of Nursing Care Quality 14(1): 16–37

Reading R, Allen C 1997 The impact of social inequalities in child health in health visitors' work. Journal of Public Health Medicine 19(4): 424–430

Redfern S, Norman 1990 Measuring the quality of nursing care: a consideration of different approaches. Journal of Advanced Nursing 15: 1260–1271

Scally G, Donaldson L 1998 Looking forward: clinical governance and the drive for quality improvement in the new NHS in England. British Medical Journal 317(7150): 61–65

Schuster MA, Asch SM, McGlynn EA, Kerr E, Hardy AM, Gifford DS 1997 Development of a Quality of Care measurement system for children and adolescents: Methodological considerations and comparisons with a system for adult women. Arch Pediatr Adolesc Med 151 1085–1092.

Shaw I 1997 Assessing quality in health care services: lessons from mental health nursing. Journal of Advanced Nursing 26: 758–764

Summers 1987 Longman dictionary of contemporary English. Longman Group UK Ltd, Essex

Tones K, Tilford S 1994 Health Education – Effectiveness, Efficiency and Equity. 2nd Edition. London: Chapman Hall.

Tarlov AR, Ware JE, Greenfield S, Nelson E, Perrin E, Zubkoff M 1989 The medical outcomes study: an application of methods for monitoring the results of medical care. Journal of the American Medical Association 262(7): 925–930

Tashakkori A, Teddlie C 1998 Mixed methodology: combining qualitative and quantitative approaches. Sage, London

Vågerö D 1994 Equity and efficiency in health reform. A European view. Social Science and Medicine 39(9): 1203–1210

Van Maanen HMT 1979 Perspectives and problems on quality of nursing care. Journal of Advanced Nursing 4: 377–389

Warden GL. Griffith JR 2001 Ensuring management excellence in the healthcare system. Journal of Healthcare Management 46(4): 228–237

Whitehead M 1993 Is it fair? Evaluating the equity implications of the NHS reforms. In: Robinson R, Le Grand J (eds) Evaluating the NHS reforms. King's Fund Institute, London, pp. 208–242

WHO (World Health Organisation) 1986 An International Conference on Health Promotion. The move towards a new public health. November 17–21, Ottawa, Canada. Copenhagen: World Health Organisation.

Williams A 1998 The delivery of quality nursing care: a grounded theory study of the nurse's perspective. Journal of Advanced Nursing 27: 808–816

World Health Organization 1986 Ottawa charter for health promotion. World Health Organization, Geneva

Further reading

Byrd M 1998 Long-term maternal-child home visiting. Public Health Nursing 15(4): 235–242

Donabedian A 1980 Explorations in quality assessment and monitoring volume: the definition of quality and approaches to its assessment. Health Administration Press, Ann Arbor, MI

Hanafin S 2003 A case study of Irish public health nursing: a model of service quality for families with infants. London, King's College London, Unpublished PhD thesis.

Joss R, Kogan M 1995 Advancing quality: total quality management in the national health services. Open University Press, Buckingham, UK

Immunisation:
ethics, effectiveness, organisation

14

Helen Bedford

Key issues

- Childhood immunisation is a highly successful public health intervention
- The unique nature of immunisation means that it has always been the subject of fiercely argued ethical debates
- Parents and health care professionals can disagree over what is in the child's best interests with respect to immunisation
- A health care professional who is well informed about immunisation issues can be highly effective in enabling parents to make an informed decision about immunisation.

Introduction

Smallpox was the first infectious disease against which immunisation was successfully practiced. Variolation, the inoculation of smallpox material into the body, was introduced into the UK in the early 18th century by Lady Mary Wortley Montagu. Although effective, this practice was not without considerable hazards since contacts of a varioliated individual might catch virulent and often fatal smallpox. Later that century Edward Jenner famously developed a vaccine derived from cow pox. The technique of administering the vaccine became known as 'vaccination' from the Latin for cow, 'vacca'. In 1979, as a result of widespread vaccination, the World Health Organization declared that smallpox had been eradicated from the world, less than 200 years after Jenner first administered a vaccine (World Health Organization 2005). This is the first and, so far, the only time in history that man has conquered an infectious disease.

At the beginning of the 21st century, children living in the UK are routinely protected with highly effective and safe vaccines against ten potentially damaging infections: diphtheria, tetanus, poliomyelitis, pertussis, *Haemophilus influenzae* type b (Hib), meningococcal C, pneumococcal, measles, mumps and rubella. Children in specific at-risk groups are offered additional vaccines including hepatitis B, BCG and influenza vaccines. Most industrialised countries have similar programmes, albeit with some variation. In the USA children are offered 12 vaccines routinely in the first 13 months of life. The majority of parents accept these vaccines for their children, with uptake in the UK in excess of 90% for the primary vaccines and the incidence of vaccine-preventable diseases is generally at an all time low. As a result of immunisation, disease rates in the USA have been reduced by 99% and the prospects for eliminating other infections are promising, with poliomyelitis the next infection targeted for global elimination (World Health Organization 2004). New vaccines on the horizon and others already in existence, such as vaccines to protect against varicella and human papillomavirus (HPV), are being considered for inclusion in the routine schedule.

Despite this outstanding success, immunisation has always been the subject of controversy and fiercely argued ethical debates. Although a simple, highly effective and safe public health intervention, which has been described as among the top-10 public health achievements of the 20th century (Centers for Disease Control and Prevention 1999), ensuring every child is fully immunised is a challenge for public health practitioners even in an industrialised country. This is, in part, a result of the difficulties of delivering equitable and accessible services to disadvantaged groups. It is ironic that the very success of the programme, which has consigned many diseases to the history books, also means that many parents no longer perceive a need for vaccines and some, often the most advantaged, reject immunisation for a variety of complex reasons. In this chapter, the current recommendations for childhood immunisation in the UK will be described, determinants of immunisation uptake will be reviewed and some ethical considerations for community public health practitioners will be discussed.

UK childhood immunisation programme

In the UK, the Joint Committee on Vaccination and Immunisation (JCVI), an independent expert advisory committee, advises the government on immunisation. Recommendations, once accepted and approved, are funded centrally and vaccines are provided free to recipients (Salisbury 2005). The role of primary health care practitioners is to deliver the programme by advising parents about it and by providing immunisation services, including the administration of vaccines according to the recommended guidelines as laid down in the Department of Health publication, *Immunisation against infectious disease* (Department of Health (DH) 2006) known as 'The Green Book'. The web-based version is regularly updated (DH 2007a), with the programme agreed in September 2006, reproduced here in Table 14.1.

The programme is constantly under review as new vaccines are developed, new formulations or uses for existing vaccines become available and issues

Table 14.1 ● Recommended UK childhood Immunisation schedule – September 2006 (from DH 2006)

Age	Vaccine	Mode of delivery
8 weeks	Diphtheria/tetanus/acellular pertussis/Inactivated polio vaccine/*Haemophilus influenzae* type b/ (DTaP/IPV/Hib), and pneumococcal	One injection One injection
12 weeks	DTaP/Hib/IPV	One injection
	Meningococcal C	One injection
16 weeks	DTaP/Hib/IPV	One injection
	Meningococcal C	One injection
	Pneumococcal	One injection
12 months	Hib/meningococcal C	One injection
13 months	Measles, mumps and rubella (MMR)	One injection
	Pneumococcal	One injection
Preschool	DTaP/IPV or dTaP/IPV (preschool booster)	One injection
	MMR (second dose) (can be give earlier)	One injection
13–18 years	Tetanus/low-dose diphtheria/IPV (Td/IPV) (school leavers' booster)	One injection

about vaccine safety or efficacy emerge as a result of post-marketing surveillance. Patterns of disease may change requiring alterations to the immunisation schedule. Examples of each of these include the withdrawal of MMR vaccines containing the Urabe mumps strain vaccine in 1992, the introduction of a vaccine to protect against meningococcal C infection (Men C) in 1999, the change from the live oral polio vaccine to the inactivated vaccine and from the whole-cell pertussis vaccine to an acellular vaccine in 2004, the discontinuation of the schools-based BCG programme in Autumn 2005, and the introduction of pneumococcal conjugate vaccine and addition of boosters of the conjugate vaccines Hib, Men C and pneumococcal in 2006.

Following introduction of the combined measles, mumps and rubella vaccine to the UK in 1988, different products were available for use. Two of these contained the Urabe mumps vaccine strain. Although active surveillance based on paediatricians' reports suggested this particular mumps strain was associated with a low risk of aseptic meningitis among recipients, a cluster of cases reported from one area suggested a much higher risk. A detailed study was conducted to examine this more closely and results showed a risk of about 1 in 11 000 cases (Miller et al 1993). A decision was made to withdraw this type of MMR vaccine from use in the UK in 1992 and only those containing the Jeryl Lynn strain have been used subsequently.

In 1999 the UK became the first country in the world to introduce a vaccine against Men C infection. The incidence of this infection had been increasing in the UK in the 1990s and the availability of a safe and effective vaccine enabled the introduction of the vaccine into the childhood schedule, as well as a mass vaccination campaign including all individuals up to 18 years of age. This has been a highly successful initiative and other countries have followed suit (Miller et al 2001a).

Although very safe and highly effective, oral polio vaccine (OPV) can occasionally result in vaccine-associated paralytic polio (VAPP) in recipients (at a rate of about 1 in 1 million) or in unimmunised contacts of a recently immunised individual, most commonly as a result of failing to wash hands after changing a nappy. OPV acts not only by protecting the individual recipient, but also by boosting immunity to polio in the community and by preventing transmission of wild virus. This is very important in situations where polio poses a significant threat. However, as polio has become rare worldwide, the threat of importation of cases to the UK is extremely low, and the risk of VAPP is less acceptable. It is on this basis that the policy in the UK changed in Autumn 2004. At the same time, a five component acellular pertussis vaccine became available. This vaccine has an efficacy similar to the traditional whole-cell vaccine and the advantage of causing fewer of the minor febrile reactions and general upset that are often associated with whole-cell pertussis vaccine. This meant that it was possible to introduce a vaccine that gives equivalent protection against five diseases with one injection rather than the previous regimen of one injection containing four vaccines and one orally administered vaccine, but with an improved safety profile (Bedford & Elliman 2004).

The incidence of tuberculosis (TB) has increased in recent years (Health Protection Agency 2005a), but the pattern of disease has changed from that when BCG vaccine was introduced. It is now less prevalent in the indigenous population and, therefore, the value of the universal schools-based programme has declined. A targeted approach is now more appropriate. In Autumn 2005, the schools-based programme ceased and, instead, vaccine is offered to high-risk groups. All babies born in areas where there is a high incidence of TB (greater than 40 per 100 000 population) should be offered BCG. Other high-risk groups include those whose parents or grandparents come from countries where TB is prevalent and those where there is close contact with TB (Department of Health 2005).

The most recent developments in the childhood programme include the introduction of a conjugate vaccine to protect against pneumococcal infection into the infant immunisation schedule. Pneumococcal infection causes the most severe form of bacterial meningitis as well as septicaemia, pneumonia and ear infections (Bedford & Lane 2006). It has been used successfully in the USA since 2001, where not only have the numbers of cases of invasive pneumococcal infection declined, but also herd immunity has led to a decline in cases of disease among the elderly (CDC 2005). In addition to this new vaccine, boosters of Hib, Men C and pneumococcal vaccine were introduced at 12 and 13 months. The need for these boosters became apparent after using conjugate vaccines for some time. It is now established that when given to very young infants, immunity is relatively short-lived and that only two doses of conjugate vaccines are needed in the primary course. To ensure longer-term protection, a booster is required in the second year of life (Southern et al 2006, Trotter et al 2004).

All these examples demonstrate that vaccine policy is constantly developing in response to research, development and changing circumstances. This should be reassuring for those delivering and receiving vaccines, but changes to the schedule can also shake confidence in the immunisation programme, and raise anxiety for parents about the safety and effectiveness of the programme. It is thus vital that health care professionals are well informed about such changes.

Unique nature of immunisation

Wider benefits and ethical issues

Immunisation is unlike almost every other intervention and it is this very fact that creates some of the ethical dilemmas associated with the practice. When adults are given medication for their cardiovascular disease, the prime beneficiary is the recipient. There is, indeed, some benefit to society in that prevention of the complications, such as a myocardial infarction, will save medical costs, but this is very much a secondary consideration. Whether or not someone is treated has little, if any, effect on the health of others. Another important difference is that patients usually seek treatment, whereas immunisation and screening programmes are actually promoted to healthy individuals by health care professionals.

Apart from a few exceptions, if enough people are immunised with an effective vaccine against an infection, the disease may be eradicated or made so uncommon that even unimmunised people have little, if any, risk of catching the disease. This 'herd immunity' is essential for protecting those people who cannot be immunised, or who don't become immune after receiving the vaccine. It also protects individuals who are not immunised because they or their parents have chosen to decline immunisation. Thus, these individuals can benefit from other people's acceptance of vaccines without themselves taking any of the associated risks, however small. Those who decline vaccination have been termed rather pejoratively, 'free-riders', but declining vaccines is not just a personal decision, it can endanger others, including those who have been immunised and who, for a variety of reasons, remain unprotected. A potent example of this involved two renal transplant patients aged 8 and 13 years. Both children had received MMR vaccine before transplantation but the second dose was contraindicated as they were then immunocompromised. Local uptake of MMR vaccine was only 61% and thus the children were not protected by herd immunity. These children acquired measles and became very ill with encephalitis, leaving one of them with significant deficits (Kidd et al 2003). However, when parents are considering immunisation, the protection of the community is not always as high a priority as ensuring that their own child is afforded the best protection. In the eyes of a minority of parents, 'best protection' involves declining immunisation for their own children.

For an individual, the safest choice is to not to be immunised but to ensure everybody else is. From a public health perspective, this is untenable. To persuade individuals to continue accepting immunisation even when levels of disease are extremely low requires both very safe vaccines and an understanding that the very reason the diseases are uncommon is because of high vaccine rates. A fall in uptake would lead to a resurgence in disease.

Vaccination programmes raise ethical issues regarding respect for parents' rights, the duties and responsibilities of health care professionals, and the role of government in formulating policies that protect society and promote public health (Alderson et al 1997). It is almost inevitable that conflicts of interest will result. This was highlighted vividly by the experience reported from Australia, when an unvaccinated 2-year-old child, injured by a wood splinter, developed tetanus. The child was successfully treated, but the parents, who objected to immunisation, declined to allow the child to have a course of tetanus vaccine. The clinicians involved not surprisingly found this case fraught with difficulties, feeling their duty to the child was severely compromised, while recognising that the parents had the authority to make this decision. In this situation they were limited to making strong recommendations that the child should be immunised (Goldwater et al 2003).

Organisation of the UK immunisation programme

In the UK, routine childhood vaccines are provided free of charge. Vaccines are purchased by the NHS and distributed by a central supplier who guarantees the maintenance of ideal conditions for the vaccines. Before vaccines can be used, each batch is subjected to independent testing for purity, potency and toxicity at the National Institute for Biological Standards and Control. Vaccines are usually delivered by primary care or in child health clinics. After a child is born, his/her details are entered into a register (usually computerised) maintained by the primary care trust (PCT). Parents are usually advised about the immunisation programme by the health visitor at, or soon after, the first visit when the baby is 10–14 days old. The nature of this advice and parents' views about it will be explored in more detail later in this chapter.

As with any treatment, *informed* consent must be obtained before immunisations are given. In many areas parents are asked to sign a consent form before they attend for immunisation, this is merely consent to be included in the programme and does not mean that consent is in place for each future immunisation. Consent should be sought on each immunisation visit. However, it is not necessary for this to be obtained in writing, a signature on a consent form does not constitute conclusive proof that informed consent has been given but is a record of the decision and discussions that have occurred (DH 2006). Disputes between parents can exercise health care professionals who worry, in the case of a child brought for immunisation by someone other than the parent, such as a childminder or grandparent, whether they should they proceed with immunisation without written consent from someone with parental responsibility (Watson 2005).

Evidence of consent may be assumed if an authorised person brings a child for immunisation in response either to an invitation, or on a day when immunisation is normally given. Providing that the health care professional follows the consent procedure, and that the person who brings the child is able to consider any further information that may be relevant and agrees to the immunisation, then the procedure should be carried out. There is no requirement for written authorisation from a person with parental responsibility for the procedure to go ahead. Only in the exceptional circumstance where there is evidence of a previous concern or disagreement about any or all of the immunisations by the parent(s), is it necessary to contact the person with parental responsibility before proceeding. In this situation, it is the duty of each health care professional to ensure that all members of the primary health care team are aware of such knowledge and information (Moreton et al 2005).

The practicalities of providing immunisation will not be covered in depth here since these are all well addressed in the 'Green Book'. The organisation of immunisation services is an important factor in ensuring high uptake, with those practices who adopt a team approach achieving higher uptakes (Peckham et al 1989). An individual in the practice or clinic should have overall responsibility for immunisation issues. This includes arranging appointments, collecting data, supply and storage of vaccines and clinical advice in difficult cases. Patient reminders and recall systems in primary care are also effective in improving immunisation rates (Jacobson and Szilagyi 2005). Innovative use of new technologies can develop such principles even further, with some practices sending text messages to parents' mobile phones to remind them of an immunisation appointment (personal communication with Dr Sean Bourke). Data collection is particularly important and this includes providing parents with a record of vaccines given. This information should be entered into the appropriate pages of the Personal Child Health Record as well as transferred to the PCT child health system. Feedback of performance uptake figures to immunisation providers reinforces the importance of data collection (Nicoll et al 1989). Professionals within the practice should be aware of who is the lead in the PCT from whom they can seek further advice. The role of the PCT lead is similar to that played previously by the district immunisation co-ordinator (Elliman & Moreton 2000).

Payment for providing immunisation services

Target payments for immunisation for GPs were introduced in 1990. The fees payable depend on the percentage of the target population who receive the vaccines and whether this percentage is above targets set by the government. Currently, 70% uptake is required for the lower payment and 90% for the higher target fee. While the system has changed somewhat under the new GP contact, the principle remains the same.

As will be discussed later, payments to GPs for immunisation can affect the relationship of trust between practitioners and their patients, although in practice the financial reward is relatively small. One GP calculated that in 2002 his six partners were paid 95p each for every immunisation given (Fitzpatrick 2004a).

Who should immunise?

The provision of immunisation has increasingly become a nursing responsibility. This is a development which is to be encouraged. The 'Green Book' advises that a doctor may delegate responsibility for immunisation to a nurse as long as he/she is willing to be professionally accountable for this work, has received training and is competent in all aspects of immunisation, including knowledge of the contraindications to specific vaccines and in the recognition and treatment of anaphylaxis. If nurses carry out immunisation in accordance with accepted PCT policy, the Trust will accept responsibility for immunisation by nurses. Similarly, nurses employed by general practitioners should work to agreed protocols (DH 2006).

Determinants of vaccine uptake

High uptake of immunisation depends on a range of inter-related factors. These include the organisation of immunisation services as described above, and knowledge and attitudes of health care professionals. Among parents, socio-economic factors as well as attitudes and perceptions are the key factors (Nicoll et al 1989, Peckham et al 1989).

The relationship between social factors and vaccine uptake is complex and there are differences in the characteristics of children whose parents accept immunisation, but do not complete the course (partial immunisers) and those whose parents reject immunisation or specific vaccines altogether (non-immunisers) (Samad et al 2006a). This latter group often has strong beliefs and are less likely to consider vaccination to be safe or to be necessary (Samad et al 2006b). Children who commence the immunisation course but do not complete are more likely to come from large families (Li & Taylor 1993), to have younger mothers (Samad et al 2006a) who are lone parents (Sharland et al 1997) and to have been hospitalised (Samad et al 2006a). Among this group are parents who do not object to immunisation, but for whom social or family pressures may mean that they do not get round to completing the course. These two groups, partial and non-immunisers, thus may require different interventions. Services for partial immunisers in particular need to be accessible and flexible. Health care professionals should consider offering opportunistic or domiciliary immunisation and reviewing immunisation status when families attend primary care for other reasons as well as in other health care settings, particularly hospitals. For non-immunisers, the intervention is more likely to be an issue of giving information that is tailored to respond to parents' questions and concerns, at a level of complexity appropriate to the individual. In practice, this may mean that some parents require a lot of detailed information, including lengthy discussions with different health care professionals as well as written material.

An important factor in determining vaccine uptake is parents' attitudes to the safety of vaccines and seriousness of diseases (Peckham et al 1989). This will be examined in more detail in the next section.

Perceptions of vaccines and diseases

Parents' attitudes are critically important, in particular concerning the safety and effectiveness of vaccines and the seriousness of diseases. These will be influenced by prior beliefs and experience as well as by the advice and information they gather from a variety of sources, including health care professionals. As might be predicted, parents who view the diseases as serious and the vaccines as safe are more likely to have their child vaccinated than parents who think otherwise (Peckham et al 1989, Sutton & Gill 1993). The solution to this would then superficially appear to be simply one of providing these parents with evidence-based information about the seriousness of disease and safety of vaccines. However, parents who have vaccinated their children also express concerns about vaccine safety, and it is clear that the relationship between perceptions and behaviour is complex (Evans et al 2001, Raithatha 2003, Salmon et al 2005).

Vaccines differ from other interventions in that they are administered to healthy individuals at the instigation of health care professionals and so there is a greater ethical imperative to show that their benefits outweigh the risks. Although there is a significant body of evidence, both from research and experience showing that most vaccines have very low rates of serious adverse reactions, the perception of risk and what is acceptable differs not only between individuals, but alters depending on levels of herd immunity and, therefore, disease in the local population. Part of the perception of risk involves the definition of safety. Vaccines are referred to in official literature as being 'very safe'. While this is true, what it really means is 'relatively safe'. Nothing is totally risk free. For vaccines, the adverse side-effects are well-documented, for example, there is a risk of febrile convulsions within 6–11 days of the MMR vaccine of 1 in 3000 doses (Farrington et al 1995), whereas the risk of convulsions with natural measles infection is reported to be 1 in 100. Clearly there are greater risks associated with the natural infection compared with the vaccine. This balance of risks changes when vaccine uptake is high and the likelihood of catching an infection diminishes, all the risks are then weighted in the direction of the vaccine. However, this is a delicate balance as any reduction in vaccine uptake can once again lead to a resurgence of disease.

Perceptions of the risks of vaccine and disease will, of course, be influenced by personal experience, but sometimes these may lead to an unpredictable decision. In one study of parents' perspectives of MMR vaccine a mother described her personal experience of measles:

> 'I had measles at six or something and it allegedly damaged my eyesight very badly but, and I wear lenses now, I am very blind but, I still would rather run the risk that G catches it sometime now and we catch it quickly enough to put them in bed and so on, than expose his immune system at the age of whatever, a year, to something [vaccination] that may or may not have serious effects on the system itself.' (Non-immuniser)

> (Evans et al 2001)

Studies report that some parents who decline to have their children immunised do so on the basis that they believe vaccines do more harm than good, that the diseases they are designed to prevent are not harmful and may even be beneficial by strengthening a child's developing immune system (Evans et al 2001, Rogers and Pilgrim 1995, Smailbegovic et al 2003). Anti-vaccination groups widely disseminate the view that the risks of vaccines are far greater than is acknowledged and, in addition to short-term risks, may have long-term side-effects. Diabetes, cancers, atopy, multiple sclerosis and autism have all been reported, albeit misguidedly, to be associated with receipt of vaccines. Severity of disease is another important factor that determines whether or not a child is immunised, but there is disagreement over the severity of some infections between the orthodox medical community and other health care providers, for example, homeopaths (Schmidt & Ernst 2003). It is argued that the death rate from measles was declining long before vaccines came in and that vaccination has had a minor and, possibly, even no part to play (Schiebner 1993). Such extreme views are not supported by the significant body of scientific evidence, but are commonly expressed, and every practitioner will have been challenged to respond to them.

Decision to immunise

The decision to immunise a child is a dynamic process and may change over time. Attitudes to vaccines and diseases are influenced by a range of other factors, prior beliefs about health and medicine, use of alternative or complementary therapies, advice from parents, friends and health care professionals, as well as the influence of the media. The experience of the immunisation process itself may also affect acceptance of further vaccines (Harrington et al 2000). These influences need to be borne in mind by community practitioners when advising parents and providing immunisation services. Evans et al (2001) reported that many parents find the decision about immunisation difficult and stressful, and parents have also been described as experiencing severe emotional distress at the prospect of their child being immunised (Harrington et al 2000). Such experiences can lead to failure to complete immunisation courses and to decline immunisation for future children. Health care professionals need to recognise that some parents may need considerable time and discussion before they feel able to make a decision and to provide services that cater for this. McMurray et al (2004) highlighted the fact that some professionals have a tendency to view a parent's attendance at clinic as an indication of informed consent when, in reality, at this point parents may still have questions and professionals should be using that opportunity to offer information and elicit questions as a matter of course. This is of particular importance since many vaccines are given by practice nurses and they too must be competent to respond to parents' questions. Parents appreciate health care professionals who are empathetic, understand that they may have concerns and who respond appropriately (Harrington et al 2000).

Sources of information used by parents

Health care professionals

Health care professionals, particularly health visitors, are consistently the most frequently cited source of advice for parents on immunisation (Bedford & Lansley 2006, Casiday et al 2006, Macdonald et al 2004, McMurray et al 2004, Pareek and Pattison 2000, Smailbegovic et al 2003, Yarwood et al 2005) and health visitors are considered by other primary care professionals to be the best source of advice about specific immunisations (Petrovic et al 2001). The nature of advice given by health care professionals was investigated in a survey of over almost 1300 health visitors, general practitioners and practice nurses conducted on behalf of the Department of Health in 2004. The majority of respondents reported giving advice to parents on the benefits of immunisation, common side-effects and the diseases that vaccines protect against. Fewer, about 60% in each group of professionals, reported discussing rare effects. In the event that a parent expressed doubts about a recommended vaccine, the most likely course of action was to refer to another colleague, usually a GP or paediatrician. However, some health professionals would provide parents with more information themselves or direct them to other sources. All three groups of professionals refer parents to the internet (BMRB Social Research 2005). In this survey the majority of health professionals used publications from the Department of Health to keep up to date on immunisation, although GPs infrequently reported using the 'Green Book', the major reference on immunisation. However, it is unclear which materials were distributed to parents on a routine basis. Nearly 20% of health visitors reported using information from parents' support groups with Justice Awareness and Basic Support (JABS) the most frequently used. This finding needs further exploration since this particular group, JABS, provides support for parents who believe their children have been damaged by vaccines and there is little information contained on its website that supports childhood immunisation.

In view of their importance to parents as a source of advice about immunisation, it is disappointing to find that studies conducted amongst health care professionals have found them to be poorly informed about vaccines (Cotter et al 2003, Harris et al 2001, Henderson et al 2004, Petrovic et al 2001), do not feel completely confident about explaining specific vaccine issues (Henderson et al 2004, Petrovic et al 2001), disagree with or have reservations with some vaccine policies (Henderson et al 2004, Petrovic et al 2001), do not use or are not aware of nationally available resources on immunisation (Cotter et al 2003, Petrovic et al 2001) or believe that single measles, mumps and rubella vaccines should be available on the NHS (Macdonald et al 2004). In addition, some health care professionals reported having lost confidence in the safety of MMR vaccine (Smith et al 2001) and have expressed reservations about giving their own child specific vaccines (Brownlie & Howson 2006, Petrovic et al 2001).

Studies among parents are also informative about the advice given by health care professionals and reveal issues that present challenges for ethical practice. On the positive side, parents value the advice from health professionals (McMurray et al 2004), and particularly welcome one-to-one advice. They view GPs in particular as individuals who can 'translate' the science and as up-to-date experts (Pareek & Pattison 2000, Petts & Niemeyer 2004). They also feel that designated times for discussing such issues should be considered, such as at postnatal support groups (Evans et al 2001). The author has taken part in several such group meetings, held in the early evening, and they have resulted in a wide-ranging discussion, aired many concerns and raised important issues that a parent may feel less able to discuss on a one-to-one basis. However, the greatest criticism of health care professionals is that they do not give sufficient information and that information given tends to be 'unbalanced' or 'biased' (Bedford & Lansley 2006,

Evans et al 2001, Guillaume & Bath 2004, Smailbegovic et al 2003, Sporton & Francis 2001, Yarwood et al 2005).

A large study of nearly 1000 parents of young children in one PCT sought to survey parents about their decision making, attitudes and use of information about MMR vaccine (Casiday et al 2006). The majority of responding parents (89%) in this survey had given their child MMR vaccine. It is their comments made about trust and health care professionals that are of particular note. Some parents felt that the health care professional 'represents the government so is unable to give impartial advice', this is of concern, since many of the parents reported a considerable level of distrust in the government, especially those who had rejected MMR vaccine. More than 1 in 5 of all the parents did not agree that the government would withdraw MMR vaccine if there was evidence of risk. More encouraging was the finding that parents were generally happy with the advice from their individual health care professional, in this case 'my doctor' than from the medical profession as a whole. This distrust of the government and of some suspicion about advice from health professionals as 'agents of the government' has been echoed in other studies among parents (Bedford & Lansley 2006, Cotter et al 2003, Evans et al 2001, Flynn and Ogden 2004, Guillaume & Bath 2004, Macdonald 2004, McMurray et al 2004, Poltorak et al 2005, Raithatha et al 2003), but has also been expressed by health care professionals (Brownlie & Howson 2006, Henderson et al 2004). Part of this mistrust has arisen as a result of the controversies over new variant CJD and genetically modified food, and the refusal on the part of the Prime Minister to publicly state whether or not his infant son had the MMR vaccine (Guillaume & Bath 2004, Petts & Niemeyer 2004). Mistrust of health professionals, or a perception that they may provide information that is biased to show immunisation only in a positive light, is also a consequence of the system of payment to GPs for immunisation (Evans et al 2001, Smailbegovic et al 2003, Sporton & Francis 2001).

Studies addressing the issue of health professionals' knowledge and of parents' reasons for declining vaccines, recommend, on the basis of their findings, that parents need up-to-date information, tailored to their needs and provided by health care professionals who are well informed (Smailbegovic et al 2003). Clearly this is fundamentally important since parents cannot begin to make an informed decision about immunisation if they do not have access to the information. Unfortunately, the organisation and provision of training on immunisation is inconsistent around the country (Cummins et al 2004). In recognition of the importance of training and with the aim of ensuring consistency in its provision across the country, the Health Protection Agency has developed national minimum standards for immunisation training and a core curriculum (Health Protection Agency 2005b).

However, it is also clear that information giving alone is not enough and to simply give more and more is not the answer. There is evidence that the information needs to be reworked and translated so that it has relevance for each parent within his/her own situation, and that the way it is communicated is crucial. This communication will be more successful if it is with a health care professional with whom the parent has already developed a relationship. Trusting the health care professional who is giving advice has been found to be a pivotal factor in determining whether or not parents accept immunisation for their child (Benin et al 2006). In view of this, and given their involvement with families from the early days after a child's birth, the health visitor is the obvious lynch pin of a successful immunisation programme.

Internet

In the past 10 years the internet has become an established source of advice about many issues. Information regarding immunisation is published on the internet by the health departments of most countries, as well as by international organizations, such as the World Health Organization and the Centers for Disease Control in the United States. Sites containing information encouraging vaccine refusal or about the dangers of vaccines are also available. Use of the internet has been cited as contributing to increasing concerns about vaccination (Nasir 2000).

In one investigation involving a search on seven leading search engines for sites on immunisation or vaccination, 43% of hits using the term 'vaccination' were antivaccination sites. One hundred of these were examined in detail and just over one half represented groups or individuals concerned exclusively with opposition to vaccination. The researchers suggested that these sites established by antivaccination groups sought to present themselves as legitimate authorities with scientific credibility and to use references to support their claims, which were often works published by themselves (Davies et al 2002).

It is difficult to establish precisely the extent to which parents use the internet for advice regarding immunisation, in one study among over 800 parents of 2-year-old children, almost 30% reported using the internet for such information (Bedford & Lansley 2006). In one US-based study, parents of children who were exempt from vaccination were three times more likely than those of vaccinated children to have used the internet for information and were also more likely to highly rate the information (Salmon et al 2005). However, it is difficult to unravel cause and effect since parents may seek advice that confirms existing views rather than reject vaccines as a direct result of the information found. Whatever the influence of the internet, health professionals involved in immunisation services need to be aware of the most reliable websites and to be aware of the content of others so that they can discuss this when parents raise issues. This can be challenging as the quote below illustrates:

> 'They're downloading this and downloading that and we can't keep up with it. I mean [. . .] many different studies that have been done on MMR you can get off the Internet. . . . . .I don't have the ability to look at all these research papers and decide.' [Health visitor]
>
> (Brownlie & Howson 2006)

It is the last part of this quote that is a cause for concern, while this health visitor may not feel able to judge the scientific credibility of the research him- or herself, there are many resources available where the studies have been closely examined and reviewed, and this sort of information would assist in advising parents (Anonymous 2003, Bandolier 2005, Booy et al 2006). This includes a review by the independent publication *Drugs and Therapeutics Bulletin*, which is particularly valuable, as parents often request an independent source of advice.

Vaccine controversies

As a disease disappears and people no longer have direct experience of the suffering it may cause, they become less convinced of the need for immunisation. Any suggestion of possible adverse effects overshadows the benefits of vaccination. It is against this background that controversies about vaccines have developed. Interestingly, they are not confined to the industrialised world. The most recent controversy occurred in the state of Kano in Nigeria. The reasons for this were complex, but here, too, mistrust of government leaders and of Western biomedicine lay at the heart of the matter. Poliomyelitis had been nearing eradication until rumours started by religious clerics spread that the vaccine contained contraceptives as part of a Western plot to halt population growth. Polio cases doubled in Nigeria in 2004 and the disease was re-introduced into 16 previously polio-free countries. Fortunately, much hard work by the government to dispel these claims has been successful and a national campaign to immunise all children under the age of five was carried out in 2005 (Renne 2006).

Perhaps the most infamous contemporary vaccine controversy in the UK is the scare over the safety of MMR vaccine. This came to a head following publication in the *Lancet* of a case series of 12 children seen in one clinic who all had bowel disease and were either diagnosed as being autistic or were suspected to have autism. In eight of these children, the parents or GP recalled that the behavioural symptoms had started soon after the child had been given MMR vaccine (Wakefield et al 1998). The authors clearly state: 'We did not prove an association between measles, mumps and rubella vaccine and the syndrome described', and a later communication from members of the research team emphasised this (Murch et al 2004).

In isolation it is unlikely that the paper would have had such a major impact. As a piece of research proving cause and effect it was not valid, as the methods were inappropriate (Chen and DeStefano 1998). However, at a press conference held the day before publication, one of the authors stated that he had sufficient doubts about the safety of MMR vaccine to suggest that children should be given individual measles, mumps and rubella vaccine with a 1-year interval between doses. In contrast, three of the other authors on the paper, all paediatricians, said: 'We emphatically endorse current vaccination policy until further data are available' (Murch et al 1998).

Since the 1998 publication many studies have been conducted, set in different countries asking different questions and using different methodologies and there is now a significant body of evidence showing no link with MMR vaccine and autism and bowel disease (Booy et al 2006). In spite of this, and the methodo-logical limitations of the 1998 *Lancet* paper, many people took publication in such a prestigious journal as evidence that MMR vaccine causes autism; this has been vocally supported by some sections of the media, with phases of intense publicity since 1998, and by parents' groups who believe their children have been damaged by vaccination. However, in 2004 and 2005 as yet more studies were published (Honda et al 2005, Smeeth et al 2004) showing no link between MMR vaccine and autism, some newspapers that were formerly blatantly anti-MMR vaccine, altered their perspective. The overall result, not surprisingly, is that many parents have been concerned about the safety of the vaccine, and uptake of MMR vaccine in England, although improving, was 82% in mid-2005. This is 10% lower than in 1995 before the controversy took hold. In some areas, for example London, uptake is considerably lower (Health Protection Agency 2005c).

One of the consequences of the MMR story is that, in an effort to protect their children whilst 'avoiding the risks of MMR vaccine', some parents have sought single vaccines. Despite pressure from many quarters, the government has refused to make this option available for parents on the NHS. There are many reasons for this: from a scientific perspective there is no good evidence to suggest that MMR vaccine is anything other than highly effective with a good safety record. On the other hand, using single vaccines in the way suggested (at yearly intervals), is untried and untested anywhere in the world and the regimen would inevitably lead to incomplete schedules and delay in achieving full protection, putting individual children at risk as well as the community (Elliman & Bedford 2001). From a policy perspective, providing a choice of vaccination strategies would be tantamount to admitting that there is a problem with the safety of MMR vaccine. However, in response to this demand, many private clinics are offering the vaccines separately. Choice has become the issue at the heart of this controversy. As Mike Fitzpatrick a London GP and father of a son with autism pointed out:

'The demand for the right to choose separate vaccines had a ready appeal to a public whose right to choose schools and hospitals, methods of childbirth and dates for surgery, had been elevated into a principle of public policy. It was readily promoted by a range of private doctors and entrepreneurs who eagerly met the demand for separate vaccines resulting from the MMR scare. Profiting handsomely from the anti-MMR campaign, the proprietors of these clinics emerged as some of the most ardent supporters of Dr Wakefield's crusade'.

(Fitzpatrick 2004b)

There is no research evidence about what happens in practice when a parent discusses the issue of separate vaccines with their health care professional. However, anecdotal experience shows that many health professionals find this an extremely challenging situation and one that raises many ethical dilemmas. There is certainly support for the provision of single vaccines by some health care professionals, with 29% of health visitors and practice nurses in one survey agreeing that single vaccines should be available on the NHS (Macdonald et al 2004).

How should parents who are adamant that they do not wish their child to have MMR vaccine and would prefer to give him/her the single vaccines be advised? Do parents have the right to choose what they consider to be best for their own child? Some would argue that it is preferable for a child to have single vaccines and be protected, than to have nothing at all. However, using the single vaccines as an alternative to MMR is not merely a question of replacing a combined vaccine with three separate vaccines as discussed above. Furthermore, the single vaccines are not licensed in this country and some have an unsatisfactory safety or efficacy record. The mumps vaccine strain, Urabe, is known to be more likely to give rise to adverse effects, while the Rubini vaccine is significantly less effective than the rubella component contained in MMR vaccine. In addition, some clinics offering the single vaccines used suboptimal methods for storing and administering single vaccines, with one GP imprisoned for forging laboratory results connected with the administration of single vaccines and subsequently struck off the UK General Medical Register (Dyer 2006).

As a result, some health care professionals have found themselves caught between two roles: 'that of the agent of the State, and that of protecting the best interest of my patients' (Fry 2002).

From personal experience of talking with parents who seek advice about MMR vaccine and the single vaccines, much of their concern is allayed by discussing the scientific evidence. Many parents have made a decision to decline MMR vaccine on the basis of what they have read in the newspapers, seen on the television or after discussion with friends. It is vital that before making such an important decision they have the opportunity to discuss it with a well-informed health care professional and to have access, if appropriate, to as much information as they need. However, in my experience many parents have not been offered information, such as the NHS leaflets and factsheets, which are freely available (DH 2007b)

Parents are surprised to hear that the *Lancet* publication, which did not show a link with autism and MMR vaccine, is the only piece of research that has caused concern about the vaccine, and are reassured that so much subsequent research has shown no link. However, even this information does not reassure all parents and when they remain convinced that they would prefer single vaccines, I equip them with a series of questions to ask the vaccine provider. These include the details of safety, testing and storage of the vaccines, the recommended interval between doses and the scientific evidence for that together with recommendations for follow-up (Health Protection Agency 2006).

Other aspects of the right to choose

Many practitioners are aware that some parents feel they should have the right to choose not only whether or not they have their child immunised, but also the manner of immunisation. This belief seems to have become more prevalent since concerns about the safety of MMR vaccine ignited. Clearly parents have the right to choose whether or not to have their child immunised, but increasingly the ability to choose how their child is immunised is being reduced. For example, rather than give their child a combination vaccine, some parents would prefer each vaccine to be given on a separate occasion. The use of combination vaccines is advantageous for many reasons, not least because an infant is subjected to fewer injections overall and receives protection at a younger age. However, there is a belief among some parents, as well as health care professionals, that giving multiple vaccines in one injection may overload the immune system (Hilton et al 2006, Macdonald 2004, Smailbegovic et al 2003,). There is no evidence to suggest this happens and studies have found no increase in serious infections following MMR vaccine (Miller et al 2003, Offit et al 2002). As there is little worldwide demand for single-vaccine preparations, manufacturers are no longer producing them and so it is also increasingly difficult to obtain vaccines in anything other than a combination. Despite the obvious advantages of combination vaccines, one might suggest that this constitutes the tail wagging the dog. Parents now have a simple choice: combination vaccines or no vaccine.

Ethical conflicts for health care professionals

Before any procedure can take place on another person, informed consent must be obtained by the health care professional. The basis for this is that the person giving consent must have all the appropriate information available to make a decision.

One of the guiding principles of the standards of proficiency for specialist community public health nurses states that:

'. . . it is essential that practice is informed by the best available evidence'.

(Nursing & Midwifery Council 2004)

This includes advice given to parents on a range of issues including immunisation. Health care professionals have a responsibility to be informed and to provide parents with evidence-based information. However, national recommendations based on this information may be in conflict with a health care professional's personal views, and what then is the place of such views?

To assist them in their decision, parents often ask their health care professional if they have had their own child vaccinated. The evidence shows that some health care professionals express doubts about giving their own children the recommended vaccines (Brownlie & Howson 2006, Petrovic et al 2001). Since the advice of individual health care professionals can be so influential, this raises the question as to whether those who do not support the immunisation programme and have not had their own child vaccinated should be giving advice in this area of practice, in a similar way that health care professionals who have a conscientious objection to termination of pregnancy need not participate in treatment, but are obliged to direct the patient/client to other sources of advice.

If parents ask for advice and are given inadequate or incorrect advice they may decide not to have a vaccine. If their child subsequently succumbs to the infection, how is the health care professional placed? There is little legal precedent, but what there is would suggest that the health care professional could be held liable.

Another issue concerns the amount of information that should be provided to allow parents to make an informed decision. Well-conducted studies have identified the adverse effects associated with specific vaccines, e.g. a risk of 1 in 32 000 of idiopathic thrombocytopenic purpura following MMR vaccine, and it is clear that such risks should be communicated (Miller et al 2001b). However, should a parent also be advised of unsubstantiated or rarer adverse reactions? For example, should parents who are unaware of the controversy over the safety of MMR vaccine be informed about it and thus raise concerns that they otherwise might not have had? The position is unclear, but all questions should be answered fully and probably the best option is to provide parents with the literature produced by the Department of Health on the relevant vaccine. It would seem unnecessary and unhelpful to raise false concerns where no evicence to support them exists.

Who can give informed consent?

As a general principle, medical intervention, whether treatment or prevention, should only take place with the *informed* consent of the recipient. Where this is a child under 16 years old, that consent may be given by someone with parental responsibility or the young person themselves, if he/she fully understands what is being offered ('Fraser competent'). If a 'Fraser competent' child gives consent, yet the parent disagrees, the child's views take precedence. Where two parents with parental responsibility disagree, it may be necessary to resort to the courts to make a decision in the best interests of the child (Dyer 2003). An adult can decide not to have treatment even though such a course of action would result in his/her death. Where a child would be denied treatment because of withholding of consent, the State can step in and over-ride the parent or competent child.

Most scientific commentators accept that vaccination has had a significant effect on the reduction of vaccine-preventable diseases. The maintenance of low levels of infectious disease requires sustained high uptake of vaccines. Yet, as we have seen, there are many factors that could jeopardise this balance. As some parents find the decision to immunise so difficult, and yet maintaining high uptake rates is critical to protect individual children, as well as society now and in the future, should society have a place in the decision to immunise? In the next section the issue of compulsion will be considered.

Should immunisation be compulsory?

Controversy has always surrounded vaccination and the concept of compulsion in this field is not new. When Edward Jenner introduced vaccination against smallpox people were so convinced of the value of vaccination that, in 1853, an Act of Parliament was passed making vaccination compulsory. This resulted in 90% of infants being immunised against smallpox. Failure to comply resulted in a fine for a parent and sometimes this sanction was exercised repeatedly for the same child. In some cases this resulted in imprisonment. A vocal antivaccination lobby grew up and in some parts of the country prosecutions were not pursued, with local officials turning a blind eye to non-vaccinating parents. As time went on, 'exemption' clauses were added to the legislation to allow some people to refuse to have their children immunised, primarily on religious grounds. Predictably, these exemptions resulted in a reduction in vaccination rates that, in turn, saw an increase in cases of smallpox. Many other countries also introduced compulsion, and it was not until the creation of the NHS in 1948 that compulsion ceased in the UK, but the immunisation programme has greatly increased in complexity since then.

In USA laws requiring immunisation for school attendance have been in place since the 1960s and 1970s, and began with the aim of preventing measles (Orenstein & Hinman 1999). All States require children entering schools to receive certain vaccines but all States permit medical exceptions and, in addition, 48 States offer religious exemptions and 19 offer personal or philosophical exemptions. However, an important disadvantage of school-entry requirements is that some parents may wait until their child has to be vaccinated rather than having them vaccinated at the earliest possible age. In the USA, after many years of low measles incidence, this led to substantial outbreaks of measles in 1989–91, which were mainly confined to preschool-aged children who remained unvaccinated (Cutts et al 1992).

In the UK, although compulsion has been discussed (Bradley 1999, Noah 1987) it has not been introduced. The discussion highlights the conflict between the rights of a child to be protected against vaccine-preventable disease and the freedom of parents to make choices about child rearing. This is generally the case unless the parent's choices or actions result in serious harm or neglect (Issacs et al 2004). In the UK, high vaccine uptake rates have been achieved through a process of informed consent rather than coercion and this is generally considered a more preferable approach. However, leaving the decision with the parent can make it difficult for some. In one large study in the late 1980s, shortly before the introduction of MMR vaccine, parents were asked if they felt that it should be a legal requirement for children to be immunised before entering school. Over half the parents agreed with this suggestion, one-quarter disagreed and one-fifth was unsure. Of the parents who agreed with the proposal, 44% had not had their children vaccinated and some even commented that such a policy would be what they needed to motivate them into vaccinating their child (Peckham et al 1989).

In countries with compulsion there is some evidence that it has a beneficial effect on vaccine-uptake rates, equally, countries such as the UK and Scandinavia achieve very high uptakes without it. In the UK, should the State step in if a parent withholds consent to vaccination? What are the consequences of the child not being immunised?

Unimmunised children may develop the disease and pass it on to someone who is susceptible because they are not immunised, whether:

- by choice
- because they are too young to be immunised (pertussis disease kills very young babies)

  or

- there is a medical contraindication (live vaccines cannot be given to children with conditions such as leukaemia).

Not only will children suffer, but there is a potential cost to the State and to parents. In USA, the chance of contracting measles is 35 times more likely in a child who has been exempted from immunisation on religious or philosophical grounds (Salmon et al 1999).

In some circumstances, the State does over-ride an individual's freedom to harm themself. Legislation has long been in place to enforce the use of seat belts and measures are taken to prevent various forms of substance abuse. In the case of immunisation, matters are complicated by the fact that the person to whom the treatment may be given, i.e. the child, is not usually the person giving consent, i.e. the parent. It is well established that there are instances when it is reasonable for the State to step in and ensure treatment is given to a child even though the parents do not consent to it. An example is the enforcement of blood transfusion where parents have religious objections to it but the child is at significant risk of permanent injury or death if he/she doesn't receive it.

Whether the State does intervene in these circumstances really depends on the size and consequences of the risk. A parent could argue that the risk of catching most vaccine-preventable diseases is small, and the consequences are usually not serious and, therefore, not immunising has little hazard as long as too many people don't adopt the same view. On this basis there is probably no place for compulsion in the UK, but it could be argued that the time for compulsion may come as we near elimination of a disease.

Conclusion

In this chapter the importance of immunisation has been discussed. This highly effective, safe and simple public health intervention not only protects individual children, but also society against infectious disease. Research into parents, and health care professionals' views about immunisation clearly highlights the ethical issues and conflicts that ensue as a result of vaccination programmes. These include the rights of parents, the roles and responsibilities of health care professionals and the role of government in introducing health policies to protect the health of society as a whole and promote health.

There are many inter-related factors determining high vaccine uptake, no intervention alone will improve or maintain levels. However, there is ample evidence to show the value of the work of community public health professionals in this area, particularly in communicating with parents about the benefits and risk of immunisation. At a time when the continued success of the immunisation programme has been threatened by controversies over vaccine safety, their role as well-informed practitioners who are able to communicate effectively and appropriately is becoming even more important.

DISCUSSION QUESTIONS

- What are the main arguments for and against a legal requirement that children in the UK should be fully immunised before they are admitted to school?
- Do you consider that a health professional who is personally opposed to immunisation and declined to have their own children immunised should be involved in the provision of immunisation services?

References

Alderson P, Mayall B, Barker S et al 1997 Childhood immunisation: meeting targets yet respecting consent. European Journal of Public Health 7: 95–100

Anonymous 2003 MMR vaccine-how effective and how safe? Drug and Therapeutics Bulletin 41(4): 25–29

Bandolier 2005 MMR vaccination and autism. Online. Available: http://www.jr2.ox.ac.uk/bandolier/Extraforbando/MMRextra.pdf

Bedford H, Elliman D 2004 Misconceptions about the new combination vaccine. British Medical Journal 329(7463): 411–412

Bedford H, Lansley M 2006 Information on childhood immunisation: parents' views. Community Practitioner 79 (8): 252–255

Bedford H, Lane L 2006 Pneumococcal vaccine and the new child vaccination schedule. Nursing Times 102(39):44, 46–47

Benin AL, Wisler-Scher DJ, Colson E, Shapiro ED, Holmboe ES 2006 Qualitative analysis of mothers' decision-making about vaccines for infants: the importance of trust. Pediatrics 117: 1532–1541

BMRB Social Research 2005 Health professionals 2004 childhood immunisation survey. Online. Available: http://www.immunisation.nhs.uk/files/hp_survey_2004.pdf

Booy R, Sengupta N, Bedford H, Elliman D 2006 Measles, Mumps, and rubella: prevention. Clin Evid Jun;(15): 448–468

Bradley P 1999 Should childhood immunisation be compulsory? Journal of Medical Ethics 25(4): 330–334

Brownlie J, Howson A 2006 Between the demands of truth and government: health practitioners, trust and immunisation work. Social Science and Medicine 62(2): 433–443

Casiday R, Cresswell T, Wilson D et al 2006 A survey of UK parental attitudes to the MMR vaccine and trust in medical authority. Vaccine 24(2): 177–184

Centers for Disease Control and Prevention 1999 Impact of vaccines universally recommended for children – United States, 1900–1998. Journal of the American Medical Association 281(16): 1482–1483

Centers for Disease Control 2005. Direct and indirect effects of routine vaccination of children with 7-valent pneumococcal conjugate vaccine on incidence of invasive pneumococcal disease – United States, 1998–2003. Morbidity and Mortality Weekly Return 54(36): 893–897

Chen RT, DeStefano F 1998 Vaccine adverse events: causal or coincidental? The Lancet 351: 611–612

Cotter S, Ryan F, Hegarty H et al 2003 Immunisation: the view of parents and health professionals in Ireland. Eurosurveillance 8(6): 145–150

Cummins A, Lane L, Boccia D et al 2004 Survey of local immunisation training in England – the case for setting national standards. Communicable Disease and Public Health 7(4): 267–271

Cutts FT, Zell ER, Mason D et al 1992 Monitoring progress toward US pre-school immunization goals. Journal of the American Medical Association 267(14): 1952–1955

Davies P, Chapman S, Leask J 2002 Antivaccination activists on the world wide web. Archives of Disease in Childhood 87(1): 22–25

Department of Health (DH) Salisbury D, Ramsay M, Noakes K (eds) 2006 Immunisation against infectious disease. The Stationery Office, London

Department of Health (DH) 2005 Changes to the BCG programme. Online. Available: http://www.dh.gov.uk/asset-Root/04/11/49/96/04114996.pdf

Department of Health (DH) 2007a Immunisation against infectious disease – The Green Book. http://www.dh.gov.uk/en/policyandguidance/Healthand socialcaretopics/Greenbook/DH_4097254

Department of Health (DH) 2007b MMR the facts. http://www.mmrthefacts.nhs.uk

Dyer C 2003 Judge overrules mothers' objections to MMR vaccine. British Medical Journal 326: 1351

Dyer O 2006 Doctor struck off after vaccine scandal. British Medical Journal 333: 276

Elliman D, Moreton J 2000 The district immunisation coordinator. Archives of Disease in Childhood 82(4): 280–282

Elliman DAC, Bedford HE 2001 MMR vaccine-worries are not justified. Archives of Disease in Childhood 85: 271–274

Evans M, Stoddart H, Condon L et al 2001 Parents' perspectives on the MMR immunisation: a focus group study. British Journal of General Practice 51(472): 904–910

Farrington P, Pugh S, Colville A et al 1995 A new method for active surveillance of adverse events from diphtheria/tetanus/pertussis and measles/mumps/rubella vaccines. The Lancet 345(8949): 567–569

Fitzpatrick M 2004a MMR and autism: what parents need to know. Routledge, London

Fitzpatrick M 2004b Anti-vaccination nation? Online. Available: http://www.spiked-online.com/Articles/0000000CA6D2.htm [accessed 11 September 2005]

Flynn M, Ogden J 2004 Predicting uptake of MMR vaccination: a prospective questionnaire study. British Journal of General Practice 54(504): 526–530

Fry R 2002 Debate crystallises dilemma facing many medical disciplines. British Medical Journal 324: 733

Goldwater PN, Braunack-Mayer AJ, Power RG 2003 Childhood tetanus in Australia: ethical issues for a should-be-forgotten preventable disease. Medical Journal of Australia 178: 175–177

Guillaume LR, Bath PA 2004 The impact of scare stories on parents' information needs and preferred information sources: a case study of the MMR vaccine scare. Health Informatics Journal 10(1): 5–22

Harrington PM, Woodman C, Shannon WF 2000 Low immunisation uptake: is the process the problem? Journal of Epidemiology and Community Health 54: 394–400

Harris T, Gibbons CR, Churchill M et al 2001 Primary care professionals' knowledge of contraindications. Community Practitioner 74: 66–67

Health Protection Agency 2005a TB surveillance. Online. Available: http://www.hpa.org.uk/infections/topics_az/tb/epidemiology/reports.htm

Health Protection Agency 2005b National minimum standards for immunisation training. Online. Available: http://www.hpa.org.uk/infections/topics_az/vaccination/training_menu.htm

Health Protection Agency. COVER programme April to June 2005. CDR Weekly 2005c; 15(28): Online. Available: http://www.hpa.org.uk/cdr/archives/2005/cdr3805.pdf [accessed 17 August 2006]

Health Protection Agency 2006 Online. Available: http://www.hpa.org.uk/infections/topics_az/vaccination/071102_MMRpreferable.htm [accessed 17 August 2006]

Henderson R, Oates K, Macdonald H et al 2004 General practitioners' concerns about childhood immunisation and suggestions for improving professional support and vaccine uptake. Communicable Disease and Public Health 7(4): 260–266

Hilton S, Petticrew M, Hunt K 2006 'Combined vaccines are like a sudden onslaught to the body's immune system': parental concerns about vaccine 'overload' and 'immune-vulnerability'. Vaccine 24(20): 4321–4327

Honda H, Shimizu Y, Rutter M. 2005 No effect of MMR withdrawal on the incidence of autism: a total population study. Journal of Child Psychology and Psychiatry 46(6): 572–579

Isaacs D, Kilham HA, Marshall H 2004 Should routine childhood immunizations be compulsory? Journal of Paediatrics and Child Health 40(7): 392–396

Jacobson VJ, Szilagyi P 2005 Patient reminder and patient recall systems to improve immunization rates. Cochrane Database of Systematic Reviews 20(3): CD003941

Kidd MI, Booth CJ, Rigden SPA 2003 Measles-associated encephalitis in children with renal transplants: a predictable effect of waning herd immunity? The Lancet 362: 832

Li J, Taylor B 1993 Childhood immunisation and family size. Health Trends 25(1): 16–19

Macdonald H, Henderson R, Oates K 2004 Low uptake of immunisation: contributing factors. Community Practitioner 77(3): 95–100

McMurray R, Cheater FM, Weighall A et al 2004 Managing controversy through consultation: a qualitative study of communication and trust around MMR vaccination decisions. British Journal of General Practice 54(504): 520–525

Miller E, Goldacre M, Pugh S et al 1993 Risk of aseptic meningitis after measles, mumps, and rubella vaccine in UK children. The Lancet 341: 979–982

Miller E, Salisbury D, Ramsay M 2001a Planning, registration, and implementation of an immunisation campaign against meningococcal serogroup C disease in the UK: a success story. Vaccine 20(Suppl 1): S58–S67

Miller E, Waight P, Farrington CP et al 2001b Idiopathic thrombocytopenic purpura and MMR vaccine. Archives of Disease in Childhood 84(3): 227–229

Miller E, Andrews N, Waight P et al 2003 Bacterial infections, immune overload, and MMR vaccine. Archives of Disease in Childhood 88(3): 222–223

Moreton J, Bedford H, Elliman D 2005 Consent for screening and immunisation procedures in children and young people. Community Practitioner 78(3): 83–84

Murch S, Thomson, Walker-Smith J 1998 Autism, inflammatory bowel disease, and MMR vaccine. The Lancet 351: 908

Murch SH, Anthony A, Casson DH et al 2004 Retraction of an interpretation. The Lancet 363: 750

Nasir L 2000 Reconnoitering the antivaccination web sites: news from the front. Journal of Family Practice 49(8): 731–733

Nicoll A, Elliman D, Begg NT 1989 Immunisation: causes of failure and strategies and tactics for success. British Medical Journal 299: 808–812

Noah ND 1987 Immunisation before school entry: should there be a law? British Medical Journal 294: 1270–1271

Nursing and Midwifery Council 2004 Standards of proficiency for specialist community public health nurses. Nursing and Midwifery Council, London. Online. Available: http://www.nmc-uk.org

Offit PA, Quarles J, Gerber MA, Hackett CJ, Marcuse EK, Kollman TR, Gellin BG, Landry S 2002 Addressing parents' concerns: do multiple vaccines overwhelm or weaken the infant's immune system? Pediatrics 109(1): 124–129

Orenstein WA, Hinman AR 1999 The immunization system in the United States – the role of school immunization laws. Vaccine 17(Suppl 3): S19–S24

Pareek M, Pattison HM 2000 The two-dose measles, mumps and rubella (MMR) immunisation schedule: factors affecting maternal intention to vaccinate. British Journal of General Practice 50: 969–971

Petrovic M, Roberts R, Ramsey M 2001 Second dose of measles, mumps and rubella vaccine: survey questionnaire of health professionals. British Medical Journal 322: 82–85

Peckham C, Bedford H, Senturia Y et al 1989 The Peckham Report. National immunisation study: factors affecting immunisation in childhood. Action Research for the Crippled Child, Horsham, UK

Petts J, Niemeyer S 2004 Health risk and communication: learning from the MMR vaccination controversy. Health Risk and Society 6(1): 7–23

Poltorak M, Leach M, Fairhead J et al 2005 'MMR talk' and vaccination choices: an ethnographic study in Brighton. Social Science and Medicine 61(3): 709–719. Published online: 2 March 2005

Raithatha N, Holland R, Gerrard S et al 2003 A qualitative investigation of vaccine risk perception amongst parents who immunize their children: a matter of public health concern. Journal of Public Health Medicine 25(2): 161–164

Renne E 2006 Perspectives on polio and immunization in Northern Nigeria. Social Science and Medicine 63: 1857–1869

Rogers A, Pilgrim D 1995 Immunisation and its discontents: an examination of dissent from the UK mass childhood immunisation programme. Health Care Analysis 3: 99–115

Salisbury DM 2005 Development of immunization policy and its implementation in the United Kingdom. Health Affairs 24(3): 744–754

Salmon DA, Haber M, Gangarosa EJ et al 1999 Health consequences of religious and philosophical exemptions from immunization laws: individual and societal risk of measles. Journal of the American Medical Association 282(1): 47–53

Salmon DA, Moulton LH, Omer SB et al 2005 Factors associated with refusal of childhood vaccines among parents of school-aged children: a case-control study. Archives of Pediatric and Adolescent Medicine 159(5): 470–476

Samad L, Tate AR, Dezateux C, Peckham C, Butler N, Bedford H 2006a Differences in risk factors for partial and no immunisation in the first year of life: prospective cohort study. British Medical Journal 332: 1312–1313

Samad L, Butler N, Peckham C, Bedford H and Millennium Cohort Study Child Health Group 2006b Incomplete immunisation uptake in infancy: maternal reasons. Vaccine (in press)

Scheibner V 1993 Vaccination-100 years of orthodox research shows that vaccines represent a medical assault on the immune system. Australian Print Group, Victoria

Schmidt K, Ernst E 2003 MMR vaccination advice over the Internet. Vaccine 21: 1044–1047

Sharland M, Atkinson P, Maguire H et al 1997 Lone parent families are an independent risk factor for lower rates childhood immunisation in London. Communicable Disease Review (11): R169–R172

Smailbegovic MS, Laing GJ, Bedford H 2003 Why do parents decide against immunization? The effect of health beliefs and health professionals. Child: Care Health and Development 29(4): 303–311

Smeeth L, Cook C, Fombonne E et al 2004 MMR vaccination and pervasive developmental disorders: a case-control study. The Lancet 364: 963–969

Smith A, McCann R, McKinlay I 2001 Second dose of MMR vaccine: health professionals' level of confidence in the vaccine and attitudes towards the to the second dose. Communicable Disease and Public Health 4(4): 273–277

Southern J, Crowley-Luke A, Borrow R, Andrews N, Miller E 2006 Immunogenicity of one, two or three doses of a meningococcal C conjugate vaccine conjugated to tetanus toxoid, given as a three-dose primary vaccination course in UK infants at 2, 3 and 4 months of age with acellular pertussis-containing DTP/Hib vaccine. Vaccine 24(2): 215–219

Sporton RK, Francis S-A 2001 Choosing not to immunize: are parents making informed decisions? Family Practice 18(2): 181–188

Sutton S, Gill E 1993 Immunisation uptake: the role of parental attitudes. In: Hey V (ed.) Immunisation Research: a Summary Volume. Health Education Authority, London

Trotter CL, Andrews NJ, Kaczmarski EB, Miller E, Ramsay ME 2004 Effectiveness of meningococcal serogroup C conjugate vaccine 4 years after introduction . The Lancet 364(9431): 365–367

Wakefield A J, Murch S H, Anthony A et al 1998 Ileal-lymphoid nodular hyperplasia, non-specific colitis, and pervasive developmental disorder in children. The Lancet 351: 637–664

Watson V 2005 Caution urged over 'assuming' consent. Community Practitioner 78(4): 154

World Health Organization 2005 Smallpox. http://www.who.int/mediacentre/factsheets/smallpox/en/

World Health Organization 2004 Eradication of Poliomyelitis. *http://www.who.int/gb/ebwha/pdf_files/EB115/B115_28-en.pdf*

Yarwood J, Noakes K, Kennedy D, Campbell H, Salisbury D 2005 Tracking mothers attitudes to childhood immunisation 1991–2001. Vaccine 23(48–49): 5670–5687

Further reading

Offit PA, Coffin SE 2003 Communicating science to the public: MMR vaccine and autism. Vaccine 822(1): 1–6

Index

365